Interdisciplinary Statistics

CLINICAL TRIALS
in ONCOLOGY

Second Edition

CHAPMAN & HALL/CRC
Interdisciplinary Statistics Series

Series editors: N. Keiding, B. Morgan, T. Speed, P. van der Heijden

AN INVARIANT APPROACH TO STATISTICAL ANALYSIS OF SHAPES	S. Lele and J. Richtsmeier
ASTROSTATISTICS	G. Babu and E. Feigelson
CLINICAL TRIALS IN ONCOLOGY	J. Crowley, S. Green, and J. Benedetti
DYNAMICAL SEARCH	L. Pronzato, H. Wynn, and A. Zhigljavsky
GRAPHICAL ANALYSIS OF MULTI-RESPONSE DATA	K. Basford and J. Tukey
INTRODUCTION TO COMPUTATIONAL BIOLOGY: MAPS, SEQUENCES, AND GENOMES	M. Waterman
MARKOV CHAIN MONTE CARLO IN PRACTICE	W. Gilks, S. Richardson, and D. Spiegelhalter
STATISTICS FOR ENVIRONMENTAL BIOLOGY AND TOXICOLOGY	A. Bailer and W. Piegorsch
DESIGN AND ANALYSIS OF QUALITY LIFE OF STUDIES IN CLINICAL TRIALS	Diane L. Fairclough

Interdisciplinary Statistics

CLINICAL TRIALS in ONCOLOGY

Second Edition

Stephanie Green
Jacqueline Benedetti
John Crowley

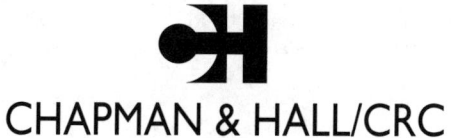

CHAPMAN & HALL/CRC

A CRC Press Company
Boca Raton   London   New York   Washington, D.C.

Library of Congress Cataloging-in-Publication Data

Green, Stephanie.
 Clinical trials in oncology / Stephanie Green, Jacqueline Benedetti, John Crowley.—2nd ed.
        p. cm. (interdisciplinary statistics series)
 Includes bibliographical references and index.
 ISBN 1-58488-302-2 (alk. paper)
 1. Cancer—Research—Statistical methods. 2. Clinical trials. I. Benedetti, Jacqueline. II. Crowley, John, 1946– III. Title. IV. Interdisciplinary statistics.
 [DNLM: 1. Clinical Trials—standards. 2. Neoplasms—therapy. 3. Clinical Trails. 4. Data Interpretation, Statistical. QZ 16 G798c 2002]
 RC267 .G744 2002
 616.99′4′00727—dc21   2002023356
                                                                         CIP

This book contains information obtained from authentic and highly regarded sources. Reprinted material is quoted with permission, and sources are indicated. A wide variety of references are listed. Reasonable efforts have been made to publish reliable data and information, but the authors and the publisher cannot assume responsibility for the validity of all materials or for the consequences of their use.

Neither this book nor any part may be reproduced or transmitted in any form or by any means, electronic or mechanical, including photocopying, microfilming, and recording, or by any information storage or retrieval system, without prior permission in writing from the publisher.

All rights reserved. Authorization to photocopy items for internal or personal use, or the personal or internal use of specific clients, may be granted by CRC Press LLC, provided that $1.50 per page photocopied is paid directly to Copyright Clearance Center, 222 Rosewood Drive, Danvers, MA 01923 USA. The fee code for users of the Transactional Reporting Service is ISBN 1-58488-302-2/03/$0.00+$1.50. The fee is subject to change without notice. For organizations that have been granted a photocopy license by the CCC, a separate system of payment has been arranged.

The consent of CRC Press LLC does not extend to copying for general distribution, for promotion, for creating new works, or for resale. Specific permission must be obtained in writing from CRC Press LLC for such copying.

Direct all inquiries to CRC Press LLC, 2000 N.W. Corporate Blvd., Boca Raton, Florida 33431.

Trademark Notice: Product or corporate names may be trademarks or registered trademarks, and are used only for identification and explanation, without intent to infringe.

Visit the CRC Press Web site at www.crcpress.com

© 2003 by Chapman & Hall/CRC

No claim to original U.S. Government works
International Standard Book Number 1-58488-302-2
Library of Congress Card Number 2002023356
Printed in the United States of America 1 2 3 4 5 6 7 8 9 0
Printed on acid-free paper

Dedications

To all the patients who have been enrolled in Southwest Oncology Group trials over the past 45 years; their participation in our trials has helped immeasurably in the struggle against cancer. (SG)

In memory of Norma Benedetti, my mother-in-law, and Stacy Trepp, whose deaths due to cancer are a constant reminder of how much work there is left to do. (JB)

In memory of my father, who died too young of pancreatic cancer. (JC)

Contents

Acknowledgments	**xiii**
1 Introduction	**1**
1.1 A brief history of clinical trials	1
1.2 The Southwest Oncology Group	6
1.3 Example trials	7
1.4 The reason for this book	9
2 Statistical Concepts	**11**
2.1 Introduction	11
2.2 The Phase II trial — estimation	19
2.3 The Phase III trial – hypothesis testing	23
2.3.1 Response as the outcome	24
2.3.2 Survival as the outcome	30
2.4 The proportional hazards model	37
2.5 Sample size calculations	39
2.6 Concluding remarks	40
3 The Design of Clinical Trials	**41**
3.1 Introduction	41
3.1.1 Objectives	42
3.1.2 Eligibility, treatments, endpoints	42
3.1.3 Differences to be detected or precision of estimates	43
3.1.4 Method of treatment assignment	43
3.1.5 Assumptions for sample size calculation	43
3.2 Endpoints	44
3.3 Phase I trials	48
3.3.1 Traditional designs	48
3.3.2 Newer Phase I designs	49
3.3.3 Phase I/II designs	52
3.3.4 Considerations for biologic agents	52

		3.3.5	Final comment	53
	3.4	Phase II trials		53
		3.4.1	The Standard Southwest Oncology Group Phase II design	54
		3.4.2	Randomized Phase II designs	58
		3.4.3	Other Phase II designs	61
	3.5	Phase III trials		62
		3.5.1	Randomization	62
		3.5.2	Two-arm trials	69
		3.5.3	Equivalence or noninferiority trials	73
	3.6	Conclusion		76
4	**Multi-Arm Trials**			**79**
	4.1	Introduction		79
	4.2	Types of multi-arm trials		80
	4.3	Significance level		83
	4.4	Power		84
	4.5	Interaction		86
	4.6	Other model assumptions		90
	4.7	To screen or not to screen		90
	4.8	Timing of randomization		92
	4.9	Conclusion		94
5	**Interim Analysis and Data Monitoring Committees**			**97**
	5.1	Planned interim analyses		97
		5.1.1	Caveats	103
	5.2	Data monitoring committees: Rationale and responsibilities		103
	5.3	Monitoring committees: Composition		107
	5.4	Examples		112
		5.4.1	Stopping early for positive results	112
		5.4.2	Stopping early for negative results	115
		5.4.3	Stopping an equivalence trial early for positive results	115
		5.4.4	Stopping based on toxicity and lack of compliance	118
		5.4.5	Emergency stopping based on unexpected toxic deaths	121
	5.5	Concluding remarks		122
6	**Data Management and Quality Control**			**123**
	6.1	Introduction: Why worry?		123
	6.2	Protocol development		128

		6.2.1	Objectives	128
		6.2.2	Background	129
		6.2.3	Drug information	129
		6.2.4	Stage definitions	129
		6.2.5	Eligibility criteria	129
		6.2.6	Stratification factors and subsets	130
		6.2.7	Treatment plan	131
		6.2.8	Treatment modification	131
		6.2.9	Study calendar	132
		6.2.10	Endpoint definitions	132
		6.2.11	Statistical considerations	133
		6.2.12	Discipline review	133
		6.2.13	Registration instructions	134
		6.2.14	Data submission instructions	134
		6.2.15	Special instructions	135
		6.2.16	Regulatory requirements	135
		6.2.17	Bibliography	135
		6.2.18	Forms	135
		6.2.19	Appendix	135
		6.2.20	Additional comments on SWOG study 8811	136
	6.3	Data collection		136
		6.3.1	Basic data items	137
		6.3.2	Data forms	140
	6.4	Protocol management and evaluation		143
		6.4.1	Registration	143
		6.4.2	Data flow	144
		6.4.3	Evaluation of data	145
		6.4.4	Publication	148
		6.4.5	Resolution of problems: Examples from SWOG 8811	148
	6.5	Quality assurance audits		149
	6.6	Training		150
	6.7	Data base management		151
		6.7.1	Data base structures	151
		6.7.2	Data collection, transmission, and entry	152
	6.8	Conclusion		154
	6.9	Appendix: Examples		155
		6.9.1	Treatment table for 8811	155
		6.9.2	Sample study calendar	155
		6.9.3	Sample flow sheet	156
		6.9.4	Sample treatment and toxicity form for a single agent treatment given every 4 weeks for 1 day	157
		6.9.5	Sample follow-up form	158

		6.9.6	Sample notice of death	159
		6.9.7	Sample checklist	160
		6.9.8	Sample tables	162

7 Reporting of Results — 165
7.1 Timing of report — 166
- 7.1.1 Phase II trials — 167
- 7.1.2 Phase III trials — 167

7.2 Required information — 168
- 7.2.1 Objectives and design — 168
- 7.2.2 Eligibility and treatment — 168
- 7.2.3 Results — 169

7.3 Analyses — 170
- 7.3.1 Exclusions, intent to treat — 170
- 7.3.2 Summary statistics: Estimates and variability of estimates — 172
- 7.3.3 Interpretation of results — 175
- 7.3.4 Secondary analyses — 178

7.4 Conclusion — 179

8 Pitfalls — 181
8.1 Introduction — 181
8.2 Historical controls — 181
8.3 Competing risks — 188
8.4 Outcome by outcome analyses — 195
- 8.4.1 Survival by response comparisons — 195
- 8.4.2 Dose intensity analyses — 199

8.5 Subset analyses — 203
8.6 Surrogate endpoints — 206

9 Exploratory Analyses — 209
9.1 Introduction — 209
9.2 Some background and notation — 210
9.3 Identification of prognostic factors — 212
- 9.3.1 Scale of measurement — 213
- 9.3.2 Choice of model — 216

9.4 Forming prognostic groups — 219
9.5 Analysis of microarray data — 224
9.6 Meta-Analysis — 226
- 9.6.1 Some principles of meta-analysis — 227
- 9.6.2 An example meta-analysis: Portal vein infusion — 228
- 9.6.3 Conclusions from the portal vein meta-analysis — 231
- 9.6.4 Some final remarks on meta-analysis — 231

9.7 Concluding remarks 232

10 Summary and Conclusions 233

Bibliography 237

Index 253

Acknowledgments

We would like to extend thanks to Bill Fortney, who made many invaluable comments and suggestions that greatly improved this book. Thanks also to Charles A. Coltman, Jr., the Chair of the Southwest Oncology Group, who has been an inspiration and a source of support and encouragement. We sincerely appreciate our families' patience and understanding of the time and effort spent in writing this book. Special thanks to Mike LeBlanc, Joth Jacobson, Janet O'Sullivan, and Anita Pang for help with the figures and tables, and to Kim Margolin, the study coordinator of SWOG 8811, who reviewed the Data Management and Quality Control chapter.

All royalties from the sale of this book will go to Cancer Research And Biostatistics, a nonprofit corporation founded to support the research activities of the Southwest Oncology Group Statistical Center.

CHAPTER 1

Introduction

It is best to prove things by actual experiment; then you know; whereas if you depend on guessing and supposing and conjectures, you never get educated.

–Mark Twain

...statistics are curious things. They afford one of the few examples in which the use...of mathematical methods tends to induce a strong emotional reaction in non-mathematical minds. This is because statisticians apply, to problems in which we are interested, a technique which we do not understand. It is exasperating, when we have studied a problem by methods that we have spent laborious years in mastering, to find our conclusions questioned, and perhaps refuted, by someone who could not have made the observations himself.

–Sir Austin Bradford Hill (1937)

1.1 A brief history of clinical trials

The history of clinical trials before 1750 is easily summarized: there were no clinical trials. The basic philosophy of medicine from the time of Hippocrates to the seventeenth century was humoralistic; the accepted version of this philosophy was due to the Greek Galen (130 AD). Since he "laid down...all that could possibly be said on medicine, he attained an authority that remained unchallenged until well into the sixteenth century. His views on cancer continued to be decisive for an even longer time." (De Moulin, 1989). Illness was caused by imbalances in blood, phlegm, black bile, and yellow bile; treatment consisted of restoring balance. Cancer was caused by a congestion of black bile; appropriate treatment was therefore rigorous purging, a strict bland diet and, for non-occult disease, poultices and possibly surgery with evacuation of melancholic blood.

No matter that the treatments did not work — after all, preoccupation with staying alive was contemptuously worldly. (Besides, there were always the miracles of Sts. Cosmas and Damian if the doctors couldn't do anything.) Not until the Renaissance were the humoralistic bases questioned. Various chemical, mechanical, and electrical causes of cancer were then proposed, and treatments devised in accordance with these causes. Sadly, these treatments were just as ineffective as the theories were inaccurate (e.g., arsenic to neutralize acidic cancer juice, diets to dissolve coagulated lymph, bloodletting or shocks to remove excessive electrical irritability). It never occurred to anyone to test whether the treatments worked.

The value of numerical methods began to be appreciated in the 1800s "when in 1806, E. Duvillard in Paris, applying a primitive statistical analysis, showed the favorable effect of smallpox vaccination on the general mortality rate" (De Moulin, 1989, from Duvillard, 1806). These early methods did uncover important epidemiologic facts, but were not so useful in judging treatment effectiveness. Although patient follow-up became the norm rather than the exception, and theories became more sophisticated, typical treatment research consisted only of reports of case series. In an early example of the hazards of such research, reports of the post-operative cure of breast cancer by two Edinburgh surgeons in the 1700s (one the student of the other) were wildly divergent: one was reported as curing 4 out of 60 patients, the other as curing 76 out of 88 (De Moulin, 1989, from Monro, 1781 and Wolff, 1907). Little wonder that it was nearly impossible to tell what worked and what did not.

If some of the treatments had not been actively harmful, perhaps it would not have mattered. Despite major advances in the understanding of disease by 1900, there were still few effective treatments. "The thick textbooks of 1900 are as sweepingly accurate on diagnosis as today's, but the chapters are all tragedies because they lack a happy ending of effective treatment" (Gordon, 1993). Still, the few medical advances (mercury for syphilis, digitalis for heart disease, iodine for goiter) and especially the advances in surgery allowed by anesthetics and antiseptics ushered in the "golden age" of Western medicine. Doctors had a priestly role as wise and trusted advisors, with warm and personal relationships with their patients (Silverman, 1992). Of course, these trusted advisors with warm personal relationships did not experiment on their patients. Thus even though most of the principles of comparative trials had been enunciated as early as 1866 by Claude Bernard — "...else the doctor walks at random and becomes sport of illusion" (Boissel, 1989, quoted from Bernard,

1866) — and despite the development of modern methods of experimental design in other scientific fields, clinical research remained limited.

In the middle of this century, treatment options began to catch up with biological advances; questions abounded, and clear answers were not coming fast enough. The first randomized therapeutic clinical trial (1946–48) was the result of a pressing medical problem (tuberculosis), a severely limited supply of a new agent (streptomycin), and frustration with the uninterpretability of 100 years of uncontrolled experimentation. Sir Austin Bradford Hill made the statistical arguments for the trial: the best way to get an answer, particularly given a streptomycin supply sufficient for only 50 patients, was a strictly controlled trial (Hill, 1990). Dr. Phillip D'Arcy Hart, an expert in the treatment of tuberculosis, gave the medical arguments. "The natural course of pulmonary tuberculosis is... so variable and unpredictable that evidence of improvement or cure following the use of a new drug in a few cases cannot be accepted as proof of the effect of that drug. The history of chemotherapeutic trials in tuberculosis is filled with errors..." He went on to note that the claims made for gold treatment, which had persisted over 15 years, provided a "spectacular example" and concluded that results in the future could not be considered valid unless tested in an adequately controlled trial (Gail, 1996, quoting from Streptomycin in Tuberculosis Trials Committee of the Medical Reseach Council, 1948).

This first trial demonstrated convincingly that a regimen of streptomycin plus bed rest was superior to bed rest alone. Not at all bad for the first attempt: 15 years and still no answer on gold with the old observational methods, 2 years with the new methods and a clear answer on streptomycin.

The trial of streptomycin for pulmonary tuberculosis "can be seen to have ushered in a new era of medicine," and Hill generally is agreed to have done "more than any other individual to introduce and foster adoption of the properly randomized controlled trial in modern clinical research" (Silverman and Chalmers, 1991). His efforts to explain and promote good clinical research were tireless and ultimately effective, particularly after the thalidomide tragedy of the 1960s demonstrated the potential harm in *not* doing carefully controlled trials.

Controlled trials in cancer in the United States were first sponsored by the National Cancer Institute (NCI) under the leadership of Dr. Gordon Zubrod. Zubrod, profoundly influenced by the streptomycin trial, employed the new methods himself (with others) in the study of penicillin in pneumonia and introduced the methods to other early leaders in the cancer clinical trials effort (Zubrod, 1982). Upon his move to the NCI, a comparative study in childhood acute leukemia was designed. This effort expanded into two of the initial cooperative cancer clinical trials groups, the Acute Leukemia Groups A and B; Group B (now Cancer and Leukemia Group B, or CALGB) had the honor of publishing the first trial (Frei et al., 1958). Zubrod was also instrumental in the formation in 1955 of the Eastern Solid Tumor Group (now the Eastern Cooperative Oncology Group, or ECOG) which published the first randomized trial in solid tumors in the United States in 1960 (Zubrod et al., 1960).

Of course not everyone was immediately persuaded that randomized trials were the best way to conduct clinical research. Jerome Cornfield, who advised Zubrod, was a major figure in the development of biostatistical methods at the NCI and an early advocate of randomization. His response to the suggestion from a radiotherapist that patients be assigned to conventional therapy or super voltage according to hospital instead of by randomization is often quoted. The quote is a very tactfully worded suggestion that the approach would be suitable if there were no other design options. He ended with an example of a sea sickness trial with treatment assigned by boat. How could the trial be interpreted if a great deal more turbulence and seasickness occurred on one of the boats? The radiotherapist got the point and randomized by patient (Ederer, 1982). Cornfield is also important for his advocacy of adequate planning, attention to quality, and especially adequate sample size: "...clinical research... is littered with the wrecks of studies that are inconclusive or misleading because they were of inadequate scope" (Ederer, 1982, quoting from a memorandum to the Coronary Drug Project steering committee).

Ever since the streptomycin trial, randomized studies have been invaluable in assessing the effectiveness of new therapies. In some cases cherished beliefs have been challenged. An early example was the University Group Diabetes Project (UGDP) which contradicted the widespread view that lowering blood sugar with oral hypoglycemic drugs prolonged life in patients with diabetes. Other examples include the National Surgical Adjuvant Breast and Bowel Program (NSABP) trials of breast cancer surgery demonstrating that more is *not* better, the Cardiac Arrhythmia Suppression Trial (CAST) demonstrating that suppression of ventricular arrhythmia by encainide or flecainide in patients having recent myocardial infarction *increases* the death rate instead of decreasing it, and the Southwest Oncology Group trial in non-Hodgkin's lymphoma demonstrating that new highly toxic combination chemotherapy regimens are *not* better than the old standard combination regimen. However, cherished beliefs die hard. Results such as these met with heavy resistance despite the randomized designs (for other examples, see Klimt, 1989); think how easy it would have been to dismiss the results if the designs had been inherently biased. Positive results are happier examples of the importance of clinical trials: the Diabetic Retinopathy Trial demonstrating dramatically reduced visual loss due to photocoagulation therapy, trials establishing the effectiveness of therapy in improving survival in patients with Wilms' tumor and other childhood cancers, beta blockers prolonging life after myocardial infarction, chemoradiotherapy substantially improving survival in nasopharygeal and gastric cancers.

Randomized trials cannot answer every treatment question. Randomization is not feasible in every setting, costs may be prohibitive, and political realities may interfere. Since only a limited number of trials can be done, some questions have to be addressed in other ways. However, controlled trials are by far the best method available for addressing difficult and controversial questions in a way that minimizes distrust of the results. Consider the 1954 Salk Vaccine trial for which at the beginning "the most urgent business was to... turn the focus away from professional rivalries, power struggles, and theoretical disputes and back to the neglected question of whether or not Salk's vaccine worked." Thomas Francis, Jr. was given the job of evaluating the vaccine because "everybody knew that when Tommy Francis talked about working up to a standard, it was one of unimpeachable thoroughness; even the most dedicated opponent to the new vaccine could never say a trial supervised by Francis was political, biased, or incomplete" (Smith, 1990). His two nonnegotiable demands before agreeing to take on the job were that the vaccine proponents would not design the trial and would have no access to the results while the trial was ongoing, and that the trial would have a randomized double-blind design instead of an observed-control design in which second graders would have gotten the vaccine and would have been compared to unvaccinated first and third graders. The results of this "textbook model of elegant clinical testing" were unquestionable. Francis's announcement that "the new vaccine was safe, effective, and potent... was a landmark in 20th century history, one of the few events that burned itself into the public consciousness because the news was good" (Smith, 1992). Unimpeachable thoroughness, nonpolitical, unbiased, complete, independent, properly designed — Francis set a very high standard indeed, and one to which all of us involved in clinical research should aspire.

1.2 The Southwest Oncology Group

There are now dozens of national and international consortia of institutions and investigators organized for the purpose of improving the survival of cancer patients through clinical research. Our own experience is with the Southwest Oncology Group, which began in 1956 in the United States as the (pediatric) Southwest Cancer Chemotherapy Study Group under the direction of Dr. Grant Taylor at the M.D. Anderson Cancer Center in Houston, Texas. In 1958 membership was extended to include investigators evaluating adult malignancies, in the early 1960s a Solid Tumor Committee was established. Since then the pediatric part of the Group split off (to become the Pediatric Oncology Group, now part of the Children's Oncology Group), the name was changed to the Southwest Oncology Group (SWOG), and the Group has expanded to include specialists in all modalities of cancer therapy and institutions in all regions of the country. Most of the studies done by the Group are designed to assess whether a regimen merits further study (Phase II), or to compare two or more regimens (Phase III). Studies in cancer control research (prevention, symptom control, quality of life) are also carried out. Currently the Group is led by the Group Chair, Dr. Charles Coltman (University of Texas, San Antonio) and the Group Statistician, Dr. John Crowley (Cancer Research And Biostatistics and the Fred Hutchinson Cancer Research Center, Seattle).

The structure of SWOG is typical of cooperative groups and includes the operations office (administration, grants management, industry contracts, meeting planning, legal matters, regulatory requirements, study development, audits); the statistical center (study development, data base management, network services, computer applications, study quality control, statistical analysis and statistical research); disease committees (brain cancer, breast cancer, gastrointestinal cancer, genitourinary cancer, gynecologic cancer, head and neck cancer, leukemia, lung cancer, lymphoma, melanoma, myeloma, sarcoma); discipline committees (such as radiotherapy, surgery, pathology, cytogenetics, bone marrow and stem cell transplantation); standing committees (such as cancer control, women and special populations, immunomolecular therapeutics); and all of the participating institutions that enter patients into trials. Group trials and related scientific investigations are proposed and developed within the disease committees under the leadership of the disease committee chairs. Committee leadership is also provided by the disease committee statistician, who is responsible for reviewing, designing, monitoring, and analyzing all studies done in the committee. Each study developed has a clinician assigned (the study coordinator) to lead the development effort, to evaluate the data after the study is open, and to be the primary author on the manuscript when the study is complete. Each study also has a protocol coordinator assigned from the operations office, who coordinates the production and review of the study protocol, and a data coordinator from the statistical center who does most of the necessary setup work for opening a study, registers patients to the study, and reviews and evaluates all of the study data. Participating physicians and clinical research associates at Group institutions are responsible for submitting protocols to their Institutional Review Boards, identifying patients suitable for studies, obtaining informed consent, assuring study participants are treated and followed according to protocol, and for correctly submitting all required data.

The Group typically has 80 to 100 actively accruing studies at any one time and 400 closed studies in active follow-up. Over 3000 physicians from more than 500 institutions participate. Since the Group began, 130,000 patients have been registered to its studies, and 2000 abstracts and manuscripts have been published. The Group's extensive clinical trials experience provides the context and examples for this book.

1.3 Example trials

We describe here a few of the trials that will be used as examples throughout the remainder of this book. SWOG 8811 (Margolin et al., 1994) is an example of a Phase II trial. The aim was to decide if the combination of 5-fluorouracil and folinic acid was worth further study in patients with advanced breast cancer. A detailed description is given in Chapters 3 and 6. The disappointing answer to the trial question, as with so many Phase II trials, was that the combination was not worth further study. As stated above, not every regimen can be tested in a comparative trial; Phase II studies serve to screen out inactive regimens and identify those most promising for randomized testing. The primary measure of activity in a Phase II trial is usually tumor response, either complete response (total disappearance of all evidence of disease) or partial response (reduction of tumor). Toxicity and survival are typical secondary endpoints.

The Phase III study SWOG 7827 (Rivkin et al., 1993) in patients with operable, node-positive, receptor-negative breast cancer is an example of a standard two-arm randomized trial designed to determine if a new regimen is superior to a standard (control). In this case the standard was 1 year of combination chemotherapy consisting of cyclophosphamide, methotrexate, 5-fluorouracil, vincristine, and prednisone (more conveniently known as CMFVP). CMFVP had been shown in a previous randomized trial to be superior to single agent melphalan as adjuvant treatment for operable, node-positive breast cancer. (Note: adjuvant means "in addition," after complete removal of visible tumor by surgery or other means.) The new arm consisted of 2 years of treatment instead of 1 year. Node-positive, receptor-negative disease is particularly aggressive, and it was thought that this subset of patients might benefit from the additional year of therapy. Aspects of this trial are discussed in Chapters 3 and 8. Trials of a standard therapy vs. a new one are the mainstay of clinical trials research and the greatest strength of the Southwest Oncology Group. The group has done dozens of such trials, from small ones in rapidly lethal disease, to our massive 18,000 participant study (SWOG 9217) testing whether the agent finasteride can prevent prostate cancer. The usual endpoints for Phase III studies are death, toxicity, and failure, with failure in the prevention setting defined as development of the disease, failure in the adjuvant setting defined as recurrence or relapse of the disease or death, and failure in the advanced disease setting defined as progression of the disease or death. (Note: the "progress" in progression is increase in tumor, not progress for the patient.)

SWOG 8412 (Alberts et al., 1992) is also a two-arm randomized trial with a standard arm, but with a twist. In this study patients with stage IV or suboptimal stage III ovarian cancer with no prior chemotherapy were randomized to receive either cyclophosphamide plus cisplatin (standard) or cyclophosphamide plus carboplatin. The aim was not to show the superiority of carboplatin, however, but rather to show that it was approximately equivalent to cisplatin. The rationale for the aim was the extreme toxicities associated with cisplatin. If carboplatin were found to be approximately equivalent to cisplatin, it would be preferred due to a better toxicity profile. SWOG 8412 is discussed in Chapters 3 and 5.

SWOG 8738 (Gandara et al., 1993) and SWOG 8300 (Miller et al., 1998), appearing in Chapters 4 and 5, are examples of Phase III studies with more than two arms. The first was a study in advanced non-small-cell lung cancer which randomized among standard dose-intensity cisplatin, high dose-intensity cisplatin, and high dose-intensity cisplatin plus mitomycin C. The aims were to test if high dose-intensity cisplatin was superior to standard and, if so, whether mitomycin C added to the efficacy of high dose-intensity cisplatin — two comparisons in one trial. The second study, in patients with locally advanced non-small-cell lung cancer, randomized to chest radiotherapy (RT) vs. chest RT plus chemotherapy vs. chest RT plus prophylactic brain RT vs. chest RT plus chemotherapy plus prophylactic brain RT. The two aims of this trial were to test if chemotherapy improved survival and to test if prophylactic brain RT improved survival — again, two comparisons in one trial. The role of the standard two-arm design in clinical trials is clear; the properties of multi-arm designs are much less well understood and are the subject of current statistical research, as discussed in Chapter 4.

1.4 The reason for this book

Our motivations for writing this book are captured by the introductory quotes. Among the three of us we have devoted over 60 years to clinical trials research. As suggested by the first quote, we want to know whether treatments work or not. Furthermore, we want the methods we use to find out whether treatments work to be unimpeachable. Unfortunately, as suggested by the second quote, as statisticians we too often find our motives and methods misunderstood or questioned — and at times actively resented. With this book, it is our hope to improve the mutual understanding by clinicians and statisticians of the principles of cancer clinical trials. Although most of the examples we use are specific to the Southwest Oncology Group, the issues and principles discussed are important in cancer clinical trials more generally, and indeed in any clinical setting.

CHAPTER 2

Statistical Concepts

To understand God's thoughts we must study statistics, for these are the measure of His purpose.

–Florence Nightingale

2.1 Introduction

A collaborative team that includes both clinicians and statisticians is crucial to the successful conduct of a clinical trial. Although the statistical study design and analyses are mainly the responsibility of the statistician, an understanding of the basic statistical principles is vital for the clinicians involved with the study. The main goal of this chapter is to present statistical concepts that are of particular application to cancer clinical trials.

The objectives of the trial, the key types of data that are collected to meet these objectives, and the types of analyses to be performed are in large part determined by the type of study being undertaken. Phase II trials are small studies early in the development of a regimen that typically focus on response and toxicity data, while Phase III trials are large comparative studies that most frequently assess survival and progression-free survival. We introduce statistical concepts within the context of these two types of studies. Phase I trials (discussed in Chapter 3) are a third type of clinical trial which involve a much smaller number of patients, and as such, are less suited for use in illustrating basic statistical principles.

First, however, there are some general characteristics of data from clinical trials that do not depend on the type of study. Outcome measures can be classified as being either categorical (qualitative) or measurement (quantitative).

1. Categorical data — outcomes that can be classified according to one of several mutually exclusive categories

based on a predetermined set of criteria. For example, RECIST criteria for tumor response (see Chapter 3) categorize patients as achieving either a CR (complete response) if all tumor sites disappear; a PR (partial response) if the sum of maximum diameters of all target lesions decreases by 30% or more from baseline; INC (increasing) if the sum increases by 20% or more, or if new sites of tumor are noted; and STA (stable) if none of the above occur. Thus, in this case, patient response can be described by one of four categories, which are then often dichotomized into two categories for analysis (CR + PR vs. others; CR vs. others).
2. Measurement data — outcomes that are measured quantities. For example, concentrations of CA-125, a tumor antigen, are routinely collected in trials of ovarian cancer. Levels of this antigen range in value from 0 to over 10,000. In this case, the data measure a quantity that takes on many possible values. An important special case of quantitative data is time to event data, such as survival time, a measurement in units of time from entry on a study until death. What distinguishes this outcome, and its analysis, from other quantitative data is the frequent presence of what statisticians call *censoring*. In a typical clinical trial, not all patients have died by the time the study is completed and analyses are performed. For patients still alive, we know that they have lived at least as long as the time from the patient's entry on the study to the time of the analysis, but we do not know the actual death time. Special statistical techniques have been developed to incorporate these censored observations into the analysis.

Three other general concepts introduced in this section are *probability, statistic,* and *distribution*. The *probability* of an outcome is how often that outcome occurs in relation to all possible outcomes. For instance, the set of all possible outcomes for a flip of a coin is $\{H, T\}$. The probability of outcome T (tails) is 1/2 if the coin is fair. If the coin is unfair (or biased) and the outcome H (heads) is twice as likely as T, the set of all possible outcomes remains $\{H, T\}$ but the probability of T is now 1/3. If the coin is flipped twice, the set of possible outcomes is $\{HH, HT, TH, TT\}$. Note that there are two events that yield exactly one tail in two flips, since the tail can be the outcome of either the first or the second flip. With the fair coin the probability of TT is $1/2 \times 1/2 = 1/4$; with the biased coin it is $1/3 \times 1/3 = 1/9$. The probability of exactly one tail is $(1/2 \times 1/2) + (1/2 \times 1/2) = 1/2$ or $(1/3 \times 2/3) + (2/3 \times 1/3) = 4/9$ for the fair and biased coin, respectively. Multiplying the probabilities on each flip to arrive at a probability for the outcomes or events such as TT or HT is justified by an assumption of independence of coin flips, i.e., that the probability of tails on the second flip is unaffected by the outcome of the first flip.

Most commonly used statistical procedures require this independence assumption. What this means is that the value of one observation provides no information about the value of any other. In particular, multiple measures from the same patient cannot be treated as if they were from two separate (independent) patients. This is because two measurements on the same patient tend to be more alike than two measurements, one from each of two different people. Treating multiple observations (such as results from multiple biopsy specimens as to the presence of the Multi-Drug Resistance gene, or MDR) as independent is a common pitfall that should be avoided. For instance, if half of all patients have MDR-positive tumors, but within a patient multiple biopsy results are nearly always the same, then for six biopsies about 3/6 would be expected to be MDR positive if all 6 biopsies were from different patients, while either 0/6 or 6/6 would be expected to be positive if all six were from the same patient.

The outcome "number of MDR positive tumors out of N tumors" is an example of a *statistic,* that is, a summary of results from N separate tumors. In general, a statistic is any summary from a set of data points. For example, in the case of measured data such as CA-125, one could summarize the measures from a group of patients using descriptive statistics such as a mean or a median. The statistics chosen to summarize a data set will depend on the type of data collected and the intended use of the information. Some statistics are merely descriptive; others, called test statistics, are used to test hypotheses after the data from an experiment are collected.

A *distribution* characterizes the probabilities of all possible outcomes of an event or all possible values of a statistic. For a single flip of a fair coin the distribution is

outcome	H	T
probability	1/2	1/2

while for the biased coin it is

outcome	H	T
probability	2/3	1/3

When a coin is flipped multiple times, a statistic often used to summarize the outcome is the number of tails observed. The distribution of this statistic is the *binomial* distribution, the most important distribution for categorical data. The distribution from an experiment of flipping a coin N times is characterized by giving the probability that the number of tails is equal to k, for every k from 0 to N. If the probability of a tail on one flip is p, and the flips are independent, the probability of a particular sequence of flips with exactly k tails (and thus $N-k$ heads) is $p^k(1-p)^{N-k}$. The rest of the exercise is to figure out how many sequences of heads and tails have exactly k tails, and add those up. For $N = 2$ and $k = 1$, we saw above that there were two such sequences, HT and TH. In general, the answer is given by the formula $\binom{N}{k} = \frac{N!}{k!(N-k)!}$, where $(\ )$ is read "N choose k" and $N!$ is N factorial, which is simply $N \times (N-1) \times \cdots \times 2 \times 1$. Thus the probability of exactly three tails in six flips of a fair coin is $\binom{6}{3}(1/2)^3(1-1/2)^{6-3} = \frac{6!}{3!3!}(1/2)^6 = 20/64 = 5/16 = 0.3125$. The entire binomial distribution for $N = 6$, and $p = 1/2$ or $1/3$ is given in Figure 2.1.

Binomial distributions apply in countless settings other than coin flips; the one of most interest to us in this book is tumor response (the number of responses in N patients taking the place of the number of tails in N flips). In the MDR example above, the binomial distribution applies only to the case where all biopsies are from different patients, since independence is a requirement for the distribution. The probability of exactly three MDR positive patients out of six, if the probability is 1/2 for an individual patient, is .3125; if all six biopsies are from the same patient this probability is close to 0. Applying the binomial distribution to the second case is clearly inappropriate.

When outcomes are categorical, the distribution can be shown in a simple table or graph, as above. When outcomes are measured, the distribution cannot be described in a table. Instead, cumulative probabilities are described by a function $F(t)$. For time to death, for example, $F(t)$ means the probability of dying before time t. The derivative of $F(t)$, denoted $f(t)$ and often called the density, can be thought of loosely as the probability of dying at t (in a sense made precise by the calculus). We also often talk more optimistically of the survival curve $S(t) = 1 - F(t)$, the probability of surviving at least

INTRODUCTION

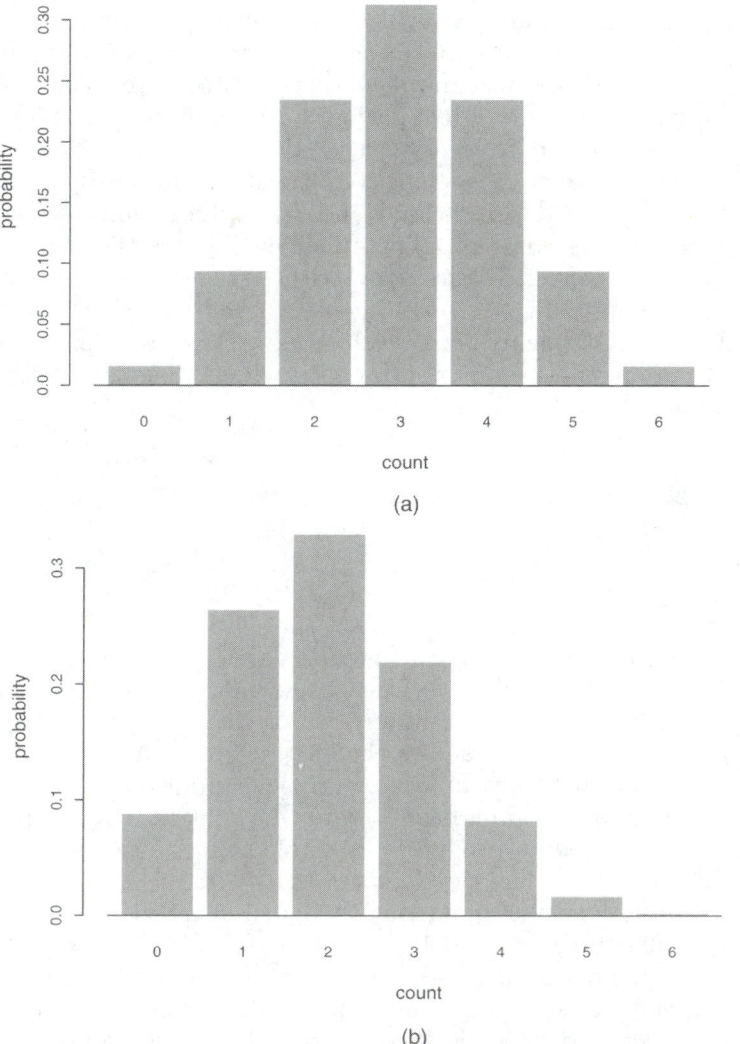

Figure 2.1. The binomial distribution for $N = 6$ and (a) $p = 1/2$, (b) $p = 1/3$.

to time t. Note that $S(0) = 1$ and $S(t)$ decreases toward 0 as t gets large. The *median* survival time, the time past which one half of the patients are expected to live, is that time m for which $S(m) = 0.5$.

Yet another quantity of interest is the *hazard function* or *hazard rate*, often denoted $\lambda(t)$. This function can be thought of loosely as the probability of death at time t given that the patient is alive just before time t: the instantaneous rate of failure. In terms of the other quantities we have described, the hazard function is given by $\lambda(t) = f(t)/S(t)$. Depending upon the type of disease, the hazard rate as a function of time can take on a variety of forms. For example, in a study involving surgery, a patient's risk of dying may be highest during the post-operative period, then decrease for a period of time. A rising hazard function is characteristic of normal mortality as one ages. In an advanced disease trial, the risk of dying may be relatively constant over the time of follow-up. These three types of hazard functions are given in Figure 2.2a, with the corresponding survival curves in Figure 2.2b.

The constant hazard case with $\lambda(t) = \lambda$ gives rise to what is called the exponential distribution, for which the survival curve is given by
$$S(t) = \exp(-\lambda t),$$
where exp is the exponential function. Under the assumption of exponential survival, the median survival m is
$$m = -\ln(0.5)/\lambda,$$
where ln is the natural logarithm. From this relationship it is easy to note that the ratio of hypothesized median survival times for two treatment arms is equal to the inverse of the ratio of the hypothesized hazards. Figure 2.3 shows the hazard function, survival curve, and median survival for an exponential distribution. Although the assumption of a constant hazard rate may not be correct in practice, it can be used to provide reasonable sample size estimates for designing clinical trials (see Chapter 3).

The most common quantitative distribution is the normal or Gaussian distribution, or bell-shaped curve. The standard normal density $f(x)$, presented in Figure 2.4, is a symmetric curve about the mean value 0. The probability of an outcome being less than x is $F(x)$, the area under the density up to x. The area under the whole curve has the value 1. The probability that an observation with this standard normal distribution is negative (zero or smaller) is $1/2$, the area under the curve to the left of 0 ($F(0) = 0.5$). The probability that an observation is greater than 1.645 is 0.05. The beauty of the normal distribution is that as sample sizes get large many common statistics that start out as non-normal attain an approximately normal distribution (or a distribution related to normal, such as the χ^2 distribution discussed in Section 2.3.1). This fact is embodied mathematically in what is known as the Central Limit Theorem. For instance, the probability of k or fewer tails in N coin flips can

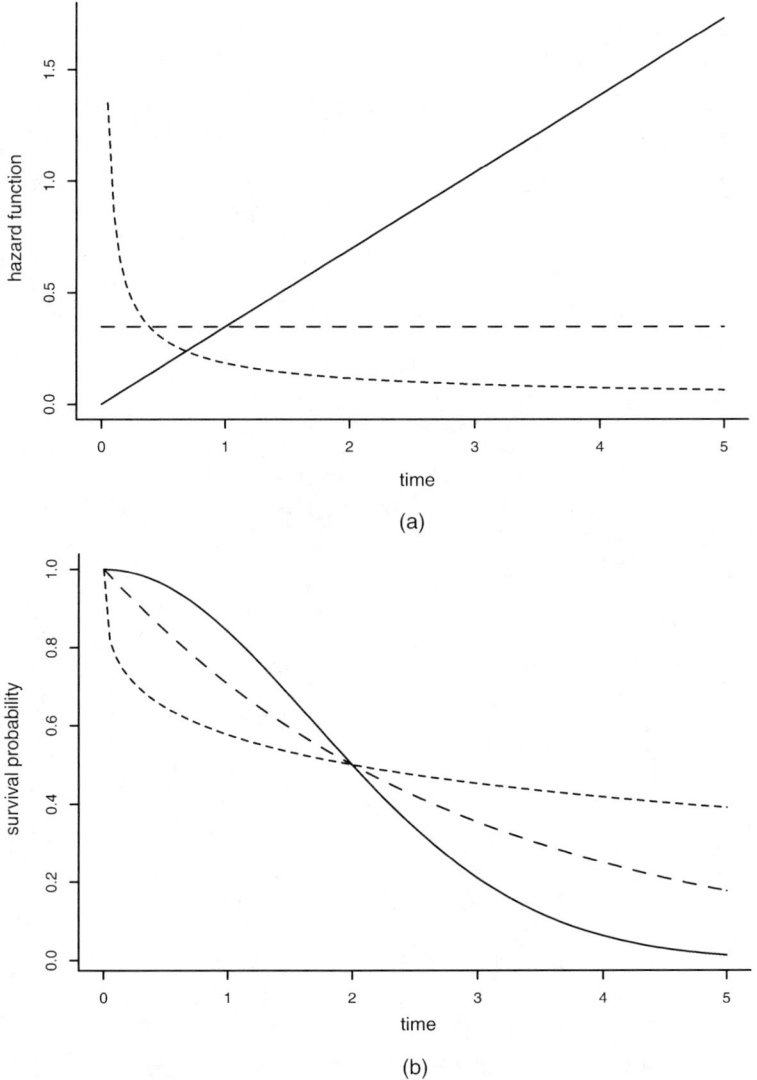

Figure 2.2. (a) Increasing (solid line), decreasing (dotted line), and constant (dashed line) hazard functions; (b) corresponding survival curves.

be found (approximately) from the normal distribution. This is useful in the development of statistical tests, and in the estimation of sample sizes (see Section 2.5).

The remainder of this chapter has been designed to present the key statistical concepts related to cancer clinical trials. For the most part, formulae will only be presented to provide insight into the use

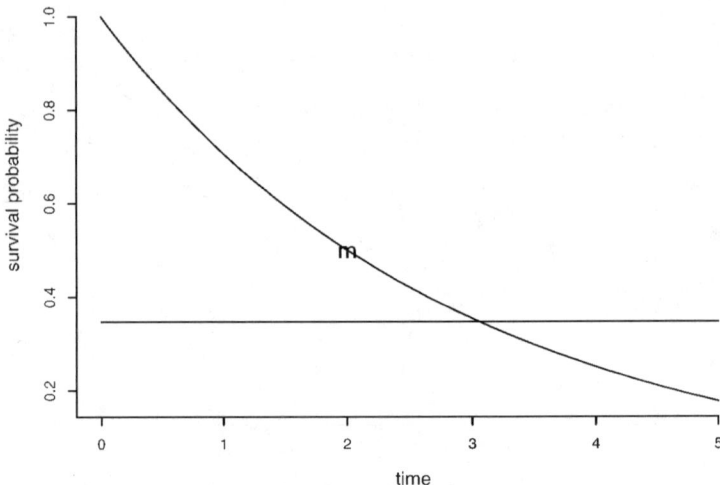

Figure 2.3. Hazard function (horizontal line), survival curve and median survival (m) for an exponential distribution.

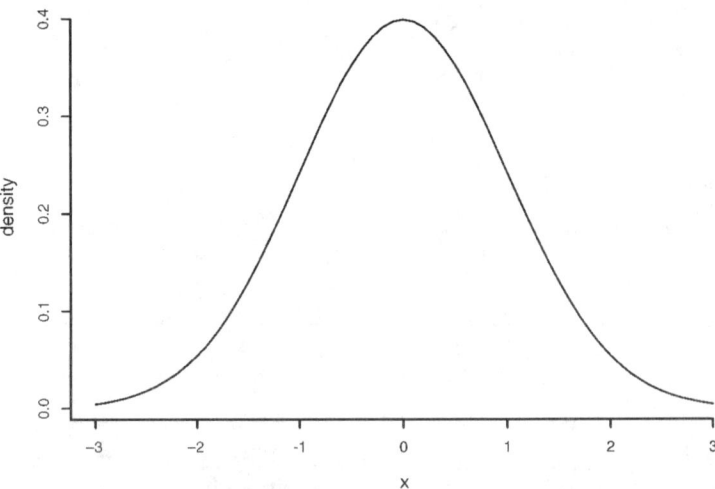

Figure 2.4. The standard normal density curve.

of certain statistical tests and procedures; it is far more important to understand *why* certain statistical techniques are used, rather than *how* to use them. We begin with examples that will be used to illustrate the key concepts.

2.2 The Phase II trial — estimation

There are two common types of Phase II trials. Trials of Investigational New Drugs (INDs) are performed to assess whether there is promise of activity for a particular disease type. Phase II pilot studies are usually done to assess the activity and feasibility of previously tested treatments, either using a new treatment schedule and/or using the drug in combination with other agents or modalities. In either case, care must be taken to explicitly define what is meant by "show some activity," "assess activity," or "evaluate feasibility."

SWOG 9134 (Balcerzak et al., 1995) was a Phase II IND trial that studied whether paclitaxel had any effectiveness in shrinking tumors of patients with soft-tissue sarcomas. Typically, the formal goal of a Phase II IND trial is to discriminate between promising and unpromising agents, based on the observed proportion responding in patients who are treated with the drug, where response is defined using a more detailed version of the response criteria mentioned in Section 2.1. The study design used for this type of trial is a two-stage design, which is detailed in Chapter 3. For our purposes here we discuss the final results, presented in Table 2.1.

The final category, NASS (no assessment, or inadequate assessment), deserves special mention. In Phase II trials, disease assessment is usually scheduled at specific time intervals, typically every 4 to 8 weeks. Particularly in Phase II trials, which often include very advanced disease patients, a patient may go off treatment prior to the definitive disease assessment, either due to toxicity, death from other causes, or refusal to continue therapy. These patients are assumed to have not responded. More discussion of this point occurs in Chapter 7.

From Table 2.1, if all responses (both CRs and PRs) are of interest, then there was a total of 6/48 patients who responded, or 0.12.

Table 2.1. Final results of Phase II paclitaxel trial.

Response	N	%
CR	1	2.1
PR	5	10.4
STA	10	20.8
INC	29	60.4
NASS	3	6.3
Total	48	100

This is said to be the estimated response probability. ("Rate" is often used instead of probability in this context, but the term is more accurately applied to concepts like the hazard.) The word "estimate" is used since this is not the true probability, but an approximation calculated from a sample of 48 individuals who were recruited for this trial. If the same trial were repeated in 48 different individuals, one would not expect that the estimated response probability for this second group of patients would be exactly 0.12, but might be smaller, or larger. If repeated trials were done, there would be a distribution of estimates of the response probability. This is due to the fact that each individual trial is made up of a sample of individuals from a larger population. In this example the larger population consists of all patients with soft-tissue sarcoma who would satisfy the eligibility criteria of the study. If we could treat the entire population of patients with paclitaxel, we would know the true response probability. What we hope, instead, is to use our sample of patients to get a reasonable estimate of the true probability, and to distinguish unpromising agents (with low true response probabilities) from promising ones. Symbolically, we denote the true response probability in the population by p, and denote the estimate of p from the sample of patients in the trial by $\hat{p}$ (here 0.12).

Accompanying this idea of an estimate of a true, but unknown, response probability is the notion of precision, or variability of our estimate. Because each estimate from a sample of individuals is not always going to produce a value that is exactly the same as the true response probability, we wish to have some assessment of how close our estimate is to the truth. This assessment depends, in large measure, on how many patients were studied. To understand this, consider the clinical trial of size 1. With one patient, an estimated response probability of either 0 or 1 is the only value that can be obtained. Yet no one would feel comfortable using that estimate as being reflective of the population. As the sample size increases, we begin to feel more confident that the resulting estimate comes close to measuring the true response probability. Thus, in a series of studies of 100 patients each, we would expect to see more precise estimates (less variability) than we would in a series of studies based on 48 patients. To illustrate this, consider Figure 2.5. These graphs are called histograms, and are a display of the frequency of values from a collection of data. Figure 2.5a displays the estimates of the response probabilities from a series of 100 studies, all based on 40 patients, while Figure 2.5b graphs the same results based on samples of size 100. In each case, the data are generated by the computer assuming the same true response probability $p = 0.20$. It can be seen that the

THE PHASE II TRIAL — ESTIMATION 21

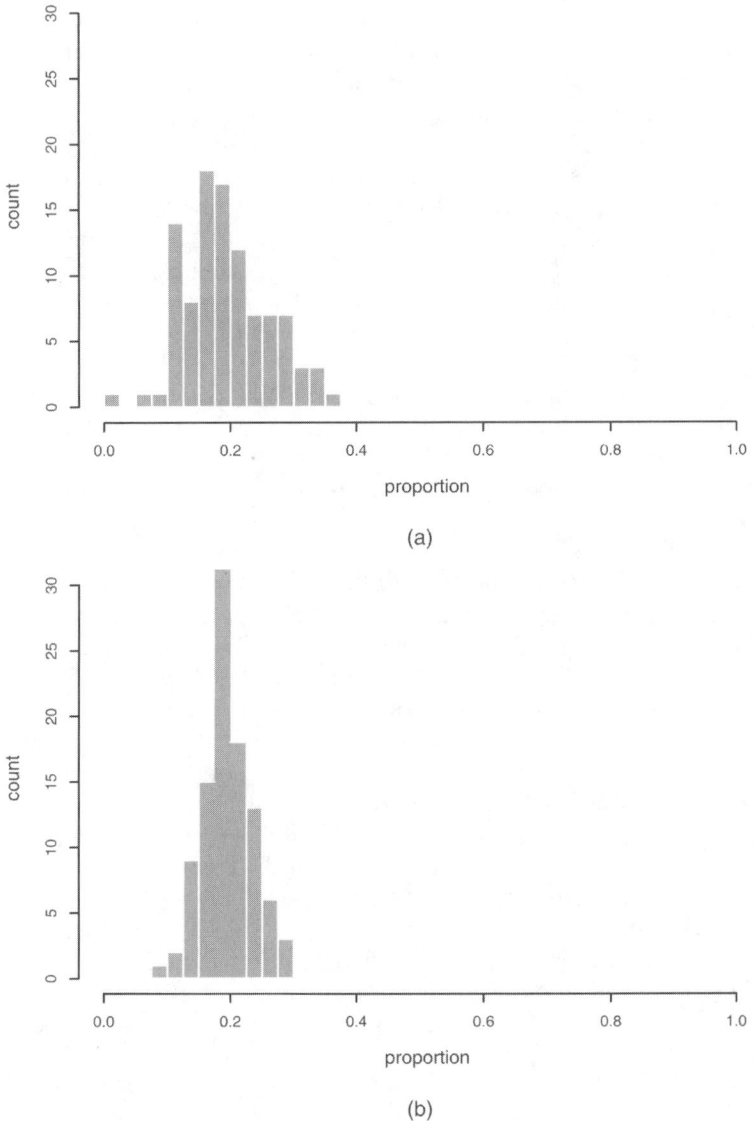

Figure 2.5. Histogram of estimated response probabilities from a series of 100 studies, each with (a) 40 patients, (b) 100 patients.

results based on trials of size 100 are more closely clustered around the value $p = 0.20$ than are the results based on a sample of size 40. Also notice that the shape of the distribution for trials of size 100 is closer to that of the normal distribution in Figure 2.4 than is the shape for trials of size 40.

The notion of precision of an estimate is often expressed as an interval of values that we could reasonably expect will include the true probability. This range of values is called a confidence interval. In the above paclitaxel example, the 95% confidence interval for the response probability is 0.047 to 0.253. This interval was obtained from some tables specifically generated for the binomial distribution (Diem and Lentner, 1970). Good approximations to this exact interval are possible when the sample size is large using the normal distribution, as explained in Section 2.1. The way we interpret this interval is to say that we are 95% confident that the true response probability (in the population) is somewhere between 0.047 and 0.253, in the sense that in a series of similar trials the 95% confidence interval will contain the true population probability 95% of the time. Investigators may choose other levels of confidence for the interval, depending upon how sure they want to be that the true value is in the interval. A 90% confidence interval may be sufficient for a Phase II trial, while 99% may be desirable when it is important to be conservative in drawing conclusions.

Suppose now that the researcher wishes to base a decision on whether to pursue treatment of soft-tissue sarcoma with paclitaxel on the results of this Phase II trial. The results of this trial, with $\widehat{p} = 0.12$, are consistent with a true response probability that is very low, or with an agent of modest activity. If the researcher was interested in finding a drug believed to have a response probability of at least 0.30, then this trial would lead the researcher to conclude that paclitaxel was not sufficiently active, and to pursue other therapies.

With a small sample size, the width of the confidence interval will be wide, implying that there is a large range of possible values for the true response probability; if the sample size is large, the corresponding confidence interval is much narrower. Table 2.2 gives the width of the confidence intervals obtained from four trials of sample sizes 20, 40, 60, and 80, all yielding the same response estimate of 20%.

Thus a confidence interval provides a measure of the precision of the estimate.

Table 2.2. Dependence of confidence interval width on sample size.

N	Confidence Interval
20	(0.06, 0.44)
40	(0.09, 0.36)
60	(0.11, 0.32)
80	(0.12, 0.30)

We have already mentioned the concept of a sample of patients from some larger population. A key aspect of any study is the reliability with which we may generalize the results we observe in our sample to the target population of interest. We discussed the impact of the size of our sample on our ability to draw reliable conclusions. Of equal importance is the similarity of our sample to the population to which we wish to apply the results of the study. For example, in the soft-tissue sarcoma trial, we may wish to test paclitaxel for use in all patients with poor prognosis soft-tissue sarcoma. However, if only patients with leiomyosarcoma are included in the Phase II trial, then the resulting response estimate may be an underestimate for patients with other histologic types, since leiomyosarcomas are traditionally unresponsive to chemotherapy. This lack of similarity in the sample and target population results in estimates that are biased; that is, they yield estimates that are not reflective of the population of interest. Care must be taken in defining eligibility criteria and in selecting patients to insure that the population sampled is representative of the population to which generalizations are to be made.

2.3 The Phase III trial – hypothesis testing

The goal of the Phase III trial is to compare treatment regimens. Early medicine based decisions on anecdotal reports of therapeutic successes or, more recently, on case series or prospective but nonrandomized trials. In these studies, groups of patients were given the therapy of interest. Results were then compared to historical knowledge or reports of patient experience with other treatments (see Chapter 1). Because of the huge potential for differences in the patient populations in these trials, biases are impossible to completely remove, making decisions based on nonrandomized trials subject to question. Since one of the major sources of bias is the unmeasurable process by which physicians and patients make treatment decisions, it is widely acknowledged that the most appropriate way to compare treatments is through a randomized clinical trial. Patients who satisfy the eligibility criteria of the trial are randomly assigned to treatment. This randomization guarantees that there is no systematic selection bias in treatment allocation. Techniques for randomization are discussed in Section 3.5. Examples of historical controls are presented in Chapter 8.

The primary objective for a Phase III trial in cancer is generally to compare survival (or occasionally disease-free or progression-free survival) among the treatment regimens. However, dichotomized categorical outcomes such as response are also often compared, and for ease of exposition we start with this dichotomous case.

2.3.1 Response as the outcome

SWOG 8412 was a study of the use of cyclophosphamide and either carboplatin or cisplatin in patients with Stage III or Stage IV ovarian cancer. One of the endpoints (though not the primary one) was the probability of response to chemotherapy among patients with measurable disease in each arm of the trial. Patients were randomized to receive either carboplatin and cyclophosphamide or cisplatin and cyclophosphamide, and were followed for survival and response. Of 291 eligible patients, 124 had measurable disease. We can record the response results of the trial in Table 2.3, called a 2 × 2 contingency table.

Note that for each treatment, we can estimate the response probability as we did for the Phase II trial above. Thus, the estimated response probability for the cisplatin arm (denoted arm A) is $\widehat{p}_A = 31/60 = 0.52$ and for the carboplatin arm (arm B) it is $\widehat{p}_B = 39/64 = 0.61$. Each estimate is based on the number of patients in the respective groups.

Because our goal here is to compare treatments, the question of interest is whether the response probability for patients receiving cisplatin differs from that for patients receiving carboplatin. We can phrase this as an hypothesis. The null hypothesis (denoted by H_0) for this illustration is that $p_A = p_B$, or in statistical shorthand, $H_0 : p_A = p_B$.

The *alternative hypothesis*, or H_1, which most often is what we are interested in establishing, can take one of two basic forms. If Treatment A is a more toxic or costly new regimen and Treatment B is a standard, the alternative hypothesis might be that the new regimen is better than the old. In statistical terms, this is written as $H_1 : p_B > p_A$. We will stay with the status quo (Treatment A) unless the new regimen proves to be better (we are not really interested in proving whether the new regimen is worse). This is known as a

Table 2.3. Responses to treatment for ovarian cancer.

	Response	No Response	Totals	Response Estimate
Arm A	31	29	60	0.52
Arm B	39	25	64	0.61
Totals	70	54	124	0.565

one-sided test. If Treatment A and Treatment B are two competing standards, we might be interested in seeing if one of the two is better. This *two-sided* alternative is denoted $H_1 : p_A \neq p_B$.

If the null hypothesis is true, then we would expect that the difference in our estimated probabilities, $\hat{p}_A - \hat{p}_B$, should be close to zero, while if there were really a difference between the two true probabilities, we would expect the difference in the estimates to be much different from zero. In a manner similar to what we did for the Phase II trial, we can create a confidence interval for the difference between the two probabilities. In this case, the 95% CI (based on the approximation using the normal distribution) is $(-0.26, 0.08)$. Because this interval contains zero, it is consistent with the hypothesis that the difference is 0; that is, that the true probabilities p_A and p_B are the same. If the interval did not include 0, the data would be more consistent with the hypothesis that the difference was nonzero.

There is another way to test the hypothesis that the two probabilities are equal. Based on the data we observe, we would like a formal way of deciding when the null hypothesis is false (and not be wrong very often). That is, are the true response probabilities p_A and p_B really different, based on estimates of 0.52 and 0.61 with these sample sizes? A statistical test of this hypothesis can be formulated in the following way. From Table 2.3, we see that overall, $70/124 = 0.565$ of the patients responded to chemotherapy. If there were no differences in the two regimens, we would expect about 0.565 of the patients receiving cisplatin to respond (or $0.565 \times 60 = 33.87 \approx 34$ patients), and about 0.435 of them (26) to fail to respond. Similarly, we would expect about 36 of the patients receiving carboplatin to respond, and 28 to fail to respond. How different is what we observe from what we would expect? A number used to summarize the discrepancy between the observed and expected values under the null hypothesis is called the χ^2 (Chi-squared). It is computed as

$$\chi^2 = \sum [(observed - expected)^2 / expected]$$

where the summation means sum over the four entries in the 2 × 2 table. The χ^2 is one example of a test statistic. It is appropriate when the data are categorical; that is, each observation can be classified, as in this example, according to characteristics such as treatment arm and response. A second requirement for the χ^2 test (and most commonly used statistical tests) is independence of observations.

If there were perfect agreement between the observed and expected values, the χ^2 value would be 0. The greater the discrepancy in the observed and expected values, the greater the value of the χ^2. In this case we would have

$$\frac{(31-33.87)^2}{33.87} + \frac{(29-26.13)^2}{26.13} + \frac{(39-36.13)^2}{36.13} + \frac{(25-27.87)^2}{27.87} = 1.08$$

A simpler but algebraically equivalent formula uses just one cell of the 2×2 table (any one) and the marginal totals. The notation is given in Table 2.4. Using the number of responses on arm A for specificity, the formula is $(r_A - n_A r/n)^2/[n_A n_B r(n-r)/n^3]$. Note that the numerator is still of the form $(observed - expected)^2$. With the data in Table 2.3, this is $124^3(31 - 60 \times 70/124)^2/(60 \times 64 \times 70 \times 54) = 1.08$. In some circumstances this formula is modified slightly to $(r_A - n_A r/n)^2/[n_A n_B r(n-r)/n^2(n-1)]$, as in the logrank test defined in Section 2.3.2; in other cases a modification known as the continuity-corrected χ^2 is used.

If we were to perform the same clinical trial again in 124 different patients, we would get a different value for the χ^2 test, since we would expect the new sample of patients to have a somewhat different set of responses. Thus, the statistic can take on a variety of values, characterized by a density as in Figure 2.6. When the null hypothesis is true, we can compute the probability that the χ^2 statistic exceeds certain values by looking at the appropriate area under the curve in Figure 2.6, or using a table of the χ^2 distribution. From Figure 2.6, we would find that the probability of observing a value of 1.08 or greater is very high (it can happen about 30% of the time) under the assumption that the two probabilities are equal (the null hypothesis is true). Thus, we would reason that there is not sufficient evidence to conclude that the drug regimens are different.

Use of the χ^2 distribution is actually an approximation that is reasonably accurate unless sample sizes are small. When sample sizes are small, the exact solution is known as Fisher's exact test. The appropriateness of the χ^2 for larger sample sizes is a useful consequence of the Central Limit Theorem discussed in Section 2.1. In fact, distributions of many statistical tests can be approximated by a standard normal or a χ^2 distribution.

Table 2.4. Notation used in χ^2 test of 2×2 contingency table.

	Response	No Response	Totals
Arm A	r_A	$n_A - r_A$	n_A
Arm B	r_B	$n_B - r_B$	n_B
Totals	r	$n - r$	n

THE PHASE III TRIAL – HYPOTHESIS TESTING

We are now ready for a more formal introduction to the idea of hypothesis testing. In the above clinical trial we wished to test $H_0 : p_A = p_B$. We performed the trial, and based on the data, made a decision about the populations. The consequences of this decision relative to the true values of p_A and p_B are summarized below:

		Truth	
		$p_A = p_B$	$p_A \neq p_B$
	Accept H_0	Correct	Type II Error
Decision			
	Reject H_0	Type I Error	Correct

The type I error probability, or α, or significance level, is the probability that we conclude in our trial that the two treatments are different, even though they really are not (false positive). The acceptable Type I error rate is decided in the planning stages of the trial. The most common significance level for testing is 0.05. In our example, if we wish to test whether the treatments are different using a 0.05 significance level, we first consider the distribution of our χ^2 statistic when there are no true differences (under the null hypothesis). How large does the χ^2 have to be before we decide that the treatments are different? As just explained, the probability under the null hypothesis that a χ^2 statistic is greater than any particular value x can be found from Figure 2.6 as the area under the curve for

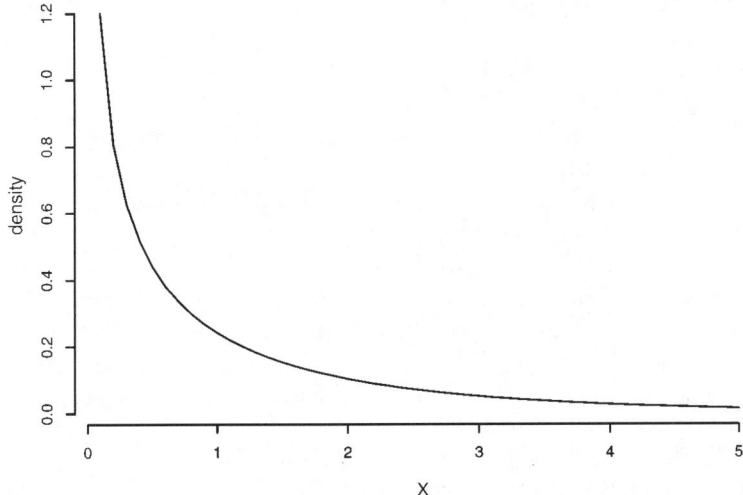

Figure 2.6. The chi-squared distribution (with 1 degree of freedom).

values of x and above, or from published tables. For $x = 3.84$ the area is 0.05. Thus if we conclude that p_A and p_B are different only when the χ^2 statistic is greater than 3.84, we know we will only be making a Type I error 5% of the time. Next we consider the observed value of our statistic, 1.08. Since it is less than 3.84, we do not conclude that p_A and p_B are different. Instead we conclude that there is insufficient evidence to reject the null hypothesis of equality. (Note that this is not the same as concluding that the two probabilities are identical, only that we cannot prove they are different.) If there had been 27 and 43 responses instead of 31 and 39, our test statistic would have been 6.2 instead of 1.08 and we would have rejected the null hypothesis and concluded that p_A and p_B were different.

You might ask how the hypothesis testing approach to deciding whether p_A and p_B are different is related to the confidence interval approach described previously. In a fundamental way they are equivalent (differences arise due to various approximations). A confidence interval can be derived directly from a test of hypothesis by considering tests of $H : p_A - p_B = \Delta$ for all possible Δ instead of just 0. If the hypothesis is not rejected (i.e., if the result would not be unusual if the true difference were Δ), then Δ is in the confidence interval; if it is rejected (if the result would be unusual if the true difference were Δ), then Δ is not in the interval. Thus a confidence interval can be thought of as the set of all possible hypothesized values for which a test does not reject the hypothesis. In particular, if 0 is in the confidence interval for $p_A - p_B$, the null hypothesis of no difference is not rejected; if 0 is not in the interval, the hypothesis of no difference is rejected.

A concept related to the significance level α of a test is the p-value, the probability under the null hypothesis of a result equal to or more extreme than the one we observed. The p-value for our example is the probability of obtaining a statistic with the value 1.08 or greater, which is 0.3. If the statistic had been 6.2, the p-value would have been 0.013. By definition the smaller the p-value the less likely the observed result under the null hypothesis. When there is little chance of having obtained an observed result under the null hypothesis, we conclude that the null hypothesis is not true. Note the correspondence between p-values and the observed value of the test statistic. The rule for rejecting the null hypothesis using a χ^2 can be stated either as "reject if the test statistic is greater than 3.84" or "reject if the p-value is less than 0.05."

As noted above, distributions of many test statistics can be approximated by the normal distribution or the χ^2 distribution, which is related to the normal distribution. Thus, p-values from many statistical tests can be approximated by finding the area to the right of an observed value using either the standard normal curve or the χ^2 distribution. Tables of the normal and χ^2 distributions can be found in any standard statistical text, for example, Rosner (1986).

For a normal distribution the area to the right of the observed value is the p-value corresponding to a one-sided test. One-sided tests are used when only a specified direction (e.g., A > B) is of interest. In this case A < B or A = B lead to the same conclusion (B is the preferred treatment), so we have a type one error only if we erroneously conclude A > B. For a two-sided test, differences in both directions, either A > B or B > A, are of interest, so we make a type I error if we conclude either A > B or B > A when there is no difference. The p-value in this case is twice the area to the right to allow for a difference of the same or greater magnitude in the other direction. For instance, the area under the normal curve above 1.96 is 0.025, so if a test statistic is equal to 1.96 the p-value for a one-sided test would be 0.025 while the p-value for a two-sided test would be 0.05. The χ^2 is inherently two sided due to the squaring of differences, which eliminates the + or − indication of direction. Note that 1.96^2 is 3.84, the value for which the p-value of a χ^2 statistic (with 1 degree of freedom) would also be 0.05. The decision of whether to perform a one-sided or two-sided test depends upon the goals of the study and should be specified during study development (see Section 7.3.3).

While we can predetermine the significance level of a test of hypothesis directly, the probability β of a type II error is dependent upon several things: (1) sample size; (2) the true difference between p_A and p_B; and (3) the significance level of the test. If the true difference is very large (for example, p_A near 1 and p_B near 0), we would expect that it would be relatively easy to determine that a difference in probabilities exists, even with a small sample size. However, if p_A and p_B are very close, though not equal, it might take a very large number of patients to detect this difference with near certainty. Thus, a trial that failed to detect a difference, but which was based on a small sample size, does not prove $p_A = p_B$, and should be reported with caution (since if the true difference is modest, a type II error or false negative result is likely).

The power of a test for a particular alternative hypothesis is defined to be $1 - \beta$, the probability of detecting a difference that is really there. Ideally, we would always like to have a large enough sample size to ensure high power for differences that are realistic and clinically meaningful. In designing clinical studies, it is important for the clinician and statistician to discuss the magnitudes of the clinical differences that would be meaningful to detect, in order to design a study with small enough error rates to make the conclusions from the results credible.

2.3.2 Survival as the outcome

In most cancer clinical trials, the primary outcome is patient survival. Patients are randomized to two (or more) groups, and followed until death. In a typical Phase III trial, there is an accrual period (often several years long), and then some additional follow-up time prior to analysis of the data. At the time of the final analysis, some patients will have died, while some patients will remain alive. For those patients who remain alive, the total time of observation will vary, depending upon when in the accrual period they were registered to the trial. The actual survival time for these patients is unknown, but we do know that they have survived at least from registration until the date of their last known contact. This represents a minimum survival time. Data of this type are described as being subject to censoring. We illustrate statistical issues related to censored data using the survival times from Table 2.5, which represent the ordered survival times for the patients on an imaginary trial. Times with a + next to them represent censored observations.

Given data of this type, we frequently wish to calculate some statistic that summarizes patient survival experience. It is not uncommon to see the average value of the uncensored survival times reported as the mean survival time. This estimate is incorrect, since it ignores the information about the patients who remain alive. A mean of all times (both censored and not) is an underestimate, since the censored observations are really minimum possible survival times. However, it, too, is often interpreted as the average survival time.

An alternative measure that may be meaningful is the survival probability at some time point of interest (e.g., at 2 years). How might this be computed? Using the data in Table 2.5, one measure would be $11/20 = 0.55$, based on the fact that 11 of 20 patients either died after 24 months or had not died. This rate is optimistic, since it assumes that all patients with censored observations less

Table 2.5. Ordered survival times (months) on an imaginary trial.

1	2	4+	6	6	7+	9	11	15+	16
17	18+	24	24+	25+	26	28	31+	32+	35+

than 2 years would have survived a full 2 years if they had been observed further. Another approach would be to ignore those patients who were censored prior to 2 years, yielding a rate of $7/16 = 0.44$. This rate was computed by deleting all patients who had censored observations prior to 24 months. This estimate is overly pessimistic, since it disregards information we do have about additional patient survival. A third approach that has been used in the literature is to ignore all patients (both alive and dead) who would not have been followed for at least 2 years. This, too, ignores valuable information.

Ideally, we wish to use as much patient information as possible. The most common method used in clinical trials is to estimate the survival experience of the patients using the Kaplan-Meier (product-limit) estimate (Kaplan and Meier, 1958). The data from Table 2.5 are expanded in Table 2.6, with the addition of calculations of the survival curve. The second column of the table gives the number of patients alive just before the given time. This number represents the number of patients at risk of dying at the next observation time. The

Table 2.6. Calculation of cumulative survival proportions for the imaginary trial data.

Time (Months)	# at Risk	# of Deaths	# Censored	Surviving This Time	Cumulative Survival
1	20	1	0	$19/20 = .95$	.95
2	19	1	0	18/19	$.95 \times (18/19) = .90$
4	18	0	1	18/18	$.90 \times (18/18) = .90$
6	17	2	0	15/17	$.9 \times (15/17) = .79$
7	15	0	1	15/15	$.79 \times (15/15) = .79$
9	14	1	0	13/14	$.79 \times (13/14) = .74$
11	13	1	0	12/13	.68[1]
15	12	0	1	12/12	.68
16	11	1	0	10/11	.62
17	10	1	0	9/10	.56
18	9	0	1	9/9	.56
24	8	1	1	7/8*	.49
25	6	0	1	6/6	.49
26	5	1	0	4/5	.39
28	4	1	0	3/4	.29
31	3	0	1	3/3	.29
32	2	0	1	2/2	.29
35	1	0	1	1/1	.29

[1]The remaining cumulative survival estimates are calculated in the same way as the above calculations.

next two columns summarize how many patients die, or are censored. For each listed time the percent surviving is simply the ratio of the number remaining alive compared to the number at risk.

The final column lists the cumulative chance of surviving. At time zero, all patients are alive, and thus the initial cumulative proportion of patients alive begins at 100%. At time 1, there is one death, and thus the proportion surviving, and the cumulative proportion surviving is 19/20, or 0.95. At the next time interval, there are now 19 patients still at risk (since one has already died). There is one death, giving a proportion surviving of $18/19 = 0.947$. Cumulatively, the probability of surviving for 2 months is the product of the probability of surviving 1 month times the probability of surviving 2 months among those surviving 1 month. Thus, this probability is estimated as $0.95 \times 0.947 = 0.90$ (which is just 18/20, the fraction surviving 2 months). At time 4, there are 18 patients at risk. One patient is censored at this point. Thus, the probability of surviving 4 months is $18/18 = 1$, and the cumulative probability remains unchanged. However, in the next time interval, the patient with the censored observation at time 4 is no longer under observation, and is dropped from the number of patients at risk. Two patients die at time 6, so that the estimate of the probability of surviving time 6 given survival past time 4 is $15/17 = 0.882$, and the cumulative chance of surviving 6 months is estimated by $0.90 \times 0.88 = 0.79$. Note that this is between the value achieved by throwing the censored observation out of all calculations ($15/19 = 0.789$) and assuming that individual is still at risk past time 6 ($16/20 = 0.80$).

The estimated cumulative proportions surviving are calculated similarly for all observation times. The (*) indicates a time at which both a death and a censored observation occurred simultaneously. In calculating the estimate, we assume that the censored observation occurs after the death (in this case, just past 24 months), and hence is treated as being in a later time period. The successive products of the individual proportions surviving give this estimate the name product-limit estimator. Using this technique, we obtain a 24-month survival estimate of 0.49.

A plot of the survival curve computed above is given in Figure 2.7. The curve is graphed as a step function, meaning it remains constant except at the death times. Statistically this is the most appropriate; attempting to interpolate between points can lead to biased estimates. The tic marks on the graph represent the censored observations.

We can now use this curve to provide point estimates of survival statistics of interest. For example, if 1-year survival is commonly

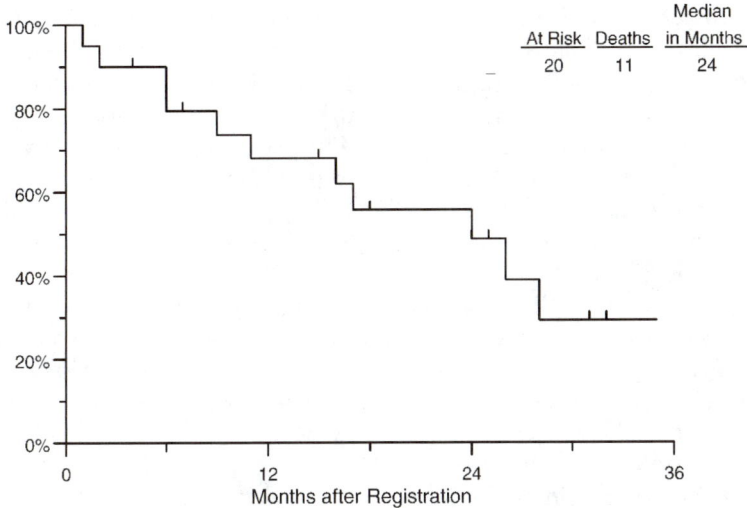

Figure 2.7. Plot of the survival curve calculated in Table 2.6.

reported, one would read up from the 12-month point on the horizontal axis, and find the estimated 1-year survival to be 0.68.

Instead of survival at some selected time, a common statistic of interest is the median survival time. This is the time at which one estimates that half the patients will have died. The median survival time is estimated from the product-limit estimate to be the first time that the survival curve falls to 0.50 or below. For our example, the survival proportion is 0.56 at 18 months, and falls to 0.49 at 24 months. Thus the median survival is estimated to be 24 months.

Approximate confidence interval formulae are available for the product-limit estimates of the proportion surviving (Breslow and Crowley, 1972) and for the median survival (Brookmeyer and Crowley, 1982). What is most important to remember is that the width of the confidence intervals increases as one estimates further out on the time scale. This is because fewer patients contribute information as time increases. Thus, one will have more confidence in the accuracy of survival estimates calculated early on than for estimates late in the study. For example, if only two patients were entered in a study longer than 5 years ago, the estimated 5-year survival probability is of questionable accuracy.

There are several common pitfalls in the interpretation of data from a survival curve. One common mistake is the attempt to interpret a final nonzero estimate of survival as a plateau. By the nature of the estimation procedure, if the final observation is a censored one, the survival curve will not reach zero. This does not imply that the probability of dying has ended, but rather that follow-up has run out. Related to this is the frequent extrapolation of the final cumulative survival past the times for which patients were observed. For example, in a study with data similar to those presented in Table 2.6, one might eyeball the curve and conclude everyone will be dead by 5 years, or one might optimistically extend the final part of the curve and conclude 29% will still be alive at 5 years. Neither extrapolation is justified since there is no information concerning the shape of the curve after 35 months.

Typically, in a Phase III clinical trial, we are not merely interested in estimating a survival curve. Our primary goal is to compare the survival curves between the treatment groups under study. Our hypotheses are usually formulated in terms of differences in survival, namely, $H_o : S_A = S_B$ vs. $S_B > S_A$, where S represents the true survival curve in the population. That is, our null hypothesis is that the two treatment regimens have the same survival, whereas the alternative is that the new treatment improves survival over the standard. One approach taken has been to compare the survival curves at a single point, e.g., to compare the 2-year survival probabilities. Historically, this was done by estimating the probability in each group and performing a test comparing these two probabilities. One problem with this is that the choice of the time point for testing is rather arbitrary. In addition, there are many situations for which the 2-year survival probabilities are the same, but the overall survival is very different. Figure 2.2b displays three situations, all giving rise to the same 2-year probabilities. One would usually prefer an overall test of the equality of the survival curves. There are a number of ways to do this. The general idea is the following: begin by ordering the survival times (and censored observations), disregarding treatment assignment. Figure 2.8 gives several examples. In these, the As represent deaths from patients receiving treatment arm A, and the Bs are the deaths from patients receiving treatment arm B. The lower case values are the respective censored observations.

If there were no effect of treatment, we would expect that the deaths that came from arm A would occur over the whole range of death times, as would the deaths from arm B (Figure 2.8a). However, if there were a treatment difference, we would expect to see some pattern, such as those seen in Figures 2.8b and c.

We can set up a test as follows. Each observation is assigned a score such as an ordered rank, with the earliest death given rank 1, the second rank 2, etc. If there is no difference in survival, we would expect that the deaths from the patients in arm A would have some small and some large scores, as would the patients in arm B. However,

(a) AB A B Aa B A BB A B Ab A B   a B   A B Bb Aa B
0   Time   3 years

(b) A A a A B A B A B b A B a B A B A B B B A B B B B
0   Time   3 years

(c) A AAa A AA   A aA   A B   A B   BbB   B BB   bBB   B
0   Time   3 years

Figure 2.8. Patterns of survival times for two treatments (A and B represent true survival times, a and b represent censored observations).

if there are differences in the groups (one has more deaths, or all of the deaths are earlier), then we would expect that one group would have more of the large (or small) scores. We can use the difference in the sums of the scores from the two groups as a test statistic. There are a number of common test statistics for censored data, each of which differs in the way the scores are determined. The most common is called the logrank test (Mantel, 1966); other test statistics, generalizations of the familiar Wilcoxon test, are given by Gehan (1965), Peto and Peto (1972), and Prentice (1978). As for the χ^2 test for discrete data, p-values can be computed for the calculated value of the logrank test for the purpose of testing the null hypothesis of equal survival in the two treatment groups.

An alternative explanation of censored data test statistics starts with 2×2 tables similar to those in Section 2.3.1. Consider the sample data in Table 2.7. All the survival times have been ordered, ignoring the treatment arm and whether or not the observations are censored.

At the time of each uncensored observation (death times), a 2×2 table is formed. The marginal totals are the number alive in each arm just before that time (the number at risk), the number who die at

Table 2.7. Survival times (months) for treatments A and B.

Time	1	2	4+	6	6	7+	9	11	15+	16
Arm	A	B	B	A	A	A	B	B	A	B
Time	17	18+	24	24+	25+	26	28	31+	32+	35+
Arm	B	A	A	B	A	B	B	A	B	A

Table 2.8. 2 × 2 table at a death time t.

	Deaths	Survivors	Total at Risk
Arm A	d_A	$n_A - d_A$	n_A
Arm B	d_B	$n_B - d_B$	n_B
Totals	d	$n - d$	n

that time, and the number who survive, and the cell entries are the number dying and the number surviving in each arm. The notation is shown in Table 2.8.

For example, at time 11 in Table 2.7, $n_A = 6$, $n_B = 7$, $d_A = 0$, and $d_B = 1$. The observed number of deaths in arm A is d_A, and the expected number under H_0, the null hypothesis of no difference, is $n_A d/n$. Define the quantity $V = n_A n_B d(n-d)/n^2(n-1)$, which is the denominator in one of the derivations of the χ^2 statistic in Section 2.3.1. For survival data measured in small units of time such as days, the number d dying at a time t will be 1, so that V reduces to $n_A n_B/n^2$. Then the logrank test is defined as

$$\left[\sum(d_A - n_A d/n)\right]^2 \Big/ \sum V$$

where the sum is over all of the times of death. With this notation, other test statistics can be defined by weighting the summands in the numerator differently:

$$\left[\sum w(d_A - n_A d/n)\right]^2 \Big/ \sum V.$$

For example, the Gehan (1965) version of the Wilcoxon test puts more weight on earlier deaths than on later ones ($w = n$, the total number at risk at the time of a death), while the logrank test weighs each table equally. The Peto and Peto (1972) and Prentice (1978) test statistics mentioned earlier also fit this formulation, with weight w being (roughly) the value of the product-limit estimate from the combined sample at time t (and thus giving more weight to earlier deaths). For more details, see for example, Crowley and Breslow, 1984. The ambitious reader can check that the value of the logrank test statistic for the data in Table 2.7 is 0.60, which when referred to tables of the χ^2 distribution gives a p-value of 0.44. (Remember to order the censored time at 24 months as just larger than the uncensored time.)

THE PROPORTIONAL HAZARDS MODEL

Although the most efficient Phase III trial is designed to compare only two treatments (Chapter 3), some trials are designed with three or more treatment arms (Chapter 4). There is a natural extension of the logrank test (and of the χ^2 test for dichotomous outcomes) that can accommodate this situation. If the null hypothesis is that there is no survival difference (or difference in response) among any of the K groups, and the alternative hypothesis is that some differences in survival (response) exist, then a single test is performed. If the null hypothesis of complete equality is rejected, then secondary analyses are performed to identify the source of the difference. Separate comparisons between all combinations of treatment pairs, without a preliminary test or other statistical adjustment, are inappropriate and should be avoided. Performing these multiple comparisons results in an overall type-I error (the probability of concluding there is a difference in *any* of these pairwise comparisons when there are no treatment differences) that is higher than the level of each individual test. There are several techniques for avoiding this problem of multiple comparisons. Further discussion of multi-arm trials is presented in Chapter 4.

2.4 The proportional hazards model

So far we have concentrated on estimating the proportion alive (or dead) at various times. Now we turn to a different characteristic of the survival distribution introduced in Section 2.1, the hazard function. Although exponential distributions (with a constant hazard rate λ) are commonly used for such purposes as sample size calculation, most often we have no idea what form the underlying hazard function, more generally denoted $\lambda(t)$, will take. No matter what that form, in Phase III trials we are usually most interested in comparing the hazards between the treatment arms (this is equivalent to comparing the survival curves). As part of that comparison, we often wish to assess whether the difference, if any, that we observe, could be due to differences among the patients in important prognostic factors. For example, if there were more high risk patients in one treatment arm than the other, we would like to know whether any survival differences were due to the high risk patients as opposed to a true treatment effect. To answer these questions, a statistical model, which is an extension of the logrank test, has been developed to accommodate other variables of interest. This model is called the Cox regression model (Cox, 1972), or the proportional hazards model. This model assumes that the hazard function for each patient is the product of some general hazard function multiplied by a term related to patient characteristics and other prognostic factors of interest. Mathematically, this function is described by

$$\lambda(t,x) = (\lambda_0(t))\exp\left(\sum_i \beta_i x_i\right),$$

or equivalently

$$\ln(\lambda(t,x)) = \ln(\lambda_0(t)) + \left(\sum_i \beta_i x_i\right),$$

where $\lambda(t,x)$ is the hazard function for a patient, x_is describe the covariates for that patient, and the βs are regression coefficients. For example, when the only covariate is treatment, coded say as $x = 0$ for treatment A and $x = 1$ for treatment B, this model states that the hazard functions for the two treatments are given by $\lambda_0(t)$ and $\lambda_0(t)\exp(\beta)$, respectively. The ratio of these hazard functions is for all t the constant $\exp(\beta)$, thus the name "proportional hazards model." The proportional hazards model can be used much as linear regression is used in other contexts, to assess the importance of prognostic factors and to compare treatments adjusted for such factors (see Chapters 7 and 9). It can account for both categorical variables, such as treatment arm assignment and sex, and for continuous measurements such as age and CA-125. The logrank test can be derived from the model when there are no covariates other than treatment; a generalization of the logrank test, adjusted for covariates, results from the larger model.

It is important to note that the proportional hazards model imposes no requirements on the form of the hazard functions, only on their ratios. An important generalization that makes even fewer assumptions is the stratified Cox model. For example, it may be that the hazard functions for covariates cannot be assumed to be proportional, but adjustment for covariates still needs to be made in a test for differences between two treatments. In this case one can define proportional hazards models for treatment, within strata defined by levels of the covariates (continuous covariates can be reduced to categories for this purpose). The model is

$$\lambda_j(t,x) = (\lambda_{0j}(t))\exp(\beta x),$$

where j indexes the strata and x identifies the treatment group. Use of this model does not allow for the assessment of whether the

SAMPLE SIZE CALCULATIONS

stratifying covariates are important with regard to survival, but it does allow for adjusted treatment comparisons, and in fact leads to what is termed the **stratified logrank test**.

2.5 Sample size calculations

Earlier in the chapter we alluded to the relationships among level, power, magnitude of differences to detect, and sample size. In this section, we discuss the issues involved in estimating sample size for clinical trials, and present one technique used in sample size determination.

Recall that there are three quantities related to sample size: level, power, and a difference one wishes to detect. Computer programs and tables exist for determining sample size estimates. It is useful, however, to consider a sample size formula, to understand how the above quantities interrelate. The derivation for these formulas can be found in standard statistical texts (see, for example, Fleiss, 1981), and will not be presented here.

When the outcomes are dichotomous, such as a response collapsed into CR + PR vs. others, the following formula can be used to obtain sample size estimates for the comparison of two treatment arms. Let p_A be the hypothesized response probability in arm A, and p_B be the response probability one hopes to detect in arm B. The average of these two probabilities is given by $\bar{p} = (p_A + p_B)/2$. The formula is

$$N = \frac{\left(z_\alpha \sqrt{2\bar{p}(1-\bar{p})} + z_\beta \sqrt{p_A(1-p_A) + p_B(1-p_B)}\right)^2}{(p_B - p_A)^2}, \quad (2.1)$$

where N is the required sample size for each treatment arm, z_α is the upper $100\alpha\%$ value from the normal distribution F ($F(z_\alpha) = 1 - \alpha$), and z_β is the upper 100β % value ($F(z_\beta) = 1 - \beta$). For $\alpha = 0.05$, $z_\alpha = 1.645$ for a one-sided test, and $z_\alpha = 1.96$ for a two-sided test (this allows for type one errors of 0.025 in each direction, for a total type one error of 0.05). If a power of 0.9 is desired, then $\beta = (1 - 0.9) = 0.1$, and $z_\beta = 1.282$.

From the above formula, note that the quantity in the denominator is the difference in the response probabilities for the two treatments. The smaller this denominator is, the larger the resulting N will be. Thus, if one wishes to be able to detect a relatively small treatment effect, a larger sample size will be required than if one is only interested in detecting large differences in the treatments.

Table 2.9. Total sample size $2N$ required to detect an increase in p_A by Δ for significance level 0.05, power 0.90, one-sided test.

p_A	$\Delta = 0.1$	$\Delta = 0.15$	$\Delta = 0.2$	$\Delta = 0.25$	$\Delta = 0.3$
0.1	472	242	152	108	80
0.2	678	326	196	132	96
0.3	816	380	222	146	104
0.4	884	402	230	148	104

Similarly, if one wishes to have greater power (causing z_β to be larger) or smaller significance level (causing z_α to be larger), the numerator will be larger, also increasing the required sample size. The numerator and thus the sample size are also larger when p_A and p_B are closer to 0.5 than to 0 or 1, since the maximum value of $p(1-p)$ is 0.25 when $p = 0.5$, and the minimum is 0 when p is 0 or 1. Table 2.9 presents the total sample size $2N$ required to detect differences from selected choices of response probabilities in a two-arm clinical trial. (A slightly different formula from Equation 2.1, due to Fleiss et al., 1980, was used.)

The table illustrates the fact that for a fixed difference $\Delta = p_B - p_A$, the sample size increases as p_A moves from 0.1 toward 0.5. For example, if $p_A = 0.1$, the total sample size is 80 to detect an increase of 0.3; however, if $p_A = 0.3$, the required total sample size is 104.

When the outcome is survival, we usually make the simplifying assumption that survival follows an exponential distribution. Formulae similar to Equation 2.1 above are used to estimate the required sample size for trials of this type. A discussion of sample size for a two-arm trial with survival as the endpoint is contained in Section 3.5.2.

2.6 Concluding remarks

One important thing to keep in mind is the distinction between a clinically significant difference and a statistically significant difference. Any numerical difference, no matter how small (and possibly of minimal, if any clinical interest), can yield a statistically significant test if the sample size is sufficiently large.

This chapter has introduced key statistical concepts and analyses. Understanding the basics will help in understanding why statisticians choose specific designs and analyses in specific settings. These choices are the subject of the rest of the book.

CHAPTER 3

The Design of Clinical Trials

Then Daniel said to the steward whom the chief of the eunuchs had appointed over Daniel, Hanani'ah, Mish'a-el, and Azari'ah, 'Test your servants for ten days; let us be given vegetables to eat and water to drink. Then let our appearance and the appearance of the youths who eat the king's rich food be observed by you, and according to what you see deal with your servants.' So he hearkened to them in this matter, and tested them for ten days. At the end of ten days it was seen that they were better in appearance and fatter in flesh than all the youths who ate the king's rich food. So the steward took away their rich food and the wine they were to drink, and gave them vegetables.

–Daniel 1: 11-16.

3.1 Introduction

It has been suggested that the biblical dietary comparison introducing the chapter is the first clinical trial in recorded history, and its designer, Daniel, the first trialist (Fisher, 1983). In this chapter we will discuss important elements of designing a clinical trial, and at the end consider how well Daniel did in designing his.

The major elements in designing a clinical trial are

1. Stating the objectives clearly
2. Specifying eligibility, treatments, and endpoints
3. Determining the magnitude of difference to be detected or the desired precision of estimation
4. Specifying how treatment assignment will be accomplished (for randomized trials)
5. Identifying distributional assumptions and error probabilities to be used for sample size calculations

3.1.1 Objectives

Identifying the primary objective requires careful thought about what key conclusions are to be made at the end of the trial. The statement "To compare A and B," for instance, is not a sufficient statement of objectives. Is the goal to identify one of the arms for further study? To reach a definitive conclusion about which arm to use in the future to treat a specific type of patient? To decide if a particular agent/route/dose has a role in treatment? To determine if A and B are equivalent? To generate evidence for or against a biologic hypothesis? Each of these objectives has different design implications.

3.1.2 Eligibility, treatments, endpoints

The eligibility criteria, the choice of treatments, and the definition of endpoints all must be suitable for the stated objectives. For eligibility, consideration should be given to which patients are likely to benefit from treatment and to the desired generalizability of the results. If eligibility criteria are very narrow, the generalizability of the study is compromised; if they are too broad, the effectiveness of treatment may be masked by the inclusion of patients with little chance of responding. For instance, very early Phase II studies are often not reproducible because they were restricted to very good risk patients. On the other hand, late Phase II studies can be unduly negative because they were conducted in heavily pretreated patients who would not be expected to respond to therapy.

The choice of treatments also has to be suitable. For instance, if the primary aim of a trial of agent A alone vs. a combination of agents A and B is to decide whether the addition of agent B improves the effectiveness of agent A, then administration of agent A should be identical on the two treatment arms; otherwise differences could be due to alterations in A as well as to the addition of B.

Endpoints should also be suitable for the objectives. For instance, if the primary aim is to identify the arm of choice for treating patients, then endpoints that best reflect benefit to the patient should be used. Tumor shrinkage in itself usually is not of direct benefit to a patient, whereas longer survival or symptom improvement is. Using convenient or short-term endpoints instead of the ones of primary interest can result in incorrect conclusions (see Chapter 8 for a discussion of "surrogate" endpoints). Some difficulties with common endpoint definitions are discussed in Section 3.2.

INTRODUCTION

3.1.3 Differences to be detected or precision of estimates

If the aim of the study is comparative, the trial should be designed to have sufficient power to detect the smallest difference that is clinically meaningful. A study is doomed to failure if it is designed to have good power to detect only unrealistically large differences. In practice, trials are often designed to have adequate power only to detect the smallest affordable difference, not the smallest meaningful difference. Consideration should be given as to whether the affordable difference is plausible enough to warrant doing the study at all, since it is a waste of resources to do a trial with little chance of yielding a definitive conclusion.

If a single arm study is being designed, consideration should be given to how precise the results must be for the information to be useful. If the confidence interval for an estimate is so large that it covers the range of values from wonder drug to dud, then the information to be gained is not particularly useful, and the conduct of the trial should be discouraged.

3.1.4 Method of treatment assignment

We will take it as given in this chapter that randomization is a necessity for comparative trials, because

1. Nonrandomized treatment assignments can never be assumed to result in comparable treatment groups.
2. It is impossible to adjust for all potential imbalances at the time of analysis, especially for the factors that lead to the selection of treatments by patients and physicians.

Chapter 8 has examples illustrating the problems of nonrandomized control groups. Decisions about randomization that must be made include what stratification factors to use, the specific randomization scheme to be employed, and whether blinding is necessary. These are considered in Section 3.5.

3.1.5 Assumptions for sample size calculation

Although historical information cannot be used for definitive treatment comparisons, it is useful in specifying the assumptions required for sample size calculations. Estimates of the characteristics of the endpoints (most often summary statistics such as the median, mean, standard deviation, etc.) are needed, as is an estimate of the rate of accrual of patients. Specifics for Phase II and III trial designs are included throughout the rest of this chapter. Phase I trials generally do not have pre-set sample size goals (see Section 3.3).

3.2 Endpoints

A few comments on endpoints are in order before we start on the specifics of trial design. Many of the common endpoints used in clinical trials are problematic in one way or another, often due to correlations among possible outcomes or due to the logical traps in complicated definitions. The examples below are commonly used endpoints in cancer trials, but the same principles hold for endpoints for any clinical study.

Survival is defined as the time from registration on study to time of death due to any cause. As described in Chapter 2, survival distributions can still be estimated when not all patients have died by using the information from censored survival times (time from registration to date of last contact for living patients) as well as from the known death times. Survival is the most straightforward and objective of cancer endpoints, but even here there can be problems. Bias can result when there are many patients lost to follow-up; examples are given in Chapter 6. If most patients are still alive at the time of analysis, estimates can be highly variable or not even defined (this was discussed in Chapter 2). If many patients die of causes other than the cancer under study the interpretation of survival can be problematic, since the effect of treatment on the disease under study is of primary interest.

Using *time to death due to disease* (defined the same way as survival, except that observations are censored at the time of death if death is due to causes other than the cancer of interest) is not a solution to the problem of competing causes of death. Even if cause of death information is reliable, which is often not the case, unbiased estimation of time to death due to disease is possible only if deaths due to other causes are statistically independent of the cancer being studied, and if it makes sense to think of removing the risk of dying from other causes. (See Chapter 8 for a discussion of competing risks.) The independence of causes of death is rarely a good assumption. Good and poor risk cancer patients tend to be systematically different with respect to susceptibility to other potentially lethal diseases as well as to their cancers. Furthermore, the cause-specific endpoint does not include all effects of treatment on survival, for example, early toxic deaths, late deaths due to leukemia after treatment with alkylating agents, death due to congestive heart failure after treatment with Adriamycin, etc. These examples all represent failures of treatment. Since it is not possible to tell which causes of death are or are not related to the disease or its treatment, or what the nature of the relationships might be, it is not possible to tell exactly what "time to death due to disease" estimates. Furthermore, if results using this endpoint are different from those using overall survival, the latter must take precedence. (A treatment generally is not going to be considered effective if deaths due to disease are decreased only at the expense of increased deaths due to other causes.) We recommend using only overall survival.

Progression-free survival (or relapse-free survival for adjuvant studies) is defined as the time from registration to the first observation of disease progression or death due to any cause. If a patient has not progressed or died, progression-free survival is censored at the time of last follow-up. This endpoint is preferred to time to progression (with censorship at the time of death if the death is due to other causes) for reasons similar to those noted above. A common problem we find with the progression-free survival endpoint is that advanced disease is often not followed for progression after a patient has been taken off treatment because of toxicity or refusal. Since early discontinuation of treatment in advanced disease typically is related to poor patient response or tolerance, in these studies we often use *time to treatment failure* (time from registration to the first observation of disease progression, death due to any cause, or early discontinuation of treatment) instead.

A variation on progression-free survival is *duration of response,* defined as the time from first observation of response to the first time of progression or death. If a responding patient has not progressed or died, duration of response is censored at the time of last follow-up. Since it can be misleading to report failure times only in a subset of patients, particularly when the subset is chosen based on another outcome, we do not recommend use of this endpoint. (Section 8.4 gives more details on this issue.)

Response has often been defined as a 50% decrease in bidimensionally measurable disease lasting 4 weeks, progression as a 25% increase in any lesion, relapse as a 50% increase in responding disease. We have often been assured that everyone knows what this means, but we find that there are so many gaps in the definitions that what everyone knows varies quite a lot. For instance, does a patient with a 25% increase in one lesion at the same time as a 50% decrease in the sum of products of perpendicular diameters of all measurable lesions have a response or not? Is the 25% increase measured from baseline, or from the minimum size? If it is an increase over baseline, does it make sense that a lesion that shrinks to 1.4 cm × 1.5 cm from 2 × 2 must increase to 2.24 × 2.24 to be a progression, while one that shrinks to 1.4 × 1.4 must only increase to 1.72 × 1.72 to be a relapse? In practice, is an increase in a previously unchanged lesion from 0.8 × 0.8 to 0.9 × 0.9 really treated as evidence of progression? If disease is documented to have decreased by 50% once, can it be assumed the decrease lasted 4 weeks, or does it have to be documented again? If nonmeasurable disease is clearly increasing, while measurable disease is decreasing, is this still a response? The previous standard Southwest Oncology Group response definition (Green and Weiss, 1992) was quite detailed to clarify these and other common ambiguities in response definitions.

Recognition of these and other issues led to an international collaboration to revise the old World Health Organization response criteria. Over several years members of the European Organization for Research and Treatment of Cancer (EORTC), the National Cancer Institute of the United States and the National Cancer Institute of Canada Clinical Trials Group developed and published (Therasse et al., 2000) new criteria called RECIST (Response Evaluation Criteria in Solid Tumors). Many previously unaddressed aspects of response assessment have now been clarified. Additionally, a key modification implemented in these definitions was the change to unidimensional measurements instead of bidimensional. Assessments of various data sets indicated the simpler definition of a 30% decrease in the sum of maximum diameters resulted in very similar response determinations as the old 50% decrease in sum of products. (Note: If an M × M lesion decreases to 0.7M × 0.7M, then there is a 30% decrease in the maximum diameter and a 51% decrease in the product of diameters.) The change to a 20% increase for progression resulted in somewhat longer time to progression in 7% of patients and shorter in 1%, but the differences were considered acceptable. (Note: If an M × M lesion increases to 1.2M × 1.2M, this is a 20% increase in maximum diameter and a 44% increase in product of diameters.)

Despite these standardizations, response remains a problematic endpoint. Nonmeasurable disease is hard to incorporate objectively, as is symptomatic deterioration without objective evidence of progression. Both problems introduce subjective judgment into response assessment. Furthermore, tests and scans are not all done on the same schedule (some infrequently), and due to cost constraints noncritical assessments may be skipped. This results in insufficient information to apply the strict definitions of response, either leaving final response determination as "unknown" (not an official RECIST category) or introducing even more subjective judgment. While response frequently is used as an indicator of biologic activity in Phase II studies (for which response monitoring tends to be more carefully done), it is not recommended as the primary endpoint in Phase III trials.

Toxicity criteria also present a variety of logical problems. Toxicities are usually graded on a 6-point scale, from grade 0 (none) to grade 5 (fatal), with mild, moderate, severe, and life-threatening in between. Toxicities that cannot be life-threatening should not have the highest grades defined (e.g., alopecia should not have a grade 4). Lesser grades also should not be defined if they are not appropriate (cerebral necrosis would not be mild, for example). Care must be taken with the boundary values when categorizing continuous values into this discrete scale, so that there is no ambiguity. All the possibilities must be covered. (If grade 1 is "mild and brief pain" and grade 2 is "severe and prolonged pain," how is a severe but brief pain classified?) Each possibility should be covered only once. (If grade 1 is "mild or brief pain" and grade 2 is "severe or prolonged pain," severe but brief pain still cannot be coded.) The Southwest Oncology Group developed detailed toxicity criteria (Green and Weiss, 1992) to address these issues and to supplement the limited list of Common Toxicity Criteria (CTC) provided by the NCI. Since then, extensive changes and additions to the CTC have been developed. These can be found on the CTEP (Cancer Therapy Evaluation Program of NCI) website (currently at http://ctep.cancer.gov/reporting/ctc.html) and are in widespread use.

Quality of life is the hardest of cancer endpoints to assess. In the past, toxicity and response have often been used as surrogates for quality of life. Toxicity certainly reflects one aspect of quality (with the exception of abnormal lab values without symptoms), but response, by itself, may not. Responses are not necessarily accompanied by benefits such as symptom relief or improvement in function, nor is an objective tumor response necessary for such benefits. There are many facets of quality of life, and the relative importance of each is a matter of individual preference. Physical and emotional functioning, plus general and treatment-specific symptoms have been identified as key aspects of quality of life in cancer patients. Another key to quality of life assessment is patient self-report. It is nice if physicians believe their patients are feeling better; it is even better if the patients think so. Detailed recommendations concerning quality of life assessment implemented in SWOG have been published (Moinpour et al., 1989). As noted in Chapter 6, however, proper assessment of quality of life is very expensive so it is not routinely incorporated into our studies.

The message to take away from Section 3.2 is that endpoint definitions require careful attention. Imprecisely defined or subjective endpoints result in inconsistent or biased interpretation by investigators, which in turn result in a compromised interpretation of the study. Precisely defined but inappropriate endpoints result in comparisons that do not answer the questions posed by the study.

3.3 Phase I trials

3.3.1 Traditional designs

The primary aim of a Phase I trial is to determine the maximum tolerated dose (MTD) of a new agent. These trials traditionally have been used for cytotoxic drugs, where it is assumed that higher doses will be more toxic, as well as more effective. For the determination of the MTD, the endpoint of interest is whether or not a patient experiences a dose limiting toxicity (DLT), where the definition of the type and level of toxicity considered dose limiting is stated in the protocol, and determined by the disease and type of drug being tested. The subjects studied generally are patients with advanced disease for whom no effective standard therapy is available. A traditionally used design is a modified Fibonacci design. Typically, three patients are entered at the first dose level, which is often chosen to be 10% of the mouse LD10 (dose at which 10% of mice die). If no patients experience DLT, three patients are entered at the next dose level; if one patient experiences DLT, three additional patients are treated at the same dose; if two or three patients experience DLT, the dose is concluded to be above the MTD and dose escalation is discontinued. If six patients are treated, escalation continues if one patient experiences dose limiting toxicity, otherwise the dose is concluded to be above the MTD and escalation ends. When a dose is concluded to be above the MTD the next lower dose is declared the MTD if six patients have already been treated at that dose. Otherwise three additional patients are treated at the next lower dose, and if zero or one have DLTs this is declared the MTD. If two or more have DLTs there is further de-escalation according to the same scheme. The design continues until the MTD is declared or until the first dose is concluded to be above the MTD.

The sequence of dose levels used for escalation in the traditional design is often chosen to increase according to the following scheme: the second dose level is 2 times the first, the third is 1.67 times the second, the fourth is 1.5 times the third, the fifth is 1.4 times the fourth, and all subsequent doses are 1.33 times the previous. (The sequence is reminiscent of a Fibonacci sequence, which starts out with two numbers, after which each subsequent number is the sum of the two previous numbers. Fibonacci was a mathematician in Pisa who published and taught during the first half of the 13th century.)

Although the traditional design generally gets the job done, it is not optimal in any sense. This design does not converge to the true MTD, confidence intervals perform poorly (nominal 80% confidence intervals do not include the correct value 80% of the time, 95% intervals are often of infinite length), and it is sensitive to both the starting dose and the dose–toxicity relationship (Storer, 1989). It is also difficult to adapt this design to agents for which different levels of toxicity are suitable (1/6 to 1/3 of patients experiencing severe toxicity is not always appropriate). Furthermore, with the traditional design many patients may be treated at low doses, which is inefficient with respect to resources. Since the usual assumption justifying Phase I designs is that both toxicity and effectiveness are increasing functions of increasing dose, implying that the MTD is also the most effective dose, ethical issues are raised. Patients volunteer for Phase I studies, in part, as a final hope of benefit. To the extent that it can be done safely, the number of patients treated at ineffective doses should be minimized. Alternatives to the traditional design have been investigated to decrease the number of patients treated at low doses and to improve the MTD estimate. Although the tiny sample sizes at each dose for most Phase I studies preclude good statistical properties, newer designs may perform better than the traditional design.

3.3.2   Newer Phase I designs

To assess the performance of designs, an explicit definition of the MTD is required. The general idea in a Phase I trial is to find a dose to recommend for Phase II testing that does not result in too many patients experiencing severe toxicity, with "not too many" often approximately 1/3. Mathematically, if $\Psi(d)$ is the function representing the probability of severe toxicity at dose d, then the MTD is the dose d_{MTD} that satisfies $\Psi(d_{MTD}) = 1/3$. Strategies to improve efficiency over the traditional design include allowing for more rapid escalation of doses than with the standard modified Fibonocci sequence, treating fewer than three patients per dose level, and modifying the sampling scheme for better estimation of the MTD.

Many proposals address the problem of too many patients being treated at low doses by accruing fewer patients at each dose, at least until DLTs start being observed. Recent proposals also are more flexible with respect to re-escalation (up and down designs). Storer (1989; 2001) developed a design that initially adds and evaluates one patient at a time. If the first patient does not have a DLT, the dose is escalated until a DLT is observed; if the first patient does have a DLT, the dose is de-escalated until no DLT is observed. At this point accrual to dose levels is done in threes, with dose level increased if no DLTs are observed, not changed if one is observed, and decreased if two or three are observed. The study ends after a fixed number of cohorts of patients has been accrued. At the conclusion of accrual, Ψ and the MTD, $\Psi^{-1}(1/3)$ are estimated using a logistic model (i.e., the probability of response as a function of dose is modeled as $\Psi(d) = \exp(\alpha + \beta d)/(1 + \exp(\alpha + \beta d))$). Simulations have shown that this procedure improves the estimate of the MTD and reduces the proportion of patients treated at low dose levels without greatly increasing the proportion of patients treated at unacceptably high doses.

Continual reassessment methods (CRM) are another approach to improving Phase I designs. These designs include model-based criteria for dose escalation and de-escalation, in a addition to a model-based estimate of the MTD. The original proposal for these designs (O'Quigley, Pepe, and Fisher, 1990) is to recalculate an estimate of the MTD after each patient is treated and assessed for toxicity, and then to treat the next patient at the dose level closest to this estimate. The final estimate of the MTD occurs after a prespecified number of patients have been treated. The most attractive aspects of this type of design are that all previous results are used to determine the next dose and that MTD estimates are improved over the traditional design. However, because CRM designs use a statistical model based on *a priori* assumptions about the dose–toxicity relationship to select the starting dose, it is possible that the first dose used is not always the lowest dose thought to be clinically reasonable. (This use of *a priori* modeling is part of branch of statistics known as Bayesian methods.) Of additional concern, these designs may result in dose escalations that skip several dose levels, in treatment of only one patient at a dose level when patient heterogeneity is high, and time delays in waiting for toxicity assessment after each patient (a problem shared with the initial stage of the Storer design). Various modifications of the basic CRM design have been proposed to address these issues, such as starting at the first dose regardless of the initial estimate, not restricting to one patient at each stage and not allowing dose levels to be skipped (Goodman et al., 1995), or using an initial stage similar to Storer's (successively higher doses given to one or two patients until toxicity is observed) to target the appropriate dose range before switching to CRM (Møller, 1995). Also see O'Quigley, 2001.

Other proposals to speed up the Phase I process involve larger dose increases early on, followed by more conservative escalations when targets are reached. Collins (1986, 1990) proposed accelerated escalation (maximum of a doubling) until a target area under the plasma concentration vs. time curve (AUC) is reached, with the target determined from mouse pharmacokinetic information. Although savings were noted in Phase I trials of several agents, this pharmacokinetically guided dose escalation (PGDE) approach has not proven practical, largely due to the drawback of real-time pharmacokinetic monitoring (Collins, 2000). Simon et al. (1997) investigate one patient per cohort and a doubling of the dose until toxicity (one patient with dose limiting toxicity or two with grade 2) is observed (intrapatient escalation allowed), followed by standard cohorts of three to six patients with smaller dose increments. The approach appears to have reasonable properties — reduced sample size, small increase in toxicity — but practical experience is needed with this design. The authors emphasize the need for careful definitions of dose limiting toxicity and of the toxicity level considered sufficiently low for intrapatient escalation.

Appropriate starting doses have also been discussed since there would be some savings if starting at higher doses could be assumed sufficiently safe. Generally, 10% of the dose at which 10% of mice die (.1MLD10) has proven very safe. In a review article by Eisenhauer et al. (2000) it was reported that only one of 57 agents had an MTD that was lower than the initial dose based on .1MLD10. It was concluded that although .2MLD10 might be suitable in certain cases with no interspecies differences in toxicology, the recent adoption of more aggressive escalation strategies means that a change would result in minimal efficiency gain.

Although various newer designs have been implemented in practice (see Berlin et al., 1998, for an example of a Storer design, Dees et al., 2000, for an example of a PGDE design, and Sessa et al., 2000 for an example of an accelerated titration design), no new standard has yet emerged. The Eisenhauer summary indicates that, although the modified Fibonacci, three-patient-per-dose-level approach should no longer be considered standard, there is no consensus on the best strategy among the various proposals. Given the limitations imposed by small samples, it is not likely that a single strategy will emerge as optimal.

3.3.3 Phase I/II designs

Occasionally additional patients are added to the patients treated at the MTD of a Phase I design and the combined group is assessed as a Phase II study. This may seem efficient, but the goals of Phase I studies and Phase II studies of efficacy are too different for sensible combination. Patients chosen as suitable for experimentation with possibly ineffective or toxic doses of an agent are going to be systematically different from those chosen as suitable to test activity of the agent. Further, the last several patients on a Phase I study, by design, have experienced a certain level of toxicity. If toxicity and anti-tumor activity are related in any way, then use of patients from the dose-finding part of a trial as part of an efficacy assessment will bias the results. More systematic approaches to assessing both toxicity and efficacy in Phase I/II designs have been proposed by Thall and Russell, 1998, and Gooley et al., 1994. Each considers choosing a dose based on two outcomes, one decreasing as a function of dose and one increasing (such as acceptable toxicity and tumor response as a function of chemotherapy dose or graft rejection and graft vs. host disease as a function of number of donor T cells). Gooley investigates three two-phase designs involving dose reduction in the event of graft vs. host disease and escalation in the event of rejections. Thall and Russell use a Bayesian approach similar to CRM designs, but with a more complicated dose function and decision scheme. Key to both papers is the use of simulation to assess the properties of proposed designs under various scenarios. The small sample properties of these complicated designs are not obvious or easily calculated and need to be carefully assessed before implementation to assure a reasonable chance of choosing an acceptable dose.

3.3.4 Considerations for biologic agents

For agents with low toxicity potential and with specific biologic targets, the standard assumptions justifying Phase I designs may not apply. As noted above, a Phase I design for a cytotoxic cancer agent generally has the objective of identifying the MTD. Since it is assumed that higher doses will be both more toxic and more effective against the cancer, toxicity is the only primary endpoint. For a biologic agent, on the other hand, the toxicity–dose curve may be quite shallow and the monotonicity assumption with respect to response may not be correct; responses may decrease or remain the same instead of increasing at high doses. The Phase I objective for this type of agent might more suitably be to identify a dose that produces biologic responses subject to acceptable toxicity. Eligibility is also problematic in that biologic response (such as immune response) can take several months to develop, and that it is patients with normal biologic function who would be expected to have reasonable responses. Thus the typical Phase I population, with short-term survival and compromised function, may not be suitable.

Given the generally poor properties of Phase I studies in general, the added complications for biologic agents mean even more uncertainty in dose selection. When toxicity can reasonably be assumed minimal over a wide range of doses, a simple solution would be to treat larger cohorts at fewer, more widely spread doses. The trial would be stopped as soon as an unacceptable toxicity was seen and lower doses with at least a specified number of biologic responses observed would be subject to further testing. If minimal toxicity is not anticipated, the Thall and Russell approach might be adapted using a dose function suitable to this setting.

3.3.5 Final comment

Since immediate access to patient outcome data is necessary for the timely and safe completion of Phase I studies, these can be difficult in a multiple-institution setting. Safety can be compromised both by the delays in getting patient data to a coordinating center, and by the innumerable possibilities for miscommunication among the clinical study coordinator, the data center, and participating institutions.

3.4 Phase II trials

Standard Phase II studies of investigational new drugs are used to screen new agents for antitumor activity and to decide which agents should be tested further. For reasons of efficiency the decisions are based on single arm studies using short-term endpoints (usually tumor response in cancer studies) in limited numbers of patients. The problem is formulated statistically as a test of the null hypothesis $H_0 : p = p_0$ vs. the alternative hypothesis $H_1 : p = p_1$, where p is the probability of response, p_0 is the probability which, if true, would mean that the agent was not worth studying further, and p_1 is the probability which, if true, would mean it would be important to identify the agent as active and to continue studying it. (See Chapter 2 for a discussion of hypothesis testing.) Typically, p_0 is chosen to be a value at or somewhat below the historical probability of response to standard treatment for the same stage of disease, and p_1 is typically somewhat above. However, keep in mind when choosing these values that response rates depend on response definitions and patient selection factors, so that the most relevant historical experience is from the same group of investigators planning the current trial. In particular, Phase II studies done at single institutions often include better-risk patients and more liberal response definitions than studies done in the cooperative groups; thus single-institution studies should not be used to determine p_0 and p_1 for a group study.

Both the choice of endpoint and the specification of null and alternative hypotheses are often done routinely in Phase II trials, with little or no thought. An endpoint other than tumor shrinkage should be considered if the assessment of response is particularly difficult or unreliable (e.g., in patients with glioblastoma); an alternative endpoint might be 6-month survival. The choice of p_0 and p_1 should be reconsidered if a review of Phase II experiences suggests changes over time. As definitions and treatments change, the old historical probabilities may not remain applicable. We found, for instance, that as our definitions of response got more stringent within SWOG, the percent of patients responding to standard treatment with doxorubicin + dacarbazine in advanced sarcoma went from 25 to 10%. Consequently, our choice of p_0 in this disease site has been changed in the last few years from 0.1 to 0.05.

3.4.1 The Standard Southwest Oncology Group Phase II design

Our standard approach to the design of Phase II trials of investigational new drugs (Green and Dahlberg, 1992) is to accrue patients in two stages, with the significance level approximately 0.05 and power approximately 0.9. A specified number of patients is targeted for a first stage of accrual, and when that target is approached the study is closed temporarily while responses are assessed. The study is stopped early if the agent appears unpromising — specifically, if the alternative hypothesis is rejected at the .02 level after the first stage of accrual. If the study is not stopped early, it is reopened to a second stage of accrual. We conclude the agent is promising only if H_0 is rejected after the second stage of accrual.

SWOG 8811, a trial of 5-fluorouracil and folinic acid in advanced breast cancer (Margolin et al., 1994), provides examples of two Southwest Oncology Group Phase II designs. This trial was designed to evaluate treatment in two subsets of patients, those with no prior chemotherapy and those who had received one previous chemotherapeutic regimen. For the trial in patients with no prior chemotherapy for advanced disease, we were interested in complete responses (complete disappearance of the tumor). The null hypothesis was specified as $H_0 : p = 0.1$ and the alternative $H_1 : p = 0.3$, because a standard cyclophosphamide, Adriamycin, 5-fluorouracil (CAF) regimen in this setting should result in a complete response probability of about 0.2. For this set of hypotheses, the Southwest Oncology Group approach requires an initial accrual of 20 patients, with an additional 15 patients to be accrued if at least two complete responses are seen in the first 20 patients. The regimen is concluded to be active if eight or more complete responses out of 35 are observed at the end of the trial. For the trial in patients with one prior chemotherapy for advanced disease, we were interested in overall response (complete or partial); the hypotheses for this subset were specified as $H_0 : p = 0.2$ and $H_1 : p = 0.4$. The standard design in this case is to accrue 25 patients initially, with 20 more patients if four or more responses are observed in the first 25, and to conclude that the regimen is worth pursuing if there are 14 or more responses in 45 patients. It should be noted that $14/45 = 0.31$ is the lowest observed proportion of patients with responses that leads to a decision in favor of the alternative true probability of 0.4 as opposed to the null hypothesized probability of 0.2.

Our approach to the design of Phase II trials has evolved in response to various practical considerations, summarized as follows.

First, for ethical reasons it is important to be able to stop subjecting patients to new agents as soon we have convincing evidence the agent is ineffective. For example, suppose in the 8811 trial in patients with no prior chemotherapy for advanced disease that there are no complete responses in the first 10 patients. The treatment is not looking as if it is benefiting patients — should the trial be stopped? The statistical problem here is judging whether or not this is convincing evidence of ineffectiveness. In this example, ten failures is probably not convincing. For instance, if you were treating with a standard regimen such as CAF, groups of ten patients would *on average* have two complete responses, but in about 11% of groups of ten there would be none. Thus it would not be very unusual to see ten nonresponders in a row even for an active regimen in breast cancer, so we would probably not decide we had sufficient evidence to conclude the new regimen inactive. Furthermore, while it is important to be able to stop a trial early when the regimen is inactive, it is also important to be conservative early, to guard against rejecting an active agent due to treating a chance series of poor risk patients. To balance this concern with that of treating the fewest possible patients with an inactive agent, at the first stage we test H_1 at the 0.02 level. This is conservative (we mistakenly reject active agents early at most 2% of the time), while at the same time making it possible to stop early when nothing is happening.

A second consideration in our choice of a standard design was that it can take a long time to complete a trial with multiple stages. Typically after the first stage of accrual we do not have enough information to determine whether the criterion for continuing to the second stage has been met, and the study has to be temporarily stopped to get this information. After closure, it can take several months for patients to complete treatment, more time for data to be submitted and records to be reviewed, and yet more time to process the reopening. For reasons of practicality, this consideration motivates the use of no more than two stages of accrual.

Third, we have rarely found circumstances under which it is important to close a Phase II cancer clinical trial early due to demonstrated *activity*. A protocol for further testing of an agent found to be active is rarely in place at the end of a Phase II trial, and additional accrual to the same protocol of a promising agent to further document the level of activity is nearly always justified. Thus we stop trials only if the alternative hypothesis is rejected (for inactivity); we do not stop early if the null is rejected (for activity).

A fourth justification for our standard design is that the percent of new agents found to be active is not high in cancer, which suggests that designs should have fairly high power and fairly low significance level. Simon (1987) summarized response results for 83 NCI-sponsored investigational agents. In the solid tumor Phase II studies the estimated response probability was greater than 0.15 in only 10% of the 253 disease–drug combinations tested. Taking 10% as an estimate of the truly active agents, conducting each trial at significance level 0.05 and power 0.9 results in 33% of the positive results being false positives (one third of the positive trials will come from rejecting the null hypothesis when it is true). Our choice of identifying at least 90% of active agents (power 0.9) at the expense of 33% of our positive results being false positives could be argued, but seems reasonable.

An appealing property of the SWOG standard designs is that decision guidelines correspond reasonably well to intuition as to what constitutes evidence in favor of one or the other of the hypotheses. Stopping at the first stage occurs when the estimate of the response probability is less than approximately p_0, the true value that would mean the agent would not be of interest. At the second stage the agent is concluded to warrant further study if the estimate of the response probability is greater than approximately $(p_0+p_1)/2$, which typically would be near the historical probability expected from other agents, and represents the value at which one might be expected to be indifferent to the outcome of the trial.

A final point to make concerning our standard design is that multi-institution studies cannot be closed after precisely a specified number of patients has been accrued. It takes time to get a closure notice out, and during this time more patients will have been approached to enter the trial. Patients who were asked and have agreed to participate in a trial should be allowed to do so, and this means there is a period of time during which institutions can continue registering patients even though the study is closing. Furthermore, some patients may be found to be ineligible after the study is closed. We try to time study closures carefully, but it is rare we get the precise number of patients called for by the design. We need designs that are flexible enough to be used when the exact sample size is not attained.

Consider the previously untreated group of study 8811 again. Recall that the design calls for 20 patients to be accrued for the first stage, with the second stage to be accrued if two or more patients have complete responses. Suppose the trial did not make it to the planned 20 patients and was stopped at 18 with one response. How should the decision to continue be made? Should you close the study because only one response was observed even though too few patients were accrued? Try to reopen the study for two more patients and see if one of these responds? The first solution is too conservative, the second impractical. Or suppose the trial was stopped at 23 with 2 responses. Should you continue because two responses were observed, or see if the two responses were in the first 20 patients? In this case the first solution is not conservative enough, while the second does not take advantage of all of the available information.

One of the advantages of the Southwest Oncology Group standard designs is that they are easily applied when the attained sample size is not the planned size. What we do is apply a 0.02 level test of the alternative at the first stage to the attained sample. If this is rejected, the trial is not continued; if it is not rejected, the trial is continued to the second stage. After the second stage, the final accrual is used as if it were the planned accrual, and the rule that would have been in place is applied accordingly. This approach has been investigated analytically and shown to have reasonable properties compared to other possible approaches to the problem (Green and Dahlberg, 1992). In the SWOG 8811 example, for the group of patients with no prior chemotherapy for advanced disease, two complete responses were observed in the first 20 patients, so accrual was continued to the second stage. The final sample size was 36 patients instead of 35, with four complete responses. Eight would have been required to reject the null hypothesis with a sample size of 36, so the regimen was concluded insufficiently active in this type of patient. For the subset of patients with one prior treatment for advanced disease, accrual was temporarily stopped after 21 patients had been entered. After all of the clinical information was submitted, it was determined that there were only two responses. This was sufficient to stop the study because $H_1 : p = 0.4$ is rejected at the 0.02 level (the p-value is 0.002).

3.4.2 Randomized Phase II designs

In some cases the aim of a Phase II study is not to decide whether a particular regimen should be studied further, but to decide which of several new regimens should be taken to the next phase of testing (assuming they cannot all be). In these cases *selection designs* may be used. Patients are randomized to the treatments under consideration, but the intent of the study is *not* a definitive comparison. The intent is to choose for further study a treatment which you are pretty sure is not worse (or at least not much worse) than the other new treatments. The decision rule from a selection design is often formulated as, "Take on to further testing the treatment arm observed to be best by any amount." The number of patients per arm is chosen to be large enough that if one treatment is superior by γ, and the rest are equivalent, the probability of choosing the superior treatment is π. This formulation means that if one of the treatments is substantially superior, it will probably be chosen for further testing. If there is not one that is substantially superior, the chosen one may not be the best, but it will probably be within at most γ of the best. It must be stressed that this design does not result in the conclusion that the selected treatment is better than the others, only that it is the best bet for further testing.

Sample sizes for selection designs were worked out both for response endpoints (Simon, Wittes, and Ellenberg, 1985) and survival endpoints (Liu, Dahlberg, and Crowley, 1993). For example, if there are two treatment arms and one wants a 90% chance (π) of selecting the better arm with respect to response when the response probability is .15 (γ) higher on one arm than the other, at most 37 patients per arm are required. If there are three arms, at most 55 per arm are required; if four arms, 67. For survival as an endpoint, γ is expressed in terms of hazard ratios (see Chapter 2 for a discussion of hazard functions and hazard ratios). The required sample sizes for a 90% chance of selecting the best arm when $\gamma = 1.5$ are 36, 54, and 64, respectively for two, three, and four arms (under the assumptions of exponential survival, maximum follow-up time approximately twice the median survival of the inferior arms, and equal amounts of time for accrual and additional follow-up).

Something to keep in mind with selection designs is that an arm is always chosen. The potential for difficulty is clear. If one of the regimens is superior, but by less than γ, the procedure may miss it and choose another. If more than one regimen is very promising, the procedure will choose only one. If all of the regimens are poor, the procedure still picks one. If at the conclusion of a study no regimens are chosen because they all looked too poor, then the assumptions on which the statistical considerations were based would no longer hold. The probability that an arm superior by γ would have been chosen would now be less than π (since an option not to choose a regimen superior by γ was added after the fact). Ignoring the design in one respect leaves open the possibility that for other outcomes it would have been ignored for other reasons. It would be impossible to figure out what might have been concluded under other circumstances, and therefore impossible to figure out what the probability of choosing a superior arm really was. If the properties of a trial are unknown, it is very difficult to interpret the trial — thus these designs should probably not be used unless one is quite committed to continued testing of the best arm in a subsequent study.

SWOG studies 8835 and 9106 are examples of how these designs can go wrong. Both studies had two-arm selection designs, SWOG 8835 with the aim of choosing either intraperitoneal (IP) mitoxantrone or floxuridine for further study in patients with minimal residual ovarian cancer, and SWOG 9106 with the aim of choosing a regimen (high dose cytoxan plus mitoxantrone plus carboplatin or high dose cytoxan plus thiotepa plus cisplatin) for a Phase III transplant trial in advanced ovarian cancer. For SWOG 8835 (Muggia et al., 1996) the survival estimate was better for floxuridine, so this was identified for further investigation. However, while the trial was ongoing, therapy with paclitaxel plus IP cisplatin was found to be useful and Phase III trials since have focused on taxane and platinum regimens. The role of IP floxuridine in ovarian cancer remains unknown. For SWOG 9106 the cytoxan, mitoxantrone, carboplatin arm had better observed survival at the end of the trial and this was used in the Phase III trial — but this was completely fortuitous because Phase III trial was opened long before the Phase II results were available (not only that, the Phase III trial was already closed before the Phase II results were known, due to poor accrual).

Occasionally control arms are included in randomized Phase II trials. The justification may be to have some assurance the arm chosen in a selection design is not worse than standard. This is a reasonable concern, but adding a control arm does not go very far in addressing it. The only assurance is that the chosen arm is probably at most γ worse than standard, but since γ is typically not very small (to keep the sample size down), one may still go ahead with an inferior agent. As well, if the improvement due to a new agent is less than γ, the standard arm might well be chosen instead and the beneficial new agent missed. Another justification may be to document that a sufficiently good risk population of patients has been accrued for a fair trial of the experimental arm. This justification does not work well either because the estimate of activity on the standard arm is too poor for adequate documentation, again due to the small sample size.

Problems arise when results of a randomized Phase II trial (particularly one that includes a control arm) look so striking that it is tempting to skip the Phase III trial. The temptation should be resisted. As discussed in Liu, LeBlanc, and Desai (1999), large observed differences are not unusual with the modest samples sizes of randomized Phase II studies. For instance, the authors investigated a typical two-arm selection design with a survival endpoint. They showed that the design will result in a hazard ratio of greater than 1.5 in 16% of trials and greater than 1.7 in 7% of trials when the survival distributions are actually the same. Differences reflected by hazard ratios of greater than 1.5, if true, would be of considerable interest, but since observed differences this large are common in the randomized Phase II setting, they cannot be considered definitive evidence in favor of the apparently superior arm.

It should also be noted that simultaneous assessment of several Phase II agents does not necessarily save time. Protocol development time is longer due to the extra complications of a multi-arm trial. Patients must be suitable candidates for all agents, restricting the eligibility pool. Apart from the obvious decrease in accrual rate to each arm due to only a fraction of the total going on each arm, there is also a decrease due to the extra effort of recruiting to a randomized trial. Accomplishing accrual to all arms will be particularly slow if there are over three arms, since sample sizes per agent are larger than for standard Phase IIs.

3.4.3   Other Phase II designs

Various other Phase II designs of two or more stages have been proposed (Fleming, 1982; Chang et al., 1987; Simon, 1987; 1989). Some (e.g., Simon, 1989) minimize the expected number of patients required on study subject to specific restraints. A problem with these designs is that sample size has to be accrued exactly, so in practice they cannot be carried out in most settings. Adaptive modifications of the designs in Fleming (1982) and Simon (1987) are possible (Green and Dahlberg, 1992).

Single stage designs (or *pilot studies*) may be acceptable if the regimen being studied consists of agents already shown to be active. In this case, the ethical concern about treating patients with ineffective treatment does not apply. Goals for pilot studies are often feasibility (e.g., Can this regimen be given in a cooperative group setting with acceptable toxicity?) or estimation (e.g., What is the 2-year survival probability to within $+/-10\%$?), in addition to the usual goal of deciding whether or not to continue testing the regimen. Sample sizes for pilot studies are typically 50 to 100 patients, depending on how precise the estimates need to be.

The selected primary endpoint is just one consideration in the decision to pursue a new agent. Other endpoints (such as survival and toxicity, if response is the primary endpoint) must also be considered. For instance, a trial with a sufficient number of responses to be considered active may still not be of interest if too many patients experience life-threatening toxicity, or if they all die quickly; or one with an insufficient number of responses but a good toxicity profile and promising survival might still be considered for future trials. Some designs for Phase II studies formally incorporate both response and toxicity into the decision rules (Bryant and Day, 1995; Conaway and Petroni, 1995; 1996). For these designs both the number of patients with tumor response and the number with acceptable toxicity must be sufficiently high to conclude the regimen should be tested further. There are a number of difficulties with these designs, perhaps most importantly with respect to the assumptions that must be made concerning toxicity–response trade-offs. These assumptions are necessarily somewhat arbitrary and cannot be assumed to reflect the preferences of either investigators or patients. In another variation on this theme, Zee et al. (1999) propose assessing both response and early progression, requiring both a high proportion of responses and a low proportion of early progressions for a successful trial. In general, for typical Phase II agents we think it best to base the design on a primary clinical endpoint, then use judgment about how secondary clinical endpoint information should be used in decisions on testing the agent or regimen further. If response does not sufficiently reflect success, an alternative primary endpoint can be used, such as *clinical benefit*, defined as either response or 6-month stability (sometimes used in breast cancer, particularly for hormonal agents). A setting where multi-endpoint designs could potentially be more useful is for biologic agents, where documentation of both clinical activity (such as disease stability if responses are not anticipated) and biologic activity (such as immune response for a vaccine) may be desired before testing the agent further.

3.5 Phase III trials

3.5.1 *Randomization*

Randomization is the cornerstone of clinical trials methodology. Without it, we would still be in the dark ages of observational studies, with no satisfactory way to assess whether any improvements observed were due to the treatment being studied or to selection factors. It now seems foolish that it was thought patients got better because of — rather than in spite of — purging, bleeding, and blistering, but recent history has also hardly been free of observational misinterpretations. Was the unquestioned use of radical mastectomy for so many years much different? Or, until randomized studies were done, was it just another untested procedure predicated on an incorrect theory of a disease process?

Stratification factors

Randomization is not quite sufficient by itself to guarantee comparable treatment arms unless the sample size is large. In small- or moderate-size studies major imbalances in important patient characteristics can occur by chance and compromise interpretation of the study. It is prudent to protect against this possibility by making sure the most important factors are reasonably well balanced between the arms. Patient characteristics incorporated into the randomization scheme to achieve balance are called *stratification factors*.

Stratification factors should be those known to be strongly associated with outcome. If the number of participating institutions is small, it may be best to stratify on this factor as well, since standards of care may differ by institution. However, any randomization scheme will fail to produce balance if too many factors are included. In general, we suggest no more than three stratification factors given the sample sizes generally used in cancer clinical trials.

If it is considered possible that the size or direction of treatment effect will be substantially different in two subsets of patients, then stratification is not sufficient. Subset analyses with sufficient sample size in each subset (in effect, two separate studies) will need to be planned from the beginning.

Randomization schemes

Various schemes are used and have been proposed to achieve both random treatment assignment and balance across important prognostic factors. The randomized block design is perhaps the most common. In this scheme, the number of patients per arm is equalized after every block of n patients; within the blocks, the assignment is random. Stratification is achieved using this scheme by having blocks within specific types of patients. For instance, if a study is to be stratified on age (<40 vs. 40−60 vs. 60+) and performance status (0−1 vs. 2), then blocked randomization would be done within each of the six defined patient groups. Note that the number of groups increases quickly as the number of factors increases. Four factors with three categories each result in 81 distinct patient groups, for example. In a moderate-size trial with multiple factors, it is likely that some groups will consist of only a few patients — not enough to complete a block — so imbalance can result.

Dynamic allocation schemes often are used to solve this problem. Instead of trying to balance treatment within small patient subsets, the treatment assigned (with high probability) is the one that achieves the best balance overall across the individual factors. Balance can be defined in many ways. A common approach is due to Pocock and Simon (1975). For example, consider a study with two factors (sex and race) and two treatment arms (1 and 2) and several patients already entered. The factors for the next patient registered are male and white. The Pocock-Simon approach involves computing, for each of the two possible treatment assignments, the number of white patients and the number of males that would result on each arm. The patient is assigned with high probability (e.g., 2/3) to the arm that would achieve the smaller overall imbalance.

Other schemes try to address ethical problems by requiring that the arm with the current best outcome be assigned to the next patient with higher probability than the other arms. This is called *adaptive allocation* or "play the winner;" see, for instance, Wei and Durham (1978). A number of problems are associated with use of these schemes. One is the possibility of too few patients being registered to one of the arms for a convincing result. A noncancer example is a trial of extracorporeal membrane oxygenation (ECMO) vs. control in newborns with severe respiratory failure (Bartlett et al., 1985). A Wei and Durham design was used, which resulted in the assignment of nine patients to the experimental arm (all lived) and one to the control arm (who died). As discussed in Royall (1991), the trial generated criticism as being unconvincing because only a single patient received standard therapy. Interpretation of the trial depended on one's perception of the efficacy of standard treatment from historical information. Royall also discusses the ethics of the trial. The investigators were already convinced of the efficacy of ECMO; use of an adaptive allocation scheme was their solution to their ethical dilemma. Is it clear, however, that it is ethical to assign a smaller percent of patients to a treatment believed inferior when it is not ethical to assign 50%? A practical problem with adaptive designs is the difficulty in continuously updating endpoints and analyzing results. Another problem is the possibility of time trends occurring at the same time that percents registered to each arm are changing, thereby introducing bias.

A point to remember in choosing a randomization scheme is that each one differs in emphasis on what is to be balanced. A randomized block design with a small number per block and no factors will result in very nearly equal numbers of patients on each arm, but does not control for chance imbalance in important prognostic factors. A block design within each type of patient defined by the factors achieves the best balance within subtypes of patients, but the number of patients per arm can be badly imbalanced. Dynamic schemes fall in between, but these do not balance within each subtype of patient (the number of males might be the same on each arm, as well as the number over 40, but males over 40 are not necessarily balanced).

Timing of randomization

In general, the best time to randomize is the closest possible time to the start of the treatments to be compared. If randomization and the time of the start of treatment are separated, patients may die, deteriorate, develop complications from other treatments, change their minds, or become unsuitable for treatment, resulting in a number of patients not treated as required. If these patients are removed from the analysis, then the patient groups may no longer be comparable, since such deviations may be more frequent on one arm than the other or reasons for deviations may be different on the arms. If all patients eligible at the time of randomization are used in the primary analysis of the study as we recommend (the *intent to treat principle* discussed in Chapter 7), then such complications add unnecessary variability. Thus it is best to minimize the problem by randomizing close to the start of treatment. For instance, in a study of adjuvant treatment for colon cancer, randomization should occur within 1 working day of the start of chemotherapy rather than at the time of surgery.

Similar considerations apply when the treatment for the two arms is common for a certain period and then diverges. For example, if there is a common induction treatment followed by high-dose therapy for one group and standard therapy for another, randomization after induction therapy eliminates the problems caused when many of the patients do not receive the high-dose therapy. If randomization is at the start of induction, these patients are either improperly eliminated from the analysis, causing bias, or add variability to the real treatment comparison, necessitating larger sample sizes.

Randomization before such treatment divergences may be required for practical reasons (to make obtaining consent easier, to add time for insurance coverage to be guaranteed, etc.) Differences in treatment arms may also begin later than the actual start of treatment on a study by choice. For instance, SWOG 7827 compared 1 year vs. 2 years of adjuvant chemotherapy (CMFVP, defined in Chapter 1) in women with receptor-negative, node-positive breast cancer (Rivkin et al., 1993). Randomization could have been done at the start of treatment or after 1 year in patients still on CMFVP. Note that the two approaches ask different questions. The first asks if 2 years or 1 year of treatment should be planned from the onset of adjuvant chemotherapy. The second asks if patients who have made it through 1 year of chemotherapy should be asked to continue for another year. To see the difference, consider Table 3.1, adapted from Rivkin et al., 1993.

Table 3.1. Compliance data by treatment and number of positive nodes for SWOG 7827.

	1–3 Positive Nodes		4+ Positive Nodes	
	1-Year Arm	2-Year Arm	1-Year Arm	2-Year Arm
No. at risk at 12 mo.[a]	86	92	83	92
Treated <6 mo.	6%	20%	10%	7%
Treated >11 mo.	86%	72%	83%	85%
No. at risk at 24 mo.		78		71
Treated >23 mo.		32%		42%

[a]No. at risk is the number of patients alive and disease free at 12 months (i.e., those who should have been treated for a year).

The decision was made on this trial to randomize at the start of treatment. Even though the first year was supposed to be identical for the two arms, some interesting differences were observed in the dropout patterns. Among patients with good-risk disease (one to three nodes involved) more on the 2-year arm dropped out in the first 6 months than on the 1-year arm, while this was not true for patients with poor-risk disease (four or more nodes involved). It is possible that knowledge of assignment to 2 years of toxic treatment was a factor in the more frequent decision of good-risk patients to drop out of treatment early, while those at higher risk of recurrence may have been more motivated (or encouraged more) to continue despite the long haul ahead. One of the conclusions from this study was that 2 years of treatment was difficult to complete. (In fact it was the main conclusion, since compliance was too poor for the trial to adequately address the benefit of adding a year of treatment.) If the study had been designed to register and randomize patients after 1 year of treatment had been completed, we can speculate that the study would have been closed early due to poor accrual, but no conclusions concerning the difficulty of completion of a planned 2-year treatment course could have been made and no exploration of early dropouts by randomized arm could have been done.

Another issue in the timing of randomization is when to obtain patient consent. Most often patients are asked to participate before randomization has occurred; part of the consent process is to agree to a random assignment of treatment. In studies of competent adults, this is the only timing we believe is appropriate. It has been argued that *randomized consent designs* are appropriate in some circumstances (Zelen, 1979). In these designs randomization occurs before patient consent, after which the patient is asked to participate according to the assigned arm. (In another proposed version of the design, only patients randomized to the experimental arm are asked for consent, while those assigned to the control arm are given control treatment without consent — the reasoning being that control treatment is all that should be expected ordinarily.) A common motivation in considering use of this design is the perception that it is easier to accrue patients to a trial if the assignment has already been made. This leads to the concern, however, that patients do not give a truly informed consent, but rather are subtly persuaded that the arm to which they are assigned is their best choice (Ellenberg, 1984). Apart from the ethical issue, there is also an analytic drawback to this design. It is often conveniently forgotten that patients are supposed to be analyzed according to the assigned arm. It is not appropriate to analyze by the arm received, or to exclude these patients from the analysis. If very many patients refuse their assigned treatment, interpretation of the study is compromised.

When to blind

Double-blinding means that neither the patient nor the clinician knows what treatment has been assigned to the patient. *Single-blinding* means only the patient does not know. *Placebo-controlled* means patients on all arms receive identical-appearing treatment, but all or part of the treatment is inactive on one of the arms. Blinded, placebo-controlled trials are expensive. Manufacture of placebos, labeling of active and inactive treatment with code numbers and keeping track of them, shipping supplies of coded treatments, communications with the pharmacies that dispense the treatments, and mechanisms for unblinding in medical emergencies all are time consuming to plan and costly to administer. There are various circumstances when blinded trials are necessary, but consider the difficulties carefully before embarking on one. One necessary circumstance is when treatment on one of the arms is commercially available (e.g., vitamins). In this case it is important for compliance that patients on each arm get an identical-appearing pill and that all patients are blinded to their assignments. This should minimize and equalize the number of patients who obtain their own supply of active drug. Whether or not the clinicians also need to be blinded depends on whether knowledge of assignment will lead to inappropriate alterations of treatment. It also depends on the endpoints. Placebos and double-blinding are necessary when important endpoints are subjective. For instance, in a double-blind antiemetic trial of placebo vs. prochlorperazine (PCP) vs. tetrahydrocannabinol

(THC) (Frytak et al., 1979), the percent of patients on the treatment arms reported as having sedation as a side effect was high — 71% on prochlorperazine and 76% on THC. Without a placebo comparison, the 71 and 76% might have been judged against 0% and the side effect judged excessive. As it was, sedation was reported in 46% of placebo patients. Coordination problems were reported for 19% of placebo patients (3% "intolerable"), and "highs" were reported in 12% of PCP patients. THC had significantly higher percentages of these two effects, but without a double-blind comparison, the results could have been criticized as reflecting biased assessments rather than true differences. Both THC and PCP had significant antiemetic effects compared to placebo. Overall unsatisfactory outcome (either repeated vomiting or CNS side effects requiring discontinuation of treatment) was reported as 54, 46, and 63%, respectively for placebo, PCP and THC (nonsignificant). Interestingly, the paper concludes THC should not be recommended for general use, but makes no comment on the usefulness of PCP.

Blinding cannot always be achieved even if considered necessary. Blinding does not work if the active treatment is highly effective with respect to one of the outcomes or if it has a distinctive side effect. This effectively unblinds the treatment arm and biased assessments of the other endpoints may result. Another circumstance where it may not be possible to blind is when a comparison involves injury or toxic effects to the patients on inactive treatment. In this case the benefits of blinding may not be sufficient to proceed, although there are a number of examples of sham surgeries being done on trials.

A recent example is a placebo-controlled study of fetal nigral transplantation in Parkinson's disease. Endpoints for this disease are subjective and placebo effects of treatment are likely, making blinding desirable. The sham surgery for this study consists of placement of steriotactic frame, general anesthesia, scalp incision, partial burr hole, antibiotics, cyclosporin, and PET studies, all of which are associated with risks to the patient. Discussion of the suitability of the design is presented by Freeman et al., 1999 and Macklin, 1999. As noted in the Freeman discussion, for a sham surgery to be considered, the question should be important and not likely to become obsolete in the near future, the current state of evidence should be promising but inconclusive, there should be no satisfactory currently available treatments, intervention should be provided in addition to any standard therapy, and the question should not be answerable with less invasive designs. These criteria are met for the study.

The ethical discussion in the two papers focuses on potential benefits to the placebo patients (including, for this trial, contribution

PHASE III TRIALS

to science, no cost standard medical treatment, later transplant at no cost if the procedure is found to be beneficial, spared other risks of transplant if found not beneficial) vs. the risks (injury or death from sham procedure, inconvenience of a procedure with no potential clinical benefit except a placebo effect). Macklin concludes that the sham surgery is not compatible with the principle of minimizing risk of harm and should not be done; Freeman et al. 1999 conclude that the risks are reasonable with respect to possible benefits. Studies are considered ethical if the risk–benefit ratio is favorable, but in an example such as this, magnitudes of risk and benefit are hard to quantify and reasonable people may disagree as to whether the ratio is favorable or unfavorable.

If a blinded trial is done, decisions must be made as to the timing and conditions for unblinding. Unblinding is clearly necessary in medical emergencies in which treatment depends on knowledge of trial assignment. Otherwise it is best not to unblind anyone until the study is published. Risks of early knowledge of treatment assignment include patients on placebo deciding to take active treatment, and clinicians receiving enough clues to be able to recognize treatment assignment in patients supposedly still on blinded treatment, leading to biased assessments of subjective endpoints.

Parting note

Randomization does not work if patients are routinely canceled (deleted from the study) after entry on a trial. If investigators and patients proceed with treatment assignments only if the randomization is to a preferred arm, then the trial is little better than a study on patients who were treated according to systematic nonrandom reasons. Due to the selection biases introduced by cancellation, all randomized trials should be conducted according to the intent-to-treat principle (Section 7.3.1).

3.5.2   Two-arm trials

The most important endpoint in judging effectiveness of treatment in a Phase III trial is survival. Quality of life may also be key, particularly when survival benefit is not anticipated. Tumor response poorly reflects survival and quality of life and is not an adequate substitute for either.

A typical objective in a Phase III trial is "to compare A and B with respect to survival in the treatment of patients with...". As discussed in Chapter 2, the null hypothesis is usually equality of survival distributions (or equivalently, of hazard functions), and the alternative is that survival is not the same. Whether or when the alternative hypothesis should be specified as one-sided or two-sided is a matter of some debate. (This issue is of practical importance, since a two-sided test of the same level requires a larger sample size than a one-sided test to achieve the same power.) Some statisticians argue that the alternative should always be two-sided because it is always possible that either arm could be worse.

We view the issue more as a decision problem. If at the end of the trial of A vs. B the conclusion is going to be either "continue to use A" or "use B," this is a one-sided setting; if the conclusion is going to be either "use A," "use B," or "use either," then it is two-sided. For instance, adding an experimental agent to a standard regimen is nearly always a one-sided setting. At the end of the trial the decision is made whether to use the extra agent or not. If the agent has either no effect or a detrimental effect on survival, the agent will not be used; if survival is improved the agent generally will be recommended for use. It would not be sensible to conclude "use either arm." Furthermore, even though the agent could be detrimental, going out of one's way to *prove* it is harmful may be unethical. On the other hand, a comparison of two standard treatments is often a two-sided setting. The decision to be made is whether one of the standards should be recommended over the other, or if either is acceptable.

Choice of significance level, power, and the difference to be detected is the major determinant of sample size (see Chapter 2). As noted at the beginning of the chapter, the difference specified to be detected should generally not be what has been observed in other studies, but rather the smallest difference it would be important to detect. A toxic treatment when the standard is no treatment might require a fairly large benefit to be worthwhile, for example. After effective treatments have been identified, however, smaller benefits may be worth detecting.

Concerning choice of significance level, the standard 0.05 is usually reasonable. Occasionally it is important to be more conservative, such as for highly controversial or highly toxic treatments. In these cases it might be prudent to have stronger evidence of effectiveness, perhaps at the 0.01 level instead of 0.05, before recommending the treatment for use.

We consider power 0.8 to be a bit low, as this means 20% of effective treatments will not be detected. (Also consider that this is 20% of the treatments effective at the specified difference. More than 20% of treatments effective at a level less than that specified will be missed.) Considering that relatively few new treatments are found to be even modestly effective in cancer, we generally recommend power 0.9.

When survival is the primary endpoint of a study, differences between arms are usually expressed as a hazard ratio, $R(t)$. The hazard ratio is the ratio of the death rates among those still alive on the two arms at each point in time (see Chapter 2). If the ratio is the same at all times, $R(t)$ is a constant R (denoted $\exp(\beta)$ in Chapter 2); this is called the *proportional hazards assumption*. Exponential survival distributions for all arms of a study give one example yielding constant hazard ratios. (As noted in Chapter 2, a hazard ratio in the exponential case is the inverse of the ratio of median survivals between the arms.) A constant hazard ratio of unity means the death rates at each point in time (and therefore the survival distributions on the two arms) are the same. If survival is very different and the proportional hazards assumption holds, R is either close to zero or very large. The most common hypotheses in Phase III trials are formulated statistically as $H_0 : R = 1$ vs. $H_1 : R > 1$ or vs. $H_1 : R \neq 1$. Rather than give formulas (the formulas are not simple) for sample size when survival is the endpoint, we will give some general ideas on how various factors change the sample size requirements. Besides level (α), power ($1 - \beta$) and R, the major influence on sample size is the amount of follow-up patients have relative to how long they live. The main point to be made is that the sample size is driven by the number of deaths expected rather than the number of patients accrued. A relatively small study of patients with rapidly lethal disease may have the same power as a very large study of patients with a low death rate and short follow-up. The number of deaths increases as median survival decreases, and as the length of time each patient is followed increases.

Table 3.2 illustrates the effect of level, power, hazard ratio to be detected, median survival, and follow-up on sample size. Assumptions used in the calculations included exponential survival distributions and accrual of 200 patients per year. The formula is described by Bernstein and Lagakos (1978).

A comparison of the sample sizes presented here compared to those based on the binomial in Table 2.9 is instructive. Researchers often have the mistaken notion that a change in the survival probabilities at a particular point in time is the same as a change in the hazard ratio. Consider a study for which a 25% increase in survival is the stated goal. If a 0.25 increase in the 1-year survival probability from 0.4 to 0.65 is desired, then according to Table 2.9, a total of 148 patients (74 per arm) would be sufficient. However, this change

Table 3.2. Sample size per arm required for a one-sided two-arm trial under various assumptions with an annual accrual rate of 200.[a]

m	R	$\alpha = 0.05$ $1 - \beta = 0.8$ $T = 1$	$\alpha = 0.05$ $1 - \beta = 0.8$ $T = 5$	$\alpha = 0.05$ $1 - \beta = 0.9$ $T = 1$	$\alpha = 0.05$ $1 - \beta = 0.9$ $T = 5$	$\alpha = 0.01$ $1 - \beta = 0.9$ $T = 1$	$\alpha = 0.01$ $1 - \beta = 0.9$ $T = 5$
1	1.25	330	260	430	360	610	530
	1.5	130	80	170	110	240	170
	2.0	60	30	80	40	110	60
5	1.25	640	430	790	570	1050	800
	1.5	310	160	390	220	510	310
	2.0	170	70	210	100	280	140

[a] R is the hazard ratio for which the specified power applies, m the median survival time in years on the control arm, α the level, $1 - \beta$ the power, and T the number of years of additional follow-up after accrual is complete.

corresponds to a hazard ratio of 2.13, implying that the median survival time more than doubles. If instead a 25% increase in median survival is desired (hazard ratio of 1.25), the sample size required per arm is several hundred.

The assumption of exponential survival distributions is common in determining sample size. Real survival distributions are never precisely exponentially distributed, but using the assumption for calculating sample size is generally adequate, provided the proportional hazards assumption still holds, at least approximately (Schoenfeld, 1983). If the proportional hazards assumption is not correct, the standard sample size calculations are not correct (Benedetti et al., 1982). For example, if survival is identical until time t before diverging (hazard ratio 1 followed by hazard ratio not equal to 1), the standard formulas do not hold. Deaths during the time the curves are identical do not provide information on the difference between the arms, so in this setting sample size is driven by the number of deaths after time t rather than the total number of deaths. Any type of clear divergence from standard assumptions will require a different type of sample size calculation.

Multiple endpoints

The above discussion addresses studies with one primary endpoint only. Generally we find that the clinical endpoint of greatest importance is easily identified; this then is primary and the one on which the sample size is based. The remaining endpoints are secondary and reported separately. Others have proposed an approach of combining all endpoints using weighted sums of differences of each endpoint of interest (O'Brien, 1984; Tang, Gnecco, and Geller, 1989;

Cook and Farewell, 1994). A problem with this approach is that the weights assigned are fairly arbitrary. The investigators make a judgment as to the relative importance of each endpoint (survival, time to progression, toxicity, various aspect of quality of life, etc.) and weight the differences observed on the treatment arms accordingly. Since no one puts precisely the same importance on all endpoints, we do not find this approach satisfactory. Instead we recommend reporting each endpoint comparison separately. If the directions of the differences do not all favor the same arm, judgments concerning which is the preferred treatment can be made according to individual preferences.

3.5.3 Equivalence or noninferiority trials

Suppose you are reading the results of a randomized clinical trial for which the primary aim was to compare two treatment arms with respect to the probability of response. The study had been designed to detect a difference of 0.15 in response probabilities. At the time of publication, 25% of the patients had responded on arm A, only 5% higher than on arm B. The results of the trial were disappointing to the investigators, so they stopped the trial early and concluded there were "no significant differences" between the arms. Does the finding of no statistically significant differences in this study establish clinical equivalence?

The answer most likely is no. *Failure to reject* the null hypothesis is not equivalent to *proving* the null hypothesis. A p-value of 0.9 does not mean we are 90% sure the null hypothesis is correct. Recall from Chapter 2 that a p-value P means that the probability of the observed result (or one more extreme) under the null hypothesis is equal to P. A small p-value means the observed result does not happen often when the true response probabilities are identical; a large one means it does happen often. If it does not happen often, the evidence contradicts the null hypothesis and we can conclude the treatments are (likely to be) different. If it does happen often, the evidence does not contradict the null hypothesis — but, unfortunately, we cannot in this case conclude the treatments are equivalent. This is because there are other hypotheses that the evidence does not contradict.

To illustrate, consider the initial example, in which the estimated response probability for arm A was 0.25 and for arm B was 0.2 (an observed difference of 0.05). Under the null hypothesis $H_0 : p_A = p_B$ (response probabilities on arm A and arm B are equal), the p-value for this observed difference depends on the sample size. Table 3.3

Table 3.3. Two-sided p-value for testing H_0, and 95% confidence interval for difference in response probabilities (normal approximation). Estimated response probabilities are 0.25 on arm A and 0.2 on arm B.

N per Arm	p-Value for $H_0 : p_A = p_B$	Confidence Interval for $p_A - p_B$
20	0.71	(−0.21, 0.31)
40	0.59	(−0.13, 0.23)
80	0.45	(−0.08, 0.18)
160	0.28	(−0.04, 0.14)
320	0.13	(−0.01, 0.11)
640	0.03	(0.00, 0.10)

gives the p-values and 95% confidence intervals for a range of sample sizes. (See Chapter 2 for a discussion of confidence intervals.) The largest p-value in Table 3.3 is 0.71, when the sample size is 20 per arm. Despite the large p-value, it is clear from the confidence interval, which covers both −0.15 and 0.15, that the evidence is consistent with a broad range of true values, and that either arm could still be substantially superior. On the other hand, the smallest p-value under the hypothesis of equality occurs at 640 per arm. With this sample size the 0.05 difference is statistically significant — but this sample size also provides the strongest evidence that the two response probabilities are similar (the confidence interval indicates arm A is better by less than 0.1).

Considering the question from another perspective, Table 3.4 shows the observed difference that would be required for the p-value to be approximately the same for each sample size, and the

Table 3.4. Proportion responding on arm B required to result in a two-sided p-value of approximately 0.7, and the 95% confidence interval for the difference in response probabilities (normal approximations). Proportion responding on arm A is 0.25.

N per Arm	Proportion Responding, Arm B	Difference, Arm B − Arm A	p-value for $H_0 : p_A = p_B$	Confidence Interval for $p_A - p_B$
20	0.20	0.05	0.71	(−0.21, 0.31)
40	0.225	0.025	0.79	(−0.16, 0.21)
80	0.225	0.025	0.71	(−0.11, 0.16)
160	0.231	0.019	0.70	(−0.07, 0.11)
320	0.238	0.012	0.71	(−0.05, 0.08)
640	0.241	0.009	0.70	(−0.04, 0.06)

corresponding 95% confidence interval. At 20 patients per arm, a p-value of 0.7 means the difference could be as large as 0.3; at 640 patients per arm, the same p-value means the difference is no larger than 0.06. The table illustrates the fact that large p-values for tests of equality provide more evidence for the null hypothesis when sample sizes are large.

It is clear from the tables that the p-value for testing equality does not in itself provide useful information concerning the equivalence of two treatments.

How could the authors legitimately claim results are approximately equivalent? One way is by using a different p-value to test a different hypothesis. The authors were interested in detecting a difference of 0.15. That can be tested by making the null hypothesis "the response probability on arm A is superior by .15 or the response probability on arm B is superior by .15" ($H_0 : p_A \geq p_B + .15$ or $p_A \leq p_B - .15$). If this hypothesis is rejected, then we can conclude that the response probabilities on the two treatment arms are within 0.15 of each other. Table 3.5 shows p-values for testing three different hypotheses, $H_1 : p_A = p_B + 0.05$ (arm A superior by 0.05), $H_2 : p_A = p_B + 0.15$ (arm A superior by .15), and $H_3 : p_A = p_B - 0.15$ (arm B superior by .15). The 95% confidence interval for the difference in probabilities is also repeated. For $N = 20$, the tests show that the outcome would not be unusual when either arm, in truth, had a response probability of 0.15 greater than the other arm. The test of the hypothesis that arm A is superior by .15 is not rejected, and the test of the hypothesis that arm B is superior by .15 is not rejected. It is not until 160 patients per arm that the hypotheses are both rejected; this is reflected in the confidence interval which excludes both -0.15 and 0.15. Table 3.5 also illustrates the fact that

Table 3.5. Two-sided p-values for tests of $H_1 : p_A = p_B + .05$, $H_2 : p_A = p_B + 0.15$ and $H_3 : p_A = p_B - 0.15$ for various sample sizes when the observed proportions responding on arms A and B are, respectively, 0.25 and 0.2.

N/Arm	H_1	H_2	H_3	Confidence Interval for $p_A - p_B$
20	1.0	0.45	0.13	(−0.21, 0.31)
40	1.0	0.28	0.03	(−0.13, 0.23)
80	1.0	0.13	0.002	(−0.08, 0.18)
100	1.0	0.09	0.001	(−0.07, 0.17)
160	1.0	0.03	0.000	(−0.04, 0.14)
320	1.0	0.002	0.000	(−0.01, 0.11)
640	1.0	0.000	0.000	(0.00, 0.10)

if you test the observed result, you always get a p-value of 1.0, which should also help convince you that large p-values do not mean much by themselves.

Designing an equivalence or noninferiority trial

The same reasoning that allows us to conclude approximate equivalence when a completed trial is sufficiently large and results are sufficiently close also allows us to design a trial with an equivalence objective (Blackwelder, 1982; Harrington, Fleming, and Green, 1982). Instead of using the standard null hypothesis of no difference, the null hypothesis is phrased instead as a small difference between the arms. The two-sided version is used for an equivalence trial. In this case the difference between arms A and B, $A - B$, is hypothesized to be Δ or $-\Delta$ (to allow for either arm to be superior) and the alternative hypothesis is that the difference is less than Δ and greater than $-\Delta$. If the null hypothesis is rejected, the conclusion is not that the arms are equivalent but that the difference between them is smaller than the specified difference Δ (in either direction). The one-sided version (the difference between arms A and B, $A - B$, is hypothesized to be Δ and the alternative hypothesis is that the difference is less than Δ) is used for a noninferiority trial. For example, a new, less toxic or less expensive treatment might be hypothesized to be slightly inferior to the standard. If this hypothesis is rejected, the conclusion is not that the new treatment is the same, but that we are reasonably sure it is not much worse (the difference is less than Δ). The alternative hypothesis for which there should be adequate power for either an equivalence or noninferiority trial is the hypothesis of equality. A point to note is that the sample size required to rule out a small difference is about the same as that required to detect a small difference. Consequently, a well-designed equivalence or noninferiority trial must be very large.

3.6 Conclusion

We opened this chapter with a discussion of a dietary trial performed by the Biblical Daniel. To conclude, let us see how Daniel's trial fared with respect to the five major design considerations listed in the introduction. The objective is pretty clear: to compare a meat and wine diet vs. a vegetable and water diet to decide which one to feed the servants from the tribe of Judah. The endpoint is less satisfactory: "appearance" after 10 days is nonspecific, highly subjective, and does not adequately measure the long-term health of the subjects. It is creditable that the endpoint was specified before the experiment was carried out, however. The treatment assignment is unacceptable. By assigning Daniel and his friends to the vegetable diet, the interpretation of the trial is compromised. Any differences in the two groups could be due to other cultural differences rather than diet. The magnitude of difference to be detected and assumptions used in sample size calculations are not specified in the biblical report; it is probably safe to assume these were not considered. So let us give Daniel 1.5 out of 5 — maybe not so bad for 2500 years ago.

CHAPTER 4

Multi-Arm Trials

On the 20th of May 1747, I took twelve patients in the scurvy, on board the Salisbury at sea. Their cases were as similar as I could have them. They all in general had putrid gums, the spots and lassitude, with weakness of their knees. They lay together in one place, being a proper apartment for the sick in the fore-hold; and had one diet common to all... Two of these were ordered each a quart of cyder a-day. Two others took two spoon-fuls of vinegar three times a-day... Two others took twenty-five gutts of elixir vitriol three times a-day, upon an empty stomach; using a gargle strongly acidulated with it for their mouths. Two of the worst patients... were put under a course of sea-water... Two others had each two oranges and one lemon given them every day. These they ate with greediness, at different times, upon an empty stomach ... The two remaining patients, took the bigness of nutmeg three times a-day, of an electuary recommended by an hospital surgeon...

The consequence was, that the most sudden and visible good effects were perceived from the use of the oranges and lemons; one of those who had taken them, being at the end of six days fit for duty.

–James Lind (1753)

4.1 Introduction

Leaping ahead a couple of millennia from Daniel, we find "the first deliberately planned controlled experiment ever undertaken on human subjects" (Stuart and Guthrie, 1953), a six-arm trial with two patients per arm. The study is a tremendous improvement over the biblical trial. It was painstakingly planned, including efforts to eliminate bias (except that two of the worst got sea water), and was reported in sufficient detail to judge the quality. Despite the pitifully small sample size, the correct conclusion that citrus prevented scurvy was reached. Lind was fortunate that one of his treatments produced a cure. We, having to live with modest treatment effects and high variability, need to consider the problems in conducting multi-arm trials.

The frequent use of the standard two-arm randomized clinical trial is due in part to its relative simplicity of design and interpretation. At its most basic, one power, one level, and one magnitude of difference to be detected have to be specified to determine sample size. Conclusions are straightforward: either the two arms are shown to be different or they are not. When more than two arms are included, complexity ensues. With four arms, there are six possible pairwise comparisons, nineteen ways of pooling and comparing two groups, and twenty-four ways of ordering the arms (not to mention the global test of equality of all four arms), for a grand total of 50 possible hypothesis tests. Some subset of these must be identified as of interest; each has power, significance level, and magnitude considerations; the problems of multiple testing have to be addressed; and drawing conclusions can be problematic, particularly if the comparisons specified to be of interest turn out to be the wrong ones.

4.2 Types of multi-arm trials

The simplest extension of the two-arm trial is to a comparison of K treatments, where no systematic relationships among the treatments exist and all comparisons are of interest. For instance, Southwest Oncology Group study 8203 compared three similar drugs — doxorubicin, mitoxantrone, bisantrene — in advanced breast cancer. None of the arms was hypothesized to be superior, and all three pairwise comparisons were of potential interest in this study.

Sometimes trials are designed with specified relationships hypothesized among the arms. Common examples in this category would be studies designed with order restrictions among the treatment arms, such as arms with increasing doses, or arms with successively added agents. Southwest Oncology Group lung study 8738 (Gandara et al., 1993) is an example of a multi-arm study with ordering — patients were randomized to receive standard-dose cisplatin (CDDP), high-dose CDDP, or high-dose CDDP plus mitomycin C, with survival hypothesized to improve with each addition to therapy.

In studies of a control vs. multiple experimental arms, one of the treatments to be compared is a standard arm or control arm while the remaining arms are promising new treatments. The intent is to determine if any of the new treatments are superior to the control arm. For example, Southwest Oncology Group lymphoma study 8516 compared standard cyclophosphamide, Adriamycin (H), vincristine (O), and prednisone (CHOP) chemotherapy to three regimens that had shown promise in nonrandomized trials: (1) methotrexate, Adriamycin (A), cyclophosphamide, vincristine, prednisone and bleomycin (MACOP-B); (2) low-dose methotrexate, bleomycin, Adriamycin, cyclophosphamide, vincristine and dexamethasone (mBACOD); and (3) prednisone, methotrexate, Adriamycin, cyclophosphamide and etoposide, combined with cytarabine, bleomycin, vincristine and methotrexate (known as ProMACE-CytaBOM); all more toxic and more expensive than CHOP — in stage II non-Hodgkin's lymphoma, to determine if the new generation regimens were superior to CHOP, and, if so, which new regimen was best (Fisher et al., 1993).

One special type of multi-arm trial is the factorial design, in which two or more treatments (possibly at multiple dose levels) are of interest alone or in combination. A factorial design assigns patients to each possible combination of levels of each treatment. Often the aim is to study the effect of levels of each treatment separately by pooling across all other treatments. Study 8300 in limited non-small-cell lung cancer provides a Southwest Oncology Group example for a factorial design (Miller et al., 1998). In this study, the roles of both chemotherapy and prophylactic radiation to the brain were of interest. All patients received radiation to the chest and were randomized to receive prophylactic brain irradiation (PBI) plus chemotherapy vs. PBI vs. chemotherapy vs. no additional treatment. PBI was to be tested by combining across the chemotherapy arms (i.e., all patients with PBI — with or without chemotherapy — were to be compared to all patients without PBI), and chemotherapy was to be tested by combining across PBI arms. Another example is given by the Children's Cancer Group study INT-133 (Meyers et al., 2001) in which children and young adults with osteogeneic sarcoma were given chemotherapy (doxorubicin, cisplatin, and high-dose methotrexate) and were randomized to biologic therapy (muramyl tripeptide (MTP)), more chemotherapy (ifosfamide), neither, or both. The trial was planned as two comparisons, ifosfamide or not, and MTP or not.

Screening designs are related to control vs. multiple experimental designs, but occur earlier in the development of the experimental regimens (see also, randomized Phase II selection designs in Section 3.4). The aim is to choose which treatments to pursue among several new ones, either by choosing the most promising regimens or eliminating the least promising. A control arm may or may not be used in a screening trial, but either way the identified regimens require further testing in future controlled trials. A Southwest Oncology Group example for this type of trial is 8905 (Leichman et al., 1995), which randomized standard 5-fluorouracil (5-FU) and six variations on standard 5-FU in advanced colorectal cancer to decide if any of the variations warranted further study.

Designs with multiple randomizations are related to factorial designs, but one or more interventions occur at later times among those still on study, or among selected subsets of patients. For instance, Southwest Oncology Group study 8600 (Weick et al., 1996) initially randomized patients with acute myelocytic leukemia to standard-dose chemotherapy vs. high-dose chemotherapy; then among standard-dose patients in complete response the study randomized again to standard dose vs. high dose.

To illustrate the issues in designing multi-arm trials, the above SWOG examples will be used, along with a simulation study (Green, 2001) that investigated a four-arm trial of an observation-only group O vs. treatment A vs. treatment B vs. A and B (AB). The simulated trial had 125 patients per arm accrued over 3 years and 3 additional years of follow-up. Survival was exponentially distributed on each arm and median survival was 1.5 years on the control arm. The sample size was sufficient for a 0.05 level test of A vs. not-A to have power 0.9 for a hazard ratio of 1.33 when there was no effect of B.

For those unfamiliar with simulations, these are experiments done on the computer. A set of random numbers is generated by the computer and transformed into random survival and censoring times; these are used as the outcomes of a "study." The transformations are chosen so that the random survival times have a particular distribution, such as the exponential distribution discussed in Chapter 2. More sets of random numbers are then generated to create more studies. Each of these can be analyzed and analysis results summarized in tables. The summaries allow us to assess the methods of analysis we use. For instance, in theory, 0.05-level tests erroneously reject the null hypothesis of no difference in exactly 5% of studies for which there are, in fact, no differences, but in practice this is just an approximation. Generating hundreds of studies allows us to see how good the approximations actually are under specific conditions.

4.3 Significance level

Multi-arm trials give rise to problems due to the inherent desire to test multiple hypotheses. Each test done in a multi-arm trial has an associated significance level. If each test is performed at level α, then there will be a probability greater than α that at least one comparison will be significant when the null hypothesis is true, resulting in an experiment-wise significance level greater than α. If many tests are done, the probability can be much greater than α. For instance, when all 50 tests mentioned in the introduction were done on 1000 simulated four-arm trials with no differences among the arms, there were significant results (at least one test significant at the 0.05 level) not in 5% of the trials, but in 28%. (In 10% of the trials, 11 or more tests were significant!)

A common approach to this problem is to start with a global test (test of equality of all arms), followed by pairwise tests only if the global test is significant. Doing a global test before allowing yourself subset tests helps limit the probability of false positive results. An alternative method is to adjust the level at which each test is performed. For example, if K tests are planned, each test could be done at level α/K. This so-called *Bonferroni correction* results in an experiment-wise level of no more than α.

In other multi-arm settings it is not necessary to adjust for all possible tests. A limited number of tests may be designated before the trial starts as being of primary interest. All other tests are considered exploratory, i.e., used to generate hypotheses to be tested in future studies, not to draw firm conclusions. Statisticians disagree on the issue of whether the primary questions should each be tested at level α, or whether the experiment-wise level across all primary questions should be α. Regardless of one's statistical philosophy, however, it should be kept in mind that if the experiment-wise level (probability of at least one false positive result in the trial) is high, a single positive result from the experiment will be difficult to interpret, and may well be dismissed by others as being inconclusive.

For lung study 8300, investigators chose to design the trial to have level 0.025 for two tests: a test of whether brain RT improved survival and a test of whether chemotherapy improved survival. No other tests were specified. It was assumed that brain RT and chemotherapy would not affect each other. Under these restrictions, the level was at most 0.05 for the experiment.

4.4 Power

For power in pairwise comparisons, the sample size calculations are the same as for a two-arm trial of the selected arms. However, keep in mind that while specified alternative hypotheses for pairwise comparisons may be reasonable, the pattern of alternatives might be implausible. For instance, in a trial of A vs. AB vs. ABC, the power to detect a difference Δ might be specified for both A vs. AB and AB vs. ABC, but 2Δ may be an implausible difference between A and ABC. If in truth the differences between A and AB and between AB and ABC are both $\Delta/2$ (for a plausible difference of Δ between A and ABC), then the trial will have inadequate power to detect either the A vs. AB difference or the AB vs. ABC differences, and the results of the trial are likely to be inconclusive.

Power and sample size considerations for ordered alternatives will depend on the method of analysis being proposed. A global test chosen to be sensitive to ordered differences can be used (Liu and Dahlberg, 1995; Liu, Tsai, and Wolf, 1996). The power in this analysis setting often refers to the power of the global test under a specific alternative. A "bubble sort" approach is also a possibility (Chen and Simon, 1994). In this method treatments are ordered by preference, e.g., A > B > C, in the sense that if survival is the same on all three, then A is the preferred treatment; B is preferred if B and C have the same survival and are better than A, and C is preferred only if it is superior to both A and B with respect to survival (preference may be due to toxicity or cost, for example). The testing is done in stages. C vs. B is tested first; B is eliminated if the test significantly favors C, otherwise C is eliminated. If C is eliminated, B vs. A is tested and B is eliminated if not significantly better than A, otherwise A is eliminated. If B is eliminated after the B vs. C comparison instead, C vs. A is tested, with C eliminated if not found to be significantly superior to A, A eliminated if it is. The treatment of choice is the one remaining. The power with this approach refers to the probability of identifying the correct treatment arm under specific alternatives. The referenced papers have details on how to determine sample size.

If an aim of the study is to combine certain arms and compare the resulting groups (e.g., combine all arms with agent A and compare to the combination of all arms without agent A), then under certain assumptions it is legitimate to calculate power according to the number of patients in the combined groups. The primary assumptions are (1) other factors and treatments are balanced across the groups (e.g., in both A and not-A there should be the same percent of patients receiving B and the same percent of good-risk and poor-risk patients) and (2) the magnitude of the effect of A vs. not-A is the same in the presence or absence of all other treatments in the trial (e.g., if there is a 33% improvement due to A in patients not receiving B, there should also be a 33% improvement due to A in patients who are receiving B). In statistical terms, this latter condition corresponds to "no interaction" (see Section 4.5). Even if both conditions are met, the power for detecting a difference due to A may be decreased if B is effective, due to the decreased number of deaths in patients treated with B. If the usual logrank test (Chapter 2) is used there is additional power loss, which can be substantial. The additional loss is due to the change in shape of survival curves when groups with different distributions are mixed. Logrank tests work best when the proportional hazards assumption is true. Unfortunately, if A vs. B differences are proportional and C vs. D differences are proportional, it does not follow that the difference between a mixture of A and C vs. a mixture of B and D is also proportional — so the logrank test no longer works as well. Use of a stratified logrank test (stratifying on the presence or absence of the other treatments) avoids this additional loss. (See Section 2.4 for a definition of stratified tests.)

The influence on the power to detect an effect of A when B is effective in a trial of O vs. A vs. B vs. AB is illustrated in Table 4.1. The table shows results from the simulation example. If, as is appropriate, a stratified logrank test is used (stratifying on the presence of B for a test of the effect of A), the influence is not large unless B is highly effective. The planned power of 0.9 for a hazard ratio of 1.33 due to A remains above 0.8 even when B is three times as effective as A. When an unstratified logrank test is used (inappropriately), the power decline is worse.

Another potential concern is joint power for both A and B. The power to detect a specified effect of A might be 0.9 and the power to detect a specified effect of B might also be 0.9, but the power to detect effects of both A and B can be considerably lower. The simulation again provides an example. If A and B are both effective with hazard ratios 1.33, the probability that both will be identified is only 0.79.

Table 4.1. Power to detect a hazard ratio of 1.33 due to A.

B Hazard Ratio	1	1.25	1.33	1.5	2	3	4
Power for A, Logrank test, Unstratified	0.92	0.90	0.89	0.88	0.82	0.76	0.70
Power for A, Logrank test, Stratified on B	0.92	0.90	0.90	0.89	0.85	0.83	0.81

4.5 Interaction

The most common analytic strategy used with factorial designs in cancer clinical trials involves collapsing over other factors to test the effect of a given factor. The simplest case is of a 2×2 factorial design, with factor A and factor B, each at two levels, such as in the example above. Collapsing over the presence or absence of B to study A and vice versa seems to be a neat trick — two answers for the price of one — until one considers how to protect against the possibility that the effect of A vs. not-A is *not* the same in the presence or absence of B. If the differences between treatments O and A, and B and AB are the same, then combining O with B and comparing to A combined with AB (using a stratified test) are proper. However, it is generally more plausible to assume A will not behave in the precisely the same way in the presence of B as in the absence of B. This is known as a *treatment interaction*. We know from our experience in the Southwest Oncology Group that such interactions do happen.

A useful way to describe interactions is by the following proportional hazards model (discussed in Chapter 2),

$$\lambda(t, x_1, x_2) = \lambda_0(t) \exp(\alpha x_1 + \beta x_2 + \gamma x_1 x_2),$$

where $x_i = 0$ or 1 depending on the absence or presence of A or B, respectively. Note that interaction in this context is a mathematical property that may or may not have any clinical meaning in the sense of drug interactions. Figure 4.1 shows the survival distributions for the four arms when A is effective treatment (α is negative), B is not effective (β is 0), and there is no interaction (γ is 0). Figures 4.2 and 4.3 illustrate the distributions when A is effective and B is not, but there are interactions. When γ is negative, the AB arm does better than A alone (positive interaction); when it is positive it does worse (negative interaction).

Testing whether there is a significant interaction (testing $\gamma = 0$ in the model) is often not a satisfactory answer. The power to detect interactions is poor, and it is not even clear how to analyze a study when a test for interaction is planned. If there is a plan to test for an interaction, there must also be a plan of how to proceed if the interaction is significant. For instance, if an interaction is significant and indicates that the combination of A and B is not good, then A and B must be tested against O separately. If both are better than O, then the question becomes which of A or B is better. Once other analyses are included in the analysis plan, the simple power calculations

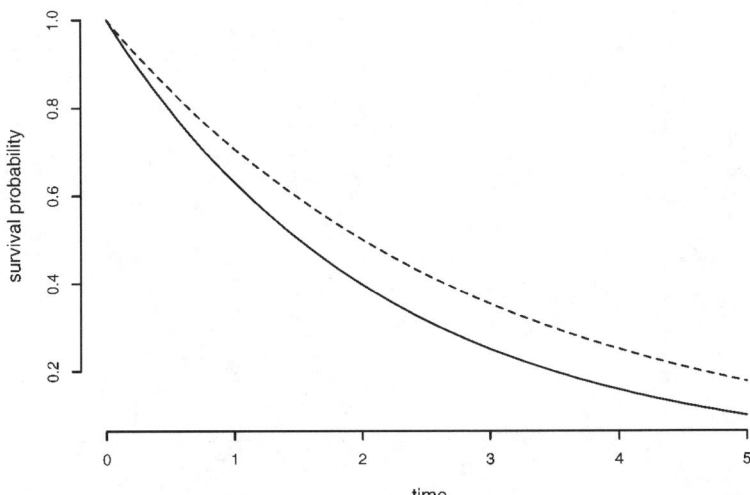

Figure 4.1. Survival distributions for a four-arm trial when A is effective, B is ineffective, and there is no interaction. Solid line represents survival distribution for Arms B and control, dotted line represents Arms A and AB.

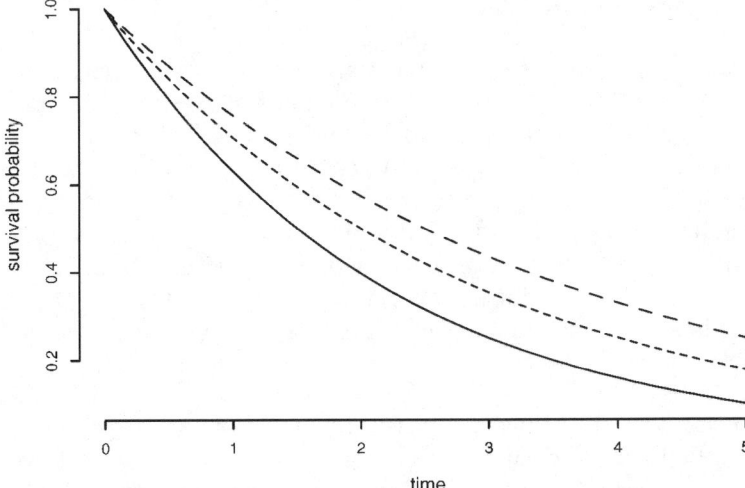

Figure 4.2. Survival distributions for a four-arm trial when A is effective, B is ineffective, and there is a positive interaction. Solid line represents survival distribution for Arms B and control, dotted line represents Arm A, and dashed line represents Arm AB.

for testing A vs. not-A no longer hold. In fact, the properties of the procedure become complex and difficult to calculate.

Possible approaches to analyzing a factorial design might include (1) pretending interactions do not exist and just testing main effects

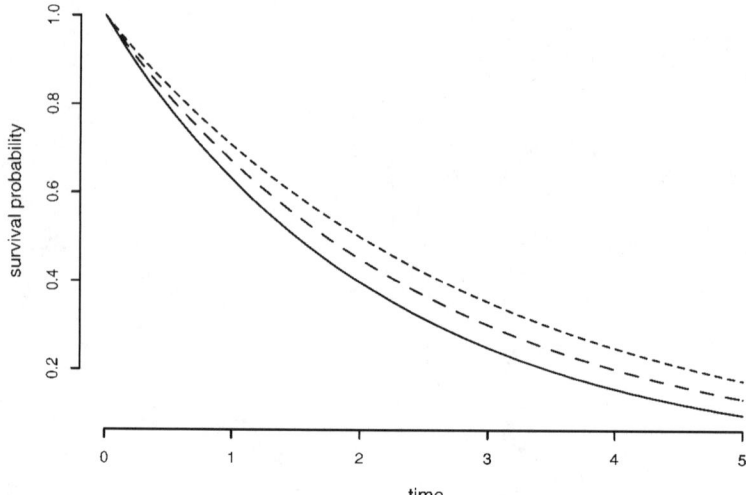

Figure 4.3. Survival distributions for a four-arm trial when A is effective, B is ineffective, and there is a negative interaction. Solid line represents survival distribution for Arms B and control, dotted line represents Arm A, and dashed line represents Arm AB.

(A vs. not-A and B vs. not-B) regardless of results (if both main effects are significant, this leads to a choice of AB), or (2) first doing a global test of the multiple arms and proceeding with other comparisons only if this test is significant, or (3) starting with a test of interaction and proceeding with subset tests if the interaction is significant or main effects if not significant.

These approaches were examined in the simulation study from the point of view of identifying the best treatment arm. The choices for the best arm are: use O, use A, use B, use AB, or use A or B but not AB. Several observations were made.

> First, overall significance levels (probability of not choosing O when all four arms are equal) for approaches 1 and 3 above (just testing main effects, or testing interactions first) are too high (0.11 and 0.13, respectively). Approach 2 (first doing a global test) does restrict the overall level, but this is at the expense of a reduced probability of choosing the correct arm when the four arms are not sufficiently different for the overall test to have high power.

> Second, when there are no interactions, then testing for one is detrimental. The probability of choosing the correct regimen is reduced if approach 3 is used instead of approach 1 when there is no interaction.

Third, if there is an interaction you may or may not be better off testing for it. If the interaction masks effectiveness of the best regimen it is better to test for interaction (e.g., when A is effective, B is ineffective and γ is positive; then the best arm is A, but the improvement due to A appears too small when the arms are combined). If the interaction enhances the effectiveness of the best arm, testing is detrimental (e.g., when A is the best arm and γ is negative; then combining arms improves power, but testing for interaction first will mean arms are combined less often).

Fourth, the power for detecting interactions is poor. Even using 0.1 level tests, the interactions were detected at most 47% of the time in the simulations.

Fifth, all approaches were inadequate for determining the best treatment arm. For each there were plausible clinical scenarios where the probability of choosing the correct arm was less than 0.5 despite the best arm having the desired 33% improvement over the control arm.

Finally, interactions that result in decreased effectiveness can wreck a study if any treatments are effective. The probability of identifying the correct regimen is poor for all methods if γ is positive and the correct arm is not the control arm. Approach 1, assuming there is no interaction, is particularly poor. (The probability is 0 in the case where A and B are both effective but the combination is not, since this approach will lead to choosing A, or to choosing B, or to choosing AB, but not to the choice of use A or B but not AB.)

Interactions and detrimental effects happen; study 8300 (Miller et al., 1998) is an unfortunate example. In this study, PBI was found to be detrimental to patient survival. Although the test for interaction was not significant, the worst arm was PBI plus chemotherapy, followed by PBI, then no additional treatment, then chemotherapy alone. Using the design criteria (test PBI at the 0.025 level combining across chemotherapy assignment, and test chemotherapy at the 0.025 level combining across PBI assignment), one would conclude that neither PBI nor chemotherapy should be used. With this outcome, however, it was clear that the comparison of no further treatment vs. chemotherapy was critical, but the study had seriously inadequate power for this test, and no conclusion could be made concerning chemotherapy.

Another example is Children's Cancer Group INT-133. The trial was planned to test the main effects of biological therapy (MTP) and additional chemotherapy (ifosfamide), and with this analysis MTP is the preferred treatment. However, inspection of all four arms revealed a significant positive interaction, as in Figure 4.2, so that the best arm appears to be the combination of MTP and ifosfamide. This is in fact the authors' stated conclusion, though one not without controversy due to the unplanned comparisons.

If power within subsets of treatments is important for any outcome, then a larger sample size is needed. In fact, to protect fully against the possibility of interaction, *more* than twice the sample size is required — four times as many patients are necessary for testing an interaction as for testing a single main effect (A vs. not-A) of the same magnitude (Peterson and George, 1993). This clearly eliminates what most view as the primary advantage to factorial designs. A theoretical discussion of factorial designs is presented in a paper by Slud (1994).

4.6 Other model assumptions

Any model assumption can result in problems when the assumptions are not correct. As with testing for interactions, testing other assumptions can either be beneficial or detrimental, with no way of ascertaining beforehand which is the case. If assumptions are tested, procedures must be specified to follow when the assumptions are shown not to be met, which changes the properties of the experiment and complicates sample size considerations.

The second SWOG lung example (8738) provides an example where some of the planned analyses were invalidated by other results. The trial was closed approximately halfway through the planned accrual because survival on high-dose CDDP was convincingly shown not to be superior to standard-dose CDDP by the hypothesized 25% (in fact, it appeared to be worse). A beneficial effect of adding mitomycin C to high-dose CDDP could not be ruled out at the time, but this comparison became meaningless in view of the standard-dose vs. high-dose comparison.

4.7 To screen or not to screen

Another design choice that can backfire is choosing a screening design instead of a full-scale trial of control vs. multiple experimental treatments. In certain settings screening trials are reasonable. One such setting is when there are multiple variations of a new regimen being considered for a comparison to a standard and insufficient resources to test all of the variations. Selection designs with survival as the primary endpoint, as described in Section 3.4.2, might be used effectively here. However, in most settings screening trials are probably not reasonable. Fewer patients are needed in a screening trial, but there are few conclusive results from such trials, the probability of error can be large, and a Phase III trial still has to be done when the screening trial is over. For any screening procedure there will be important settings in which it does not work well, unless the sample size is greatly increased.

SWOG trial 8905, with its seven variations on 5-FU in advanced colon cancer, is an example of a screening trial that did not work well. This may have been an appropriate setting for a selection approach as described above; unfortunately, the goals were more ambitious, testing was more complicated, and results were largely inconclusive. The seven arms were: (1) 5-FU intravenous (IV) push (standard treatment), (2) low-dose leucovorin plus 5-FU IV push, (3) high-dose leucovorin plus 5-FU IV push, (4) 28-day continuous infusion 5-FU, (5) leucovorin plus 28-day continuous infusion 5-FU, (6) 5-FU 24-hour infusion, and (7) N-phosphonoacetyl-L-aspartate disodium (PALA) plus 5-FU 24-hour infusion.

The design (described as a phase II-III screening design) called for 80 patients per arm, with comparisons of each of the six variations vs. standard 5-FU, plus comparisons of arms 4 vs. 5 and 6 vs. 7. Each test was to be done at the two-sided 0.05 level, with power 0.67 for each to detect a 50% improvement in survival due to one of the arms. Any of arms 4 to 7 with no responses after the first 20 patients accrued were to be dropped (Phase II part). There was sufficient experience with arms 2 and 3 that a Phase II aspect was not required for these. After the Phase II testing was complete, four interim analyses and a final analysis were planned for each two-way comparison remaining (Phase III part). It was anticipated that a large confirmatory trial would follow using the regimens showing encouraging survival trends.

Various difficulties with the design are evident. The overall level is a problem with so many pairwise 0.05 level tests. If only one of the eight primary comparisons in this trial was significant, it would be difficult to claim that the result was particularly encouraging. The overall power is a problem as well. Suppose there were 50% improvements for 1 vs. 2, 4 vs. 5 and 6 vs. 7. Since these comparisons involve different patients, results are independent (see Chapter 2) and the power to detect all three differences is calculated by multiplying $.67 \times .67 \times .67$, resulting in a power of only 0.3. Another problem is that the design did not specify how early stopping or the final conclusion would be handled if the two-way tests, taken together, were inconclusive (e.g., 7 significantly better than 1, but not significantly better than 6, and 6 not significantly better than 1).

The trial results were inconclusive. No encouraging trends were observed (let alone statistically significant differences). Only arm 7 could fairly clearly be ruled out as ineffective (Leichman et al., 1995). A follow-up study to compare arms 4 and 6 (which did at least have very slightly better survival than the remaining arms) was recently completed, and is undergoing final analysis. Unfortunately, without a standard 5-FU control arm in the new trial, no conclusion regarding improvement over standard therapy will be possible.

SWOG trial 8905 can be contrasted with SWOG trial 8516, a successful full-scale Phase III study of control (CHOP) vs. multiple experimental treatments (MACOP-B, ProMACE-CytaBOM, and mBACOD) in patients with non-Hodgkin's lymphoma. The design of this trial called for 250 patients per arm. All three experimental arms had avid supporters; any small-scale screening trial to choose what to compare to standard CHOP would likely have resulted in long-term controversy. Because a large trial of all of the competitors was done, results were conclusive that the new generation regimens offered little if any improvement over standard CHOP.

4.8 Timing of randomization

Clinical trials with an induction randomization (to get patients into response) and a maintenance randomization (to improve survival after response to induction) are related to factorial designs. If the comparisons of A vs. B for induction therapy and C vs. D for subsequent maintenance therapy are both of interest, a decision has to be made as to when to randomize to C and D. A trial designed with randomization to C and D done at a later time than the one for A vs. B asks a different question from one designed to randomize C and D at the same time as A and B. With respect to C and D, the first asks: "Given patients have completed induction, are still eligible and agree to continue, should C or D be given next?" The second asks: "Which of the planned sequences — A followed by C, A followed by D, B followed by C, or B followed by D — is the best sequence?" (See also, Section 3.5.)

Unless nearly everyone goes on to the maintenance treatment, results using either approach can be difficult to interpret. When randomizations are separated in time, it can be difficult to answer long-term questions about the first randomization. Problems of potential treatment interactions (as for factorial designs but starting later in time) are compounded by patient selection biases related to how different the patients from A and B are who make it to the second randomization. For the same reasons, if A is found to be better than B and C better than D, it cannot necessarily be concluded that A followed by C is the optimal sequence. For instance, if D is highly effective after both A and B, and more A patients agree to randomization, then the long-term comparison of A vs. B will be biased in favor of A. Or, if A is a better therapy (patients survive longer on A alone than B alone and more patients make it to randomization), but patients induced with B do better on D, the interaction plus the excess of A patients at the second randomization could result in the conclusion that A followed by C is superior, even though B followed by D might be the best sequence.

If both randomizations are done up front, then noncompliance can be a major problem — if patients do not get C or D as assigned, they must still be analyzed according to the assignment. For instance, if there are many refusers and more good-risk patients refuse to go through with C while more poor-risk patients refuse D, then any differences observed between C and D will be due both to treatment and to the type of patient who chooses to comply with treatment. Although it is still a valid test of the planned sequence, it can be very difficult to interpret. Comparing only those who get the assigned treatment is not valid. Baseline characteristics are balanced only at the time of the initial randomization; if patients are omitted later based on outcome (compliance is an outcome), all benefits of randomization are lost. If the patients who got D were good-risk patients and those who got C were poor risk, D is going to look good regardless of effectiveness. (See also Chapter 8.)

The SWOG leukemia committee addressed these difficulties in study 8600 by specifying separate randomizations for induction and consolidation, a short-term endpoint for the induction treatment (complete response (CR)) and a long-term endpoint for maintenance (survival). The objectives of the study (comparing high, and low-dose chemotherapy with respect to induction of CR, and testing whether maintenance therapy with high-dose chemotherapy improves survival of patients in CR) can be achieved by the design. Long-term comparisons of induction and sequence questions, although of interest, are not listed as objectives, as they cannot be addressed adequately by the design.

In Children's Cancer Group study INT-133 the patients were randomized to the four arms up front, even though one of the interventions (MTP) did not start for 12 weeks. There was only a 3% dropout by 12 weeks, and patients were analyzed as randomized.

Myeloma study 8229 (Salmon et al., 1990) had objectives difficult to address in a single design. Comparisons with respect to long-term endpoints of both induction therapies and maintenance therapies were specified. Both randomizations were done prior to induction therapy. Of approximately 600 patients randomized to induction, only 180 went on to more than 75% remission and their randomized maintenance assignments, 100 to vincristine, melphalan, cyclophosphamide and prednisone (VMCP) and 80 to sequential hemi-body RT plus vincristine and prednisone (VP). By the design, VMCP and RT should have been compared using all 600 patients according to their assigned arms, but with 420 patients not receiving the assignments, this would have been uninterpretable. The 100 VMCP patients were compared to the 80 RT patients, but due to all the possible selection biases, this analysis also could not be interpreted adequately.

4.9 Conclusion

The main points of the chapter can be summarized as follows.

First, when there are more than two treatment arms, many questions are asked and many tests are done. Multiple tests mean multiple opportunities for errors. Limiting the probability of error when a large number of errors is possible requires a large number of patients.

Second, power calculations depend on model assumptions. More arms require more assumptions. If the assumptions are wrong, the calculations are in error, and the trial may not have adequate power to answer anything of interest. Unfortunately, assumptions are often wrong. Thus, the more arms, the higher the likelihood that the trial will provide no answers.

Third, interactions are common. In fact, it seems plausible that A does *not* work the same way in the presence of B as in the absence of B for most treatments B. When there are interactions, the ability to identify the best treatment arm from a factorial design can be severely compromised. There is a school of thought, led by some statisticians, that advocates the use of factorial designs on the grounds that they deliver something for nothing (two for the price of one in the case of the 2 × 2 factorial). In our opinion this is tantamount to selling snake oil. Factorial designs were developed in agriculture and were heavily used in industrial settings when several factors at several levels must be considered with a limited number of experimental units (often no more than two per group) in a short amount of time (and never with censoring). In this setting, highly structured (factorial or fractional factorial) designs provide the only hope of getting any answers at all. The medical setting could hardly be more different.

For the best chance of a straightforward conclusion at the end of a study, use a straightforward design. A series of two-arm trials will not ask many questions, but will provide answers to most of them (if sample sizes are adequate); a series of multi-arm trials of the same total sample sizes will ask many questions, but can easily result in clear answers to none. If accrual is slower than expected, a two-arm trial might succeed in answering one question while a multi-arm trial may answer none.

If there are compelling reasons to consider multi-arm trials, keep in mind the potential problems due to multiple testing, interactions, other incorrect assumptions and noncompliance. Make sure the objectives can be accomplished by the design. Consider what might be salvageable from the study if the assumptions are wrong. Allow room for error by increasing the sample size over that required for the simplest assumptions — this could make the difference between a wasted effort and a surprising result.

CHAPTER 5

Interim Analysis and Data Monitoring Committees

The trouble with people is not that they don't know but that they know so much that ain't so.

–Josh Billings (pseudonym for **Henry Wheeler Shaw**)

5.1 Planned interim analyses

Suppose you are conducting a trial of standard fractionation RT vs. hyperfractionated RT in lung cancer and the data are looking interesting halfway through the trial. You decide to do a test and find the logrank test of survival has p-value 0.05. Is it legitimate to stop the trial at this point and conclude that hyperfractionation is superior to standard fractionation?

The answer is no. As explained in Chapter 2, if the difference between two treatment arms is tested at the end of the trial at the 0.05 level, the chance of concluding they are different when, in fact they are not, is 5%. If this same trial is tested halfway through, by plan, as well as at the end, the chance at the half way point is also 5%. But if you consider the chance of concluding that there is a difference at either time, then the chance is greater than 5%. (If the first analysis is done not by plan but just because the results look interesting, then the overall chance of concluding that there is a difference at either time is much greater than 5%.)

Analysis of data during the conduct of a trial is called an *interim analysis*. Interim analyses are dictated by the ethical imperative that a study be stopped if there are dramatic results in favor of one treatment over another. However, frequent analysis of the data can seriously compromise the trial. Only well-planned interim analyses allow appropriate monitoring while maintaining the integrity of the trial design.

To illustrate the effect of interim analyses, a computer simulation of 100 two-arm trials designed to have a final analysis at year 4 and an interim analysis at year 2 was performed. In all 100 trials, the results on the treatment arms were generated from the identical distribution. Five of the simulated studies had differences significant at the 0.05 level at year four, and five had significant differences at year 2 (Fleming, Green, and Harrington, 1984). This is what was expected according to the definition of level 0.05. (And no, there was no cheating. It did indeed come out with exactly the expected number of differences!) The interesting point of this simulation was that none of the studies significant at the 2-year analysis were the same as the studies significant at 4 years. Thus, of the 100 studies, a total of 10 showed significant differences despite no true difference between the treatment arms, yielding an overall Type I error of 10%, not 5%. The 2-year p-values for the studies with apparently significant differences at 2 years were 0.02 in three cases and 0.01 in two; by year 4 these had increased to 0.83, 0.53, 0.13, 0.21, and 0.17. The simulation illustrates both that many early positive results will become negative with further follow-up if there are no true differences, and that the Type I error rate with multiple tests is high. If you test twice, you are going to make a mistake almost 10% of the time instead of 5%; if more testing is done, the chance is even higher, up to as much as 25% when testing is done frequently.

Figure 5.1 shows a real example of a trial from the Southwest Oncology Group inappropriately closed early. Figure 5.1a shows how the study looked at the time the apparently inferior arm was dropped. There appeared to be a striking benefit to treatment arm A in the good-risk subset of patients. This was based on only a few patients and very short follow-up. Further follow-up saw additional deaths in the good-risk arm A patients, and even further follow-up showed that no long-term survivors were in the group. Figure 5.1b shows current results. Differences are no longer of interest. The example illustrates that the patterns of early data can be deceptive.

There are other similarly sobering examples from the literature. The European Organization for the Treatment of Cancer (EORTC) published a case study of the problems created by the lack of stopping guidelines in a 2 × 2 factorial trial of the addition of chemotherapy (cyclophophamide, methotrexate, and 5-FU (CMF)) and/or hormonal therapy to radiotherapy in patients with early breast cancer (Sylvester, Bartelink, and Rubens, 1994). Despite the lack of a formal plan, ten formal analyses were done at the statistical center, six during the accrual period to the trial. Beginning with the second analysis the results were shared with the study coordinator,

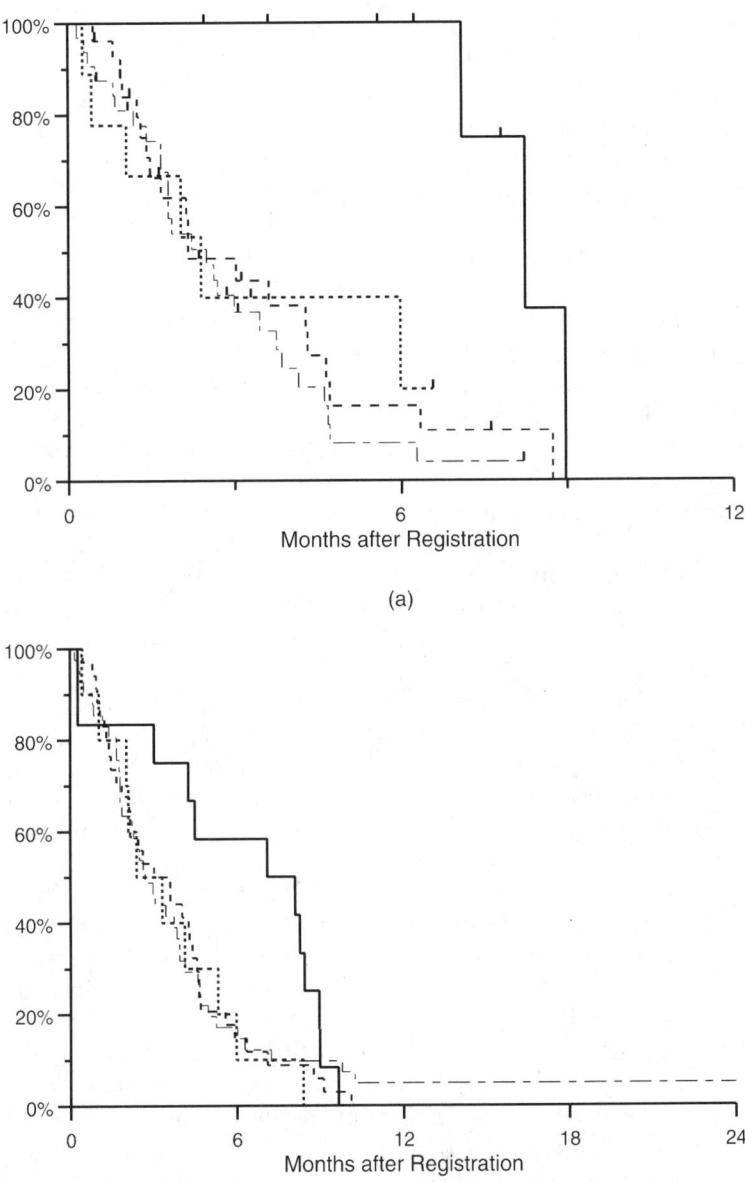

Figure 5.1. A trial inappropriately closed early: (a) interim analysis; (b) final analysis. Solid line represents good risk patients on Treatment A; short dashed line represents good risk patients on Treatment B; intermittent dashed line represents poor risk patients on Treatment A; heavy dashed line represents poor risk patients on Treatment B. (From Green, S., Fleming, T., and O'Fallon, J., *Journal of Clinical Oncology*, 5:1477–1484, 1987. With permission.)

and beginning with the third, with a larger group of investigators involved with the trial. Accrual began to slow, as it apeared that CMF was effective, and the trial was closed. By the time of publication, however, there was no longer a significant effect of chemotherapy on survival. As a result of these and other similar experiences the EORTC now has formal stopping guidelines in their protocols, and a system of data monitoring similar to that described below for the Southwest Oncology Group.

The effects of premature analysis and publication in the absence of a formal monitoring plan plague the interpretation of a recent study in esophageal cancer. This study of pre-operative chemotherapy (with 5-FU and cisplatin) and radiotherapy vs. surgery alone (Walsh et al., 1996) was planned for 190 patients to have 80% power to detect a difference of 20% in 2-year survival probabilities. The publication states, "Early indications of a clinically relevant difference between treatments suggested that an interim analysis should be undertaken. The trial was closed 6 years after it began because a statistically significant difference between the groups was found." The final accrual was 113 patients. Not surprisingly, many find these results unconvincing, but it has proved difficult to mount a confirmatory trial.

The statistical solution to the interim testing problem is to use designs that allow for early stopping but that still result in a 0.05 overall probability of a false positive conclusion. One way to accomplish this is to use designs that limit the number of times the data are tested, and that are very conservative when interim tests are done. Instead of stopping a trial whenever a p-value is 0.05, stop only when p-values are considerably below 0.05 at a few prespecified times (Haybittle, 1971). Southwest Oncology Group standards for stopping trials early are to use one to three interim analyses with small and approximately equal probabilities of stopping at each interim time (Crowley, Green, Liu et al. 1994). Sample designs are shown in Table 5.1. For instance, the first row in the table specifies a design with one planned interim analysis. For this design the study would be stopped early if the difference were significant at the 0.01 level. Otherwise the study would be continued to completion, and the final analysis done at the 0.045 level to adjust for the fact that one analysis had already been done. The overall level for this design, and for all of the designs in the table, is approximately 0.05.

In addition, we stop trials early not only when we have highly significant positive results, but also when we have highly significant negative results (done by testing the alternative as a null hypothesis, as suggested at the end of Section 3.5.3). If there is convincing

Table 5.1. Sample designs with an overall significance level of 0.05, using up to three interim analyses.

Interim Level 1	Interim Level 2	Interim Level 3	Final Level
0.01			0.045
0.005	0.005		0.045
0.01	0.015		0.04
0.005	0.005	0.005	0.045
0.005	0.01	0.01	0.04

evidence early on that an experimental regimen is not going to be useful, then the trial should be stopped, particularly if the experimental regimen is more toxic. We do not believe it is necessary to prove a more toxic experimental regimen is actually more lethal than standard treatment before deciding it should not be pursued, only that it is unlikely to have the hoped for benefit. This is the clearest example we know of the virtue of one-sided (asymmetric) testing. A two-sided approach would stop only if the new treatment were significantly worse; a one-sided approach would lead to an earlier end based on the new treatment not being better.

Generally, interim analyses should be planned after intervals during which a reasonable number of events are expected to occur. (If nothing is going to happen between analyses, there is no point in planning a test.) It is not necessary to have precisely equal numbers of events between analyses, as is sometimes stated, however. If the specified interim levels are used after times of not-quite-equal information, the final level needed to achieve an overall 0.05 level can be calculated at the end of the study. Most of the time recalculation will not be necessary, though, as the final level needed to achieve an overall level of 0.05 is quite insensitive to deviations in the timing of analysis (Crowley et al., 1994). Other analysis implications for trials with interim analyses are discussed in Chapter 7.

Other designs for interim testing include a "spending function" approach (Lan and DeMets, 1983) and a conditional power or stochastic curtailment approach (Anderson, 1987; Lan, Simon, and Halperin, 1982; Spiegelhalter, Freedman, and Blackburn, 1986). The first approach provides a way to determine what the interim testing levels should be without prespecifying the testing times: the level is equal to the area under the curve between two points of a specified function for which the total area under the curve is 0.05. The horizontal axis is the amount of information accrued over time (not time itself) and the two points are (1) the amount of information at the last analysis and (2) the amount of information at the current analysis. Problems with this approach include needing an estimate of what the total information at the end of the trial will be and the numerous approximations needed to arrive at the interim level. To us this seems an overly precise and complicated answer to the question.

The second approach allows early stopping when the probability of a significant result (given the current results) becomes small. When it starts to become clear that a trial is not going to result in a significant difference, it is tempting to cut it short and go on to the next concept. However, since we believe that convincingly negative results are just as important as convincingly positive results, we do not recommend this approach. Unfortunately, as for large p-values, "is not going to be significant" is also not equivalent to proving equality (Section 3.5.3).

The concept of "not becoming significant" can be translated statistically as "conditional power is poor" (i.e., the power to detect a difference is poor given the results so far). Suppose in our example in Section 3.5.3 that the trial had been stopped after 100 patients per arm had been accrued. Table 5.2 shows the conditional power for various outcomes if the total planned sample size is 160 per arm, along with the 95% confidence interval for the observed difference. Despite very poor conditional power when the observed difference is 0.05 or under, the confidence interval only excludes the hypothesized difference of 0.15 when the observed response probability is nearly identical. If the reported difference in response probabilities exceeds 0.03, it is not possible to make a definitive recommendation concerning therapy. The results are consistent either with arm A being better, or with either arm being acceptable. The trial at this point is equivocal, particularly if arm B is less toxic.

Table 5.2. Conditional power (probability of rejecting the null hypothesis of equality) under the alternative hypotheses (1) arm A superior with respect to response probability by 0.15 or (2) arm B superior with respect to response probability by 0.15 are true. Assume 100 per arm were accrued out of a total of 160 per arm planned for the trial.

N per Arm	Arm A, Arm B Response Estimates	Conditional Power (Arm A by .15)	Conditional Power (Arm B by .15)	95% Confidence Interval
100 of 160	0.25, 0.25	0.08	0.08	$(-0.12, 0.12)$
100 of 160	0.25, 0.22	0.21	0.02	$(-0.09, 0.15)$
100 of 160	0.25, 0.20	0.34	0.01	$(-0.07, 0.17)$
100 of 160	0.25, 0.15	0.73	0.00	$(-0.01, 0.21)$

5.1.1 Caveats

No method of interim analysis works if an extra analysis is done because results look interesting. "Looks interesting/does not look interesting" amounts to an interim analysis in itself. If this is done repeatedly with the possibility of a formal test each time (whether or not the test is done), the number of interim analyses becomes far greater than the number specified in the design. All of the careful probability calculations used to specify multi-stage designs are based on the assumption that analysis time is independent of outcome.

Another word of advice is to base the interim analyses on the longest term primary outcome. Early closure based on a short-term endpoint will leave you with insufficient power to test the longer-term endpoints and may result in an equivocal conclusion (see also Section 8.6 on surrogate endpoints).

5.2 Data monitoring committees: Rationale and responsibilities

Specifying a design with planned interim analyses is only a partial solution to the problem of inappropriate early stopping discussed above. Studies with stopping rules can still be ended early through the mechanism of investigators deciding not to enroll any more patients on trial. Despite appropriate stopping guidelines, if investigators are shown early results they might decide not to participate any more for a variety of reasons. If trends are emerging, the current best arm might be considered preferable to randomization; if current results are similar, the less toxic arm might be preferred; if subset results are striking, only selected patients might be entered; or if results look generally poor on both arms, the investigators might use different treatments altogether. This sort of informal study closure can be avoided by not presenting interim results to investigators, and having the necessary study monitoring performed by a data monitoring committee that has confidential access to results.

We have some evidence that informal and inappropriate stopping does occur when results are routinely reported, and that use of a data monitoring committee minimizes such problems. Prior to 1985, Southwest Oncology Group trials were conducted without formal stopping guidelines or monitoring committees. Results of each ongoing trial were reported frequently, both at the semi-annual Group meetings and at national oncology meetings. Studies were closed by the vote of investigators active in the disease committee. We

Table 5.3. Accrual during successive 6-month intervals for two trials.

Interval	1	2	3	4	5	6	7	8
SWOG trial	52	36	26	16				
NCCTG trial	24	15	20	21	15	29	25	24

examined 14 of our trials conducted under these circumstances, and compared them to 14 trials matched on disease site from the North Central Cancer Treatment Group which did have a monitoring committee policy (Green, Fleming, and O'Fallon, 1987). A variety of problems were discovered in the Southwest Oncology Group trials. Declining accrual occurred in five; two were inappropriately closed early; three studies were reported early as positive, but final results were not as convincing. Two trials did not even have set accrual goals. In contrast, NCCTG experienced minimal problems in the conduct of its trials. An accrual example from our investigation (the same study as in Figure 5.1) is shown in Table 5.3. SWOG accrual declined precipitously from 52 in the first 6-month interval to 16 in the final interval, due to what appeared to be convincing results (Figure 5.1a). The study was closed early. After further follow-up results were no longer convincing (Figure 5.1b). The matching study in NCCTG accrued steadily at about 20 per 6-month interval. Accrual on this study was completed and the final results were conclusive.

Of course we have to admit that since this comparison was not randomized, differences between the Groups other than the monitoring committee approach could account for the problems noted in the SWOG studies. Still, the comparison is interesting.

The statistical difficulty discussed is just one of the critical aspects of study monitoring. The most important monitoring function is protection of patients from harm. It is also the most difficult, since most of the ethical ambiguities of clinical trials arise from this principle. How much evidence is required before it becomes unethical to treat with a possibly less effective or more toxic regimen? Much has been written on the subject (Byar et al., 1976; Gilbert, McPeek, and Mosteller, 1977; Mackillop and Johnston, 1986; Hellman and Hellman, 1991; Passamani, 1991). These and other essays may make clear what some of the ethical questions are, but answers remain elusive. We offer just a couple of comments. First, there is no gold-standard statistical cutoff for a single endpoint that determines when results become convincing. Results of a study with 200 patients are not appreciably different when the last patient is omitted. A study with p-value 0.005 is barely more convincing than one with 0.0051. Stopping rules for a primary endpoint do not cover situations when unexpected or highly significant results emerge in secondary endpoints. The best statistics can do is provide guidelines that limit the number of mistaken conclusions. Second, it is important to consider both potential harm to patients on the study and potential harm to all future patients at risk for getting the treatments studied. Yes, the next patient on a trial with a trend is at risk for receiving the currently inferior arm. On the other hand, if the trend is false, it is not just the next patient registered at risk for the inferior arm, it is all future patients treated according to the published incorrect conclusion. The difficulty is particularly acute in oncology since relatively few new agents and regimens are found to be improvements — which means that a high percentage of early positive trends will, in fact, be false positives. Only additional accrual can clarify whether emerging differences are real or not.

Deciding when there is sufficient evidence of harm to stop all or part of a trial can be painfully difficult. It is at least reasonable to expect that a small group committed to careful review of all aspects of a trial will make better decisions than large groups acting informally based on impressions of the data.

While there is general agreement that the primary responsibilities of a data monitoring committee are participant safety and study integrity, there is less agreement on the specific responsibilities. For instance, the majority of cancer cooperative groups agree that data monitoring committees do not review or approve the study design or evaluate the performance of individual study centers (George, 1993), but both of these functions have been common in data monitoring committees of trials sponsored by the National Eye Institute (Hawkins, 1991). In some sense every aspect of study conduct affects safety and integrity. The number of oversight responsibilities assigned to a data monitoring committee will depend on what other resources and structures are available to the investigators (e.g., steering committee, operations office, statistical center, advisory board, sponsoring institution).

Even the specifics of the most basic task of the data monitoring committee, evaluation of interim results for evidence of benefit or harm, are not necessarily obvious. Questions (and our personal answers) include:

- How often should the data monitoring committee review interim data? (The answer to this should depend on how fast additional information becomes available on a trial. We generally recommend monitoring advanced disease studies, or any other study with rapidly accumulating events, every 6 months. Yearly monitoring may be sufficient for adjuvant or slowly accruing studies.)

- Should the primary outcome data be reviewed each time or should they be reviewed only at times of planned interim analyses? (All data, including primary outcome data, should be reviewed each time, since the unexpected does occur.)
- Should treatment arms be blinded to the data monitoring committee or not? (Definitely not. If A looks better than B, the decision to continue could well be different if A is the control arm instead of the experimental arm.)
- Should a data monitoring committee decision that evidence is sufficient to close a trial be final, or should it be advisory only? (We would say advisory, but rarely overturned.)
- If advisory, advisory to whom — the funding agency? an executive group? the investigators? (Reports should go to the individuals with ultimate responsibility for the integrity of the trial.)
- Should a data monitoring committee be able to make major design changes to a trial? (No, the data monitoring committee may offer suggestions but design is the responsibility of the principal investigators. On the other hand, major design changes initiated by the principal investigators should be approved by the data monitoring committee.)
- Are a data monitoring committee's duties over when study accrual is complete, or should the data monitoring committee also decide when results are to be reported? (It should also decide when results are to be reported. Additional follow-up generates additional data that still need to be monitored.)
- How much weight should be accorded to outside information vs. current information on the study being monitored? (Definitive outside information cannot be ignored, but this begs the question of what is definitive. A single trial of moderate size probably is not definitive; two large trials probably are; a meta-analysis probably is not; see Chapter 9.)
- How much should results of secondary endpoints influence the decision to continue or not? (Not much unless toxic death is considered secondary.)
- How scary do results have to be to stop at a time other than a planned interim analysis? (Very scary, or the purpose of interim analyses is defeated.)
- When do accrual problems justify early closure? (When results will not be available until after they are no longer of interest.)
- Should confidential information ever be provided to other data monitoring committees or planning groups? (Sometimes. If study conduct will not be compromised by limited release of information, it might be reasonable to let investigators planning

new trials know of potential problems or benefits to treatment arms they are considering. Risk to the ongoing trial includes leaked information or intelligent guesses as to the current status; risk to the new trial includes choosing an inappropriate arm based on early results that do not hold up.)

Every monitoring committee functions differently because no one has the same ethical, scientific, or practical perspectives. This means different committees might well come up with different answers to the same monitoring issues. To ensure some balance of opinions, it is best to have a variety of knowledgeable people as members of the committee.

5.3 Monitoring committees: Composition

We have suggested what is needed on a committee: variety, knowledge, and balance of opinion. To assure variety and knowledge, at least one person on the committee should thoroughly understand the biologic rationale for the trial, know the clinical experience for the regimens being used, understand the statistical properties of the design, know the operational constraints on the trial, have a broad understanding of important questions and ongoing research in the disease being studied, and have the study patients as the major focus of concern. Extremes of opinion will unbalance a committee as a whole, and either lean it toward extreme decisions or make it impossible to reach decisions at all. In particular, all members of a data monitoring committee must at least believe it is ethical to start accrual to the trial, and no one should be in a position of having a strong vested interest in the outcome.

Vested interest is a particularly troublesome concept. How it is defined and the degree to which it is tolerated have shifted significantly in the last decade. Complete independence has lately been proposed as the only valid model for monitoring committees (Walters, 1993; Fleming, 1992). Independence means, in part, that no one on the committee has a major financial interest in the trial. We agree (although the definition of major is unclear). It is also being construed to mean that no one has an academic interest in the trial either (for instance, an early report of a positive result could enhance a career or reputation). Here we are in less agreement. Unfortunately, this interpretation of independence tends to bar from the committee those responsible for the science and the conduct of the trial, and this directly conflicts with the knowledge requirement. The people who know the most about the justification, background, conduct, etc. of a trial are the ones running it. The next most knowledgeable people are the ones running competing trials, also often viewed as a conflict. Finding thousands of knowledgeable people with no academic conflicts for the hundreds of randomized cancer trials going on all the time is a daunting prospect.

Many also believe that no investigators who are entering patients on a trial should be on the data monitoring committee (DeMets et al., 1995). However, the case can be made that it is only such investigators who can really appreciate and grapple with the tension between the rights of patients on the trial and the benefits to future patients that might accrue (Harrington et al., 1994).

Certainly there are cases for which any appearance of possible conflict of interest would severely compromise a study. Highly visible and controversial trials must be protected from the appearance of bias or the results will not be accepted. Such high profile trials will likely motivate data monitoring committee members to keep themselves well informed and to participate actively. On the other hand, low profile and noncontroversial trials with only modest potential impact (most cancer treatment trials qualify) do not generate enough interest for appearance of conflict to be of great concern. They also do not generate enough interest to inspire independent monitors to spend a lot of time on them.

We now have had over 15 years of experience with data monitoring committees in SWOG. The evolution of these committees is instructive. The Board of Governors of the Southwest Oncology Group first voted to establish a monitoring committee policy in July 1985, after various presentations and lengthy discussions with Group members. The suggestion that reporting could be detrimental generated a lot of debate, with objections centering on ethical issues. Some clinicians felt it was their individual responsibility to judge whether interim evidence warranted their continued participation in the trial. It was not clear to them that the committee would have sufficient first-hand information to make decisions in the best interests of the patients. There was also concern that interest in participation would decline if results were not provided, with a corresponding decrease in accrual and meeting attendance.

Ultimately the Group agreed that all Phase III studies should have monitoring committees and that explicit early stopping/reporting guidelines should be included in all Phase III study designs. Interim response and survival results were provided only to data monitoring committee members, and it was this committee that decided when the study should be closed and reported. Membership for this first generation of monitoring committees included, for each study, the study statistician and the study coordinator, the study discipline coordinators if any, the disease committee chair, the Group Chair and Group Statistician, a member of the Group who was not directly involved in the study, and an NCI representative.

Every 6 months an evaluation was prepared by the statistician, study coordinator, and disease committee chair and distributed to committee members before the semi-annual group meetings, along with recommendations on whether to close the study and whether to report the results. Committees were not to recommend early closure at times other than planned interim analyses unless factors such as poor accrual, unacceptable toxicity, or information from other studies made it necessary. Monitoring committee members indicated any disagreement by mail. Problems were resolved by conference calls or, if necessary, at a meeting scheduled for the semi-annual group meeting. If disagreement persisted, the Group Chair would make the final decision.

Our experience with this model for monitoring committees was positive. Of the first 13 randomized trials opened and completed after the monitoring policy was established (Green and Crowley, 1993), all 13 trials had specific accrual goals and early stopping and reporting guidelines. Only 10 formal meetings had to be convened at Group meetings for all of these. In all cases where a decision was necessary, a consensus was reached. Accrual patterns were fairly stable after initial increases. Accrual was appropriately terminated early for three trials. Four other trials completed accrual but were reported early due to definitive results at interim analyses. No study had misleading early results reported. It appeared that the major problems identified concerning study conduct in old Group studies had largely been resolved and appropriate early decisions were being made.

Of course we did not always get it completely right. Certain omissions in the initial policy attempt were identified and addressed. For instance, on studies coordinated by SWOG but involving several other cooperative groups (intergroup studies), representatives from the other participating groups were added due to some early communication problems. It became clear that each group needed reassurance from one of its own members that continued participation on a trial was justified. Drug company representatives, on the other hand, were specifically excluded from monitoring committees after an initial unsatisfactory experience. While the knowledge of such individuals may be great, the conflict of interest considerations are greater. ("The last priority [in the conduct of trials] ... is to make a profit and to pay dividends to shareholders" (Rockhold and Enas, 1993).) We also found it necessary to add specific language concerning member conduct. After two breaches, a strongly worded paragraph on confidentiality was added to the policy:

> Premature disclosure of confidential data monitoring committee interim therapeutic results by a member of the data monitoring committee will result in censure of that member by the Board of Governors. Censure options include loss of authorship in the study presentation and publication, decertification of status as a current and future study coordinator and/or removal from the leadership in the disease committee of record.

With only an occasional exception (noted in the examples below) monitoring for subsequent trials using the modified policy proceeded smoothly. But times change. Highly political AIDS research (Ellenberg, Finkelstein, and Schoenfeld, 1992), and fraudulent data and monitoring mismanagement discovered in high-profile breast cancer trials (Altaman, 1994; Goldberg and Goldberg, 1994; Christian et al., 1995) focused a lot of attention on clinical trials and how they are monitored. In 1992 NCI mandated changes to the Group monitoring committee structures to

> ...ensure that DMCs for NCI sponsored phase III therapeutic trials are operative, independent of trial investigators and clearly free of conflict of interest. Because clinical trials are under increasing public scrutiny, we must use procedures that protect our research against the appearance of impropriety. If we do not do this, then our excellent system for determining what treatments work and do not work may be threatened. (Simon and Ungerleider, 1992.)

It was recognized that creating committees for all 175 randomized trials sponsored by the NCI would not be practical. Thus each group was instructed to create a single committee to oversee all Phase III trials coordinated by the group. The initial membership requirements included the Group Chair and Group Statistician, but was otherwise left fairly open (Simon, 1994). Not long after it was decided this was not sufficiently independent. Since nearly all members of the first committee designated under this model were Group leaders, the appearance of conflict (Group vs. patient interests) remained. A subsequent version of the requirements explicitly excluded the Group Chair from the committee and required that the data monitoring committee chair be perceived as not representing the interests of the Group. Experience with this model was also not entirely satisfactory.

The drift away from highly knowledgeable members was too great and committee decisions were overturned.

The current iteration still excludes the Group Chair from the committee but does allow a different Group leader to be chair. The Membership and Responsibilities part of SWOG policy now states:

> A single Data and Safety Monitoring Committee (DSMC) will be established to monitor all Southwest Oncology Group phase III therapeutic trials. The DSMC will be appointed for three year terms (renewable once) by the Group Chair, with the approval of the Cancer Therapy Evaluation Program (CTEP) of the National Cancer Institute (NCI), and will include members both from within the Group and from outside the Group. A majority of the DSMC will be outside members, and at least one outside member will be a patient advocate and at least one will be a statistician. The Group Statistician and two representatives of CTEP will be non-voting members. The Group Chair may not be on the DSMC.
>
> Each of these trials will also have a Study Committee, composed of the study coordinator, study statistician, any discipline coordinators, and the disease committee chair. The Study Committee for Intergroup trials will also have a representative from each of the participating Groups.
>
> The Data and Safety Monitoring Committee will be responsible for reviewing interim analyses of data prepared by the study statistician and for recommending whether the study needs to be changed or terminated based on these analyses. The DSMC will also determine when the results of the study should be published or otherwise released to the public. The DSMC will also review any major modifications to the study proposed by the Study Committee (e.g. dropping an arm based on toxicity or reports of other trials, or changing the accrual goals). The Study Committee will be responsible for monitoring the data from the study for toxicity, feasibility, and accrual. This committee will also be responsible for initiating minor changes in the study such as clarifications and eligibility refinements, and may request that the DSMC initiate major changes as discussed above.

The new model does address concerns about potential scientific conflict of interest or misconduct by the Group leadership or by individual study chairs. With the creation of study committees, there is still ongoing careful monitoring for toxicity and procedural problems. We have some concern, however, that a monitoring committee formulated this way will not have the time, nor sufficient knowledge about each individual study and its larger scientific context, to be able to make adequately informed decisions on all 25+ studies being monitored. Furthermore, the information the committee receives comes from a single individual involved in the trial (the study statistician) instead of from several. Much as we would like to believe ourselves free of bias, the potential for conflict of interest (or even just mistakes) is clear.

5.4 Examples

We conclude this chapter with several examples of monitoring committees in action. The following studies illustrate some of the circumstances under which trials are terminated early and some of the factors monitoring committees consider in their deliberations.

5.4.1 Stopping early for positive results

SWOG 8795 (Lamm et al., 1995) was a randomized trial of intravesical Bacillus Calmette-Guerin (BCG) vs. mitomycin C in the treatment of superficial bladder cancer. Recent comparisons of BCG with other intravesical agents (thiotepa, doxorubicin) had demonstrated superiority of BCG. Previous randomized trials had failed to show mitomycin C was an improvement over thiotepa or doxorubicin, but other (small) trials had failed to show BCG an improvement over mitomycin C. Since mitomycin C had the highest estimated complete response probability of chemotherapeutic agents studied in early bladder cancer, a trial of BCG immunotherapy vs. mitomycin C was felt by most members of the genitourinary committee to be justified. The primary endpoint in this study was disease-free survival in the subset of patients with resected T_a or T_1 transitional cell disease with no carcinoma-in-situ. The design called for 663 patients in order to have power 0.9 to detect a 35% improvement due to either arm (i.e., hazard ratio of 1.35 or $1/1.35 = 0.74$). Stopping guidelines called for interim analyses after $1/4$, $1/2$, and $3/4$ of the expected information at two-sided levels 0.005, 0.01, and 0.01 levels, with the final analysis to be done at the 0.045 level, using the logrank test.

At the first interim analysis, the logrank p-value was 0.001 (Figure 5.2a) in favor of BCG. Toxicity on BCG was more frequent and severe than on mitomycin C (28 vs. 39% with no toxicity and 31 vs. 16% with grade 2–3), but there were no grade 4 toxicities. This is the one study where a consensus on closure was not reached and the final decision had to be made by the Group leadership. Arguments against stopping included (1) recurrence of superficial lesions with no worsening of severity is not life-threatening, so the difference did not prove there would be long-term benefit to the more toxic BCG (a reasonable argument) and (2) no trial would be available to patients if this one closed (not so clearly reasonable — we do hope that patients get superior care on a clinical trial, but this may instead be an example where Group interests and patient interests are not necessarily

EXAMPLES

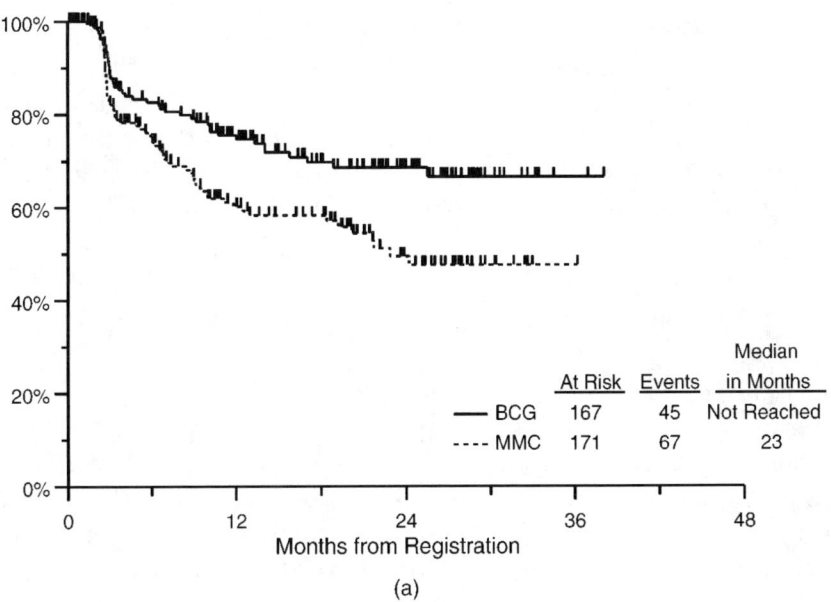

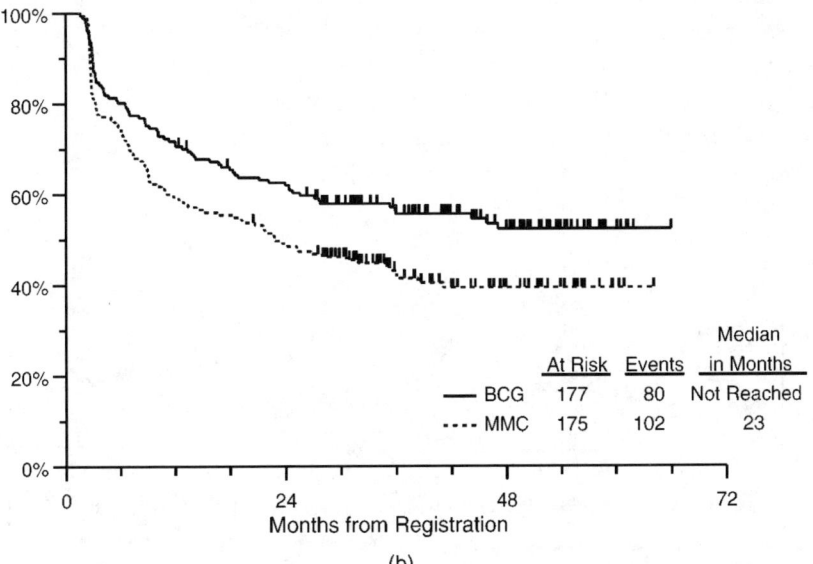

Figure 5.2. Recurrence-free survival in SWOG bladder cancer trial 8795: (a) at time of first interim analysis; (b) after closure and additional follow-up.

the same). Arguments in favor of stopping were (1) a striking difference in the stated primary endpoint was observed and the stopping guideline was met, (2) the study confirmed other evidence that BCG was efficacious in superficial bladder cancer and (3) the degree of toxicity was not unacceptable. The trial was stopped in favor of BCG. At the time of publication, differences had decreased (Figure 5.2b) as would be expected, but were still significant at $p = 0.02$.

SWOG 8892 (Al-Sarraf et al., 1998) was a trial of radiotherapy (RT) vs. RT plus cisplatin and 5-FU for patients with stage III or IV nasopharyngeal cancer. The study was based on survival as the primary endpoint and was planned for a total of 270 patients, with three interim analyses at level 0.005. At the first interim analysis, after an accrual of 138 patients, and a p-value <0.005, the trial was closed and the conclusion was reached that combined chemotherapy/RT was better that RT alone (Figure 5.3a). This result held up at the time of final analysis (Figure 5.3b). However, estimates of improvement are biased high after early stopping, since stopping is more likely when, by chance, results look a little better than they actually are. Because the trial results were so extreme with such a modest sample size, we performed a simulation to investigate whether the estimated treatment effect at final analysis was a misleading over-estimate (LeBlanc and Crowley, 1999). The answer is that the treatment difference was over estimated as expected, but not by an important amount.

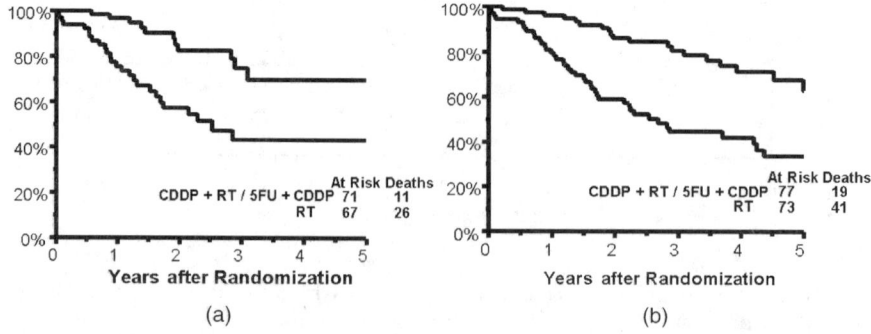

Figure 5.3. Survival in SWOG nasopharyngeal cancer trial 8892: (a) at time of first interim analysis; (b) after closure and additional follow-up.

EXAMPLES   115

5.4.2   Stopping early for negative results

Study 8738 (Gandara et al., 1993) was a trial of high-dose cisplatin, with or without mitomycin C, vs. a control arm of standard-dose cisplatin in patients with advanced non-small-cell lung cancer. The design called for 200 patients per arm, to achieve power of 0.825 to detect hazard ratios of 1.25. Interim analyses were planned at 1/3 and 2/3 of the expected information, at one-sided 0.005 levels. The final analysis was planned for level 0.045. At the first interim analysis, roughly halfway through the planned accrual, the alternative hypothesis for the comparison of high-dose to standard-dose cisplatin was rejected with a p-value of 0.003 (Figure 5.4a). While neither the null nor the alternative hypothesis regarding the high-dose cisplatin plus mitomycin C arm could be rejected, the rationale for the use of high-dose cisplatin, with or without mitomycin C, had been called into question. Furthermore, the two high-dose arms had significantly more toxicity than the standard-dose arm. The monitoring committee decided the whole trial should be closed at this point. At the time of publication the results were still negative (Figure 5.4b).

Early stopping for unconvincing negative results can have serious consequences for other ongoing trials. The Cancer and Leukemia Group B (CALGB) reported their trial of high-dose chemotherapy followed by autologous transplant for patients with breast cancer and 10 or more positive nodes when only 60% of the expected total number of events had occurred (Peters et al., 1999). The authors stated that their results were negative but inconclusive, but that clinicans and patients needed to see the results for their own decision making. A similar trial was underway in the Southwest Oncology Group (SWOG 9623). Figure 5.5 shows the accrual pattern to that trial, with a sharp dropoff after the CALGB results were presented. SWOG 9623 had to be closed in early 2001 due to poor accrual, and the question of the value of high-dose chemotherapy for this patient population will now not be as definitively answered as it might have been.

5.4.3   Stopping an equivalence trial early for positive results

Southwest Oncology Group study 8412 (Alberts et al., 1992) was designed to test equivalence of intravenous cisplatin plus cyclophosphamide vs. intravenous carboplatin plus cyclophosphamide in stage III-IV ovarian cancer. Early experience with carboplatin suggested it was substantially less toxic than its analog cisplatin, so the goal of the trial was to demonstrate that cisplatin's anti-tumor effects were

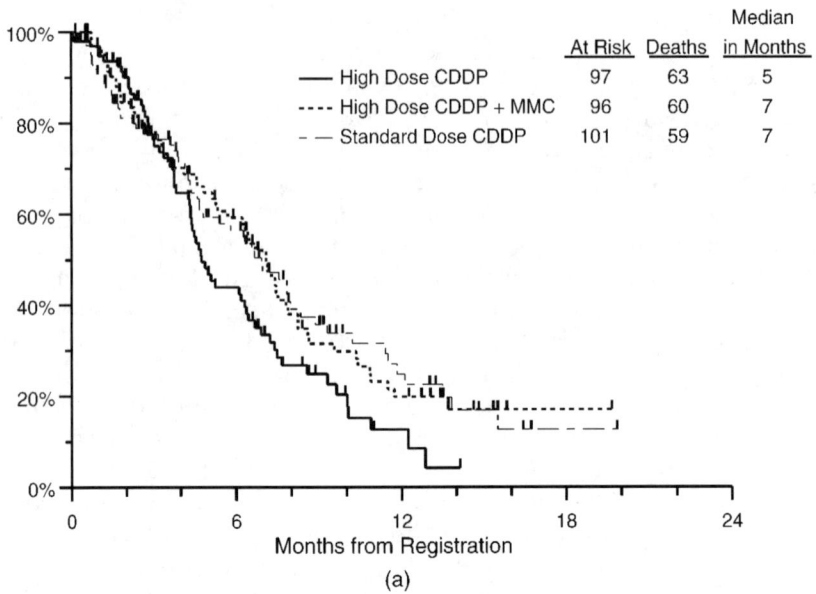

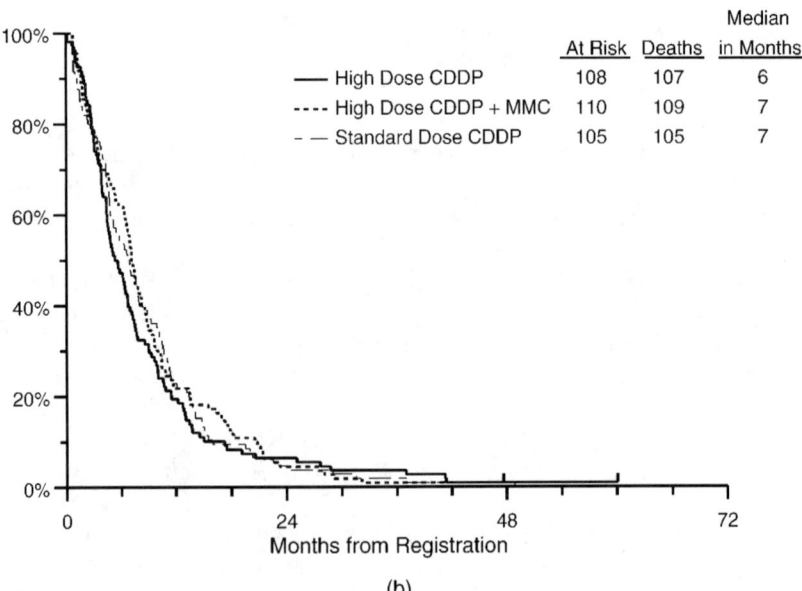

Figure 5.4. Survival in SWOG lung cancer trial 8738: (a) at time of closure; (b) after additional follow-up.

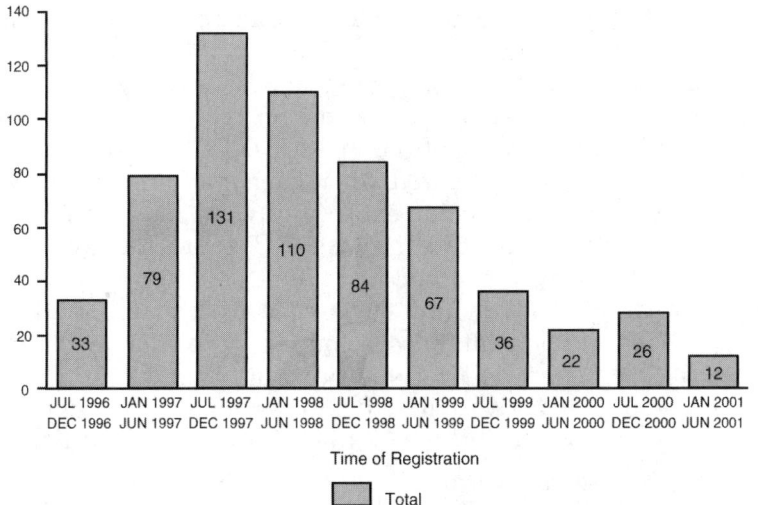

Figure 5.5. Accrual pattern to SWOG breast cancer trial 9623. A negative but 'inconclusive' trial was reported by another group in May of 1999, adversely affecting accrual.

not substantially superior. The null hypothesis was a 30% improvement due to cisplatin, and the trial was designed to have sufficient power to reject this hypothesis if the treatment arms were equivalent.

The first major decision of the monitoring committee for this trial was to consider a change of primary endpoint from pathologic complete response (CR) to survival. A problem with pathologic CR was that we were not getting complete information. Too many patients with clinical CRs were not getting second-look surgeries, so pathologic CR could not be determined. Two patients with clinical evidence of disease had second-look surgeries anyway (despite it not being required) and no disease was found. Both facts suggested an analysis based on pathologic CR would be biased. Furthermore, even if pathologic CR had been determined completely, differences would not necessarily imply patients were better or worse off long term. The change to survival was made and the stopping guidelines were modified accordingly.

At the time of the first formal interim analysis (at approximately 1/4 of the anticipated number of deaths), a 30% improvement in survival due to the cisplatin arm was ruled out at the specified level for early stopping; in fact, at this point the carboplatin arm appeared superior with respect to survival. The decision to stop the trial was not clear-cut, however. The apparent lack of survival benefit due to cisplatin and the clear superiority of carboplatin with respect to most of the severe cisplatin toxicities had to be weighed against an increase in thrombocytopenia on the carboplatin arm, inconclusive results with respect to response and time to failure, and no long-term survival information. Discussion in the monitoring committee included observations from investigators treating patients on the trial that they were relieved when their patients were randomized to carboplatin and so could expect less vomiting. Discussion also included thoughtful comments from the NCI representative concerning the risk of an equivocal trial after further follow-up if the study was closed early. A less helpful suggestion from some of the members was to report the trial but continue randomizing anyway. (This would have been contrary to the data monitoring committee policy of not reporting on active trials. It also seems inconsistent to conclude results are convincing enough to report but not to stop treating with the inferior agent.) After a formal meeting and two rounds of letters, it was decided that results were sufficiently convincing to stop accrual and to report the trial.

Figure 5.6a shows how the results looked at the time we closed the trial and Figure 5.6b shows the results at the time of publication. The results remained inconsistent with a 30% improvement due to cisplatin. Note the similarity to Figure 5.4, which illustrates stopping for a negative result. In each case we were able to stop because the hypothesized better arm looked worse instead. The results most likely were exaggerated due to the random ups and downs that occur during the course of any trial, and in each study the difference decreased by the final analysis. Results remained convincingly negative for each, however, due to the conservative approach to stopping.

5.4.4 Stopping based on toxicity and lack of compliance

Limited small-cell lung cancer study 8812 (Bunn et al., 1995; Kelly et al., 1995) was designed originally to test whether the addition of interferon to brain radiotherapy improved survival in responders to induction therapy. Formal interim analyses were to be performed after approximately 400 and 600 responders had been accrued. A secondary goal was added in protocol development to determine if a decrease in the number of severe infections in patients receiving induction therapy (RT plus concurrent etoposide (VP-16) and cisplatin) could be accomplished by adding granulocyte/macrophage colony-stimulating factor (GM-CSF) to stimulate granulocyte production. The early stopping guideline for this endpoint called for an

EXAMPLES

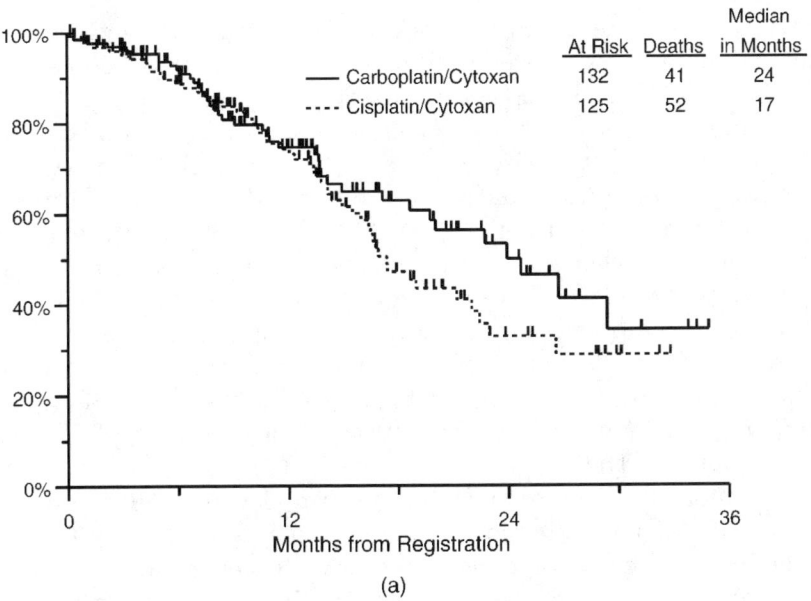

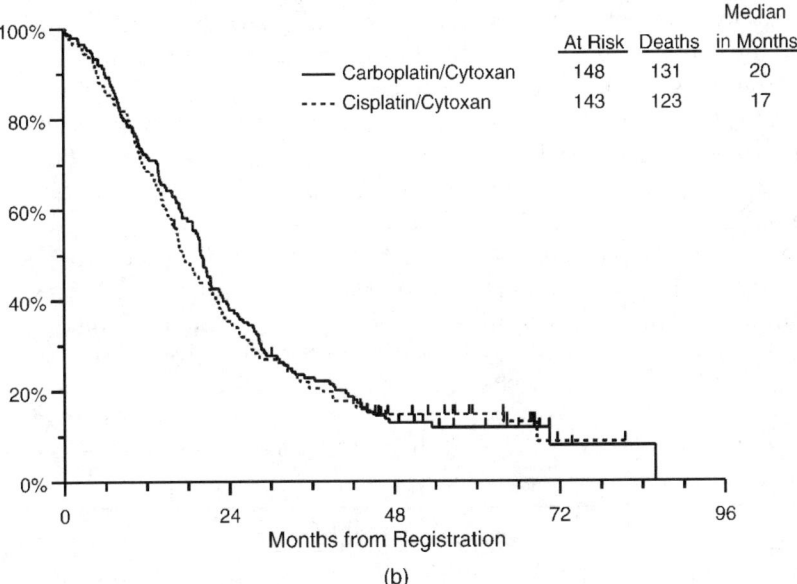

Figure 5.6. Survival in SWOG ovarian cancer trial 8412: (a) at time of closure; (b) after additional follow-up.

interim analysis after 160 patients had been evaluated for infection; the final analysis for this endpoint was to be done after 350 patients.

The induction chemotherapy used on this trial was a regimen from a pilot study with some minor modifications. Modifications included dropping vincristine, changing agents for the final cycles of treatment, modification of doses, different days of administration, and a different retreatment interval. Any one of these might have been minor; together they turned out not to be. In retrospect, a new pilot study would have been prudent. Trouble was evident early; 5 months after opening the study was temporarily closed due to severe hematologic toxicity. It was reopened 2 months later with reduced doses of chemotherapy. Severe toxicities were reduced but not eliminated, and it started to become clear that GM-CSF was causing some of the problems.

The monitoring committee had been reviewing information regularly. Emergency early closure was not necessary, but by the time of the interim analysis for the infection endpoint, results were clear. There was an unanticipated and striking increase in the number of patients with grade 4 thrombocytopenia on the GM-CSF arm (Table 5.4). There was also a possible increase in the number of severe infections, despite a small decrease in granulocytopenia (although this may have been due in part to misdiagnosis of radiation pneumonitis). The GM-CSF arm was closed.

Accrual to the no GM-CSF arm and randomization to maintenance were continued for another 6 months. At this time the monitoring committee closed the rest of the trial with only 125 patients on the maintenance randomization due to severe compliance problems. One half of all patients on interferon were refusing therapy before relapse despite only moderate toxicity. The question of whether survival was improved by patients taking interferon as long as they could stand it was not considered of sufficient interest to continue the trial.

Table 5.4. Infection and hematologic toxicity at time of interim analysis for study 8812.

	No GM-CSF(%)	GM-CSF(%)
Grade 4 Granulocytopenia	19	14
Grade 4 Leukopenia	11	10
Grade 4 Thrombocytopenia	4	30
Fatal Infection	0	4

5.4.5 Emergency stopping based on unexpected toxic deaths

One of the mechanisms of tumor resistance to therapy is thought to be development of a multidrug resistant tumor phenotype (specifically, expression of p-glycoprotein, a membrane protein involved in the transport of toxins from cells). Southwest Oncology Group study 9028 (Salmon et al., 1998) was designed to test the hypothesis that standard therapy plus agents to block transport of drugs from cells would be more effective than standard therapy alone in the treatment of multiple myeloma. Patients were randomized to receive either vincristine, doxorubicin, and dexamethasone (VAD) or VAD plus verapamil and quinine (VQ) to overcome multidrug resistance.

A difficulty in evaluation of multiple myeloma patients is determination of cause of death. Patients who die due to disease often die of multiple organ (renal, cardiac, pulmonary, hematologic) failure, which makes it difficult to distinguish death due to disease from death due to various organ toxicities. SWOG 9028 opened to accrual on October 1, 1990, and several deaths of patients on VAD plus VQ were reported to the Statistical Center over the summer of 1991. The study coordinator reviewed the charts and judged that these deaths, primarily due to renal failure in patients with poor renal function at diagnosis, were possibly related to verapamil. An amendment was prepared to reduce the dose of verapamil in these poor-risk patients, and the data monitoring committee was notified of this action. By the time the committee met, in late October, the evidence implicating verapamil was more clear, though the survival difference was not statistically significant, and the VAD plus VQ arm was closed to further accrual. Patients still being treated with VAD plus VQ were switched from sustained action to standard formulation verapamil in December, following a report implicating the sustained action formulation (Pritza, Bierman, and Hammeke, 1991). After further deliberation by the investigators, all patients were taken off verapamil in February of 1992.

Clearly some things will not wait for a semi-annual meeting of a data monitoring committee. The data monitoring committee was important in agreeing that previous actions were appropriate and in recommending further action, but if statistical center staff and the study coordinator had waited to do evaluations until it was time for the data monitoring committee to meet, other patients on this trial would likely have died of toxicity. Could actions have been taken even sooner? We have all spent time worrying about this, but think the answer is probably not much sooner. The initial deaths looked like typical myeloma deaths so earlier detection of the problem was not likely. The excess of deaths in poor-risk patients was alarming, but the difference between the arms could have been due to chance. Since the study hypothesis was still sound, a first approach of reducing the verapamil dose in poor-risk patients seemed justified. Perhaps the dates for discontinuing accrual, changing to standard formulation, and dropping verapamil altogether could have been earlier — but not early enough to have changed the management of any of the patients who died.

5.5 Concluding remarks

Paul Meier (1975) has written that "although statistics has a role, the ethical problem of continuing or stopping an experiment is not primarily statistical. Neither is it especially a medical problem or a legal one. It is, in fact, a political problem, and I see no sensible way to cope with it outside a political framework." A few years ago we would have disagreed; now we are inclined to admit there is some truth to the contention. Still, we think there is room for a variety of models for monitoring committees to accommodate the political as well as the scientific and ethical issues. An interesting discussion of the dynamic of one such committee in the highly charged political atmosphere of HIV/AIDS is given in Armitage (1999). If we *start* with the assumption that most people will make judgments out of self-interest, no model will work.

CHAPTER 6

Data Management and Quality Control

The quality of the data never stopped me from doing a quality analysis.

**–(Quote from a famous statistician.
We think it best not to say which one.)**

6.1 Introduction: Why worry?

As the old adage goes, garbage in, garbage out. Simply put, faulty data compromise studies. Survival estimates are biased if patients are lost to follow up; early results are biased by inclusion of patients who will later be found to be ineligible and by missing information; response estimates are biased if tumor assessments are missed; variability is increased if patients are not treated according to protocol, making it more difficult to detect treatment differences. The following three examples are illustrative.

Figure 6.1 shows the Kaplan-Meier estimate of survival from a sample of 10 patients, five of whom were lost to follow-up. The lost patients are censored at the time they were last known to be alive. The bottom curve shows the estimate for the extreme in which all five lost patients died right after being lost, while the top curve shows the extreme in which all lost patients actually survived until the time of analysis at 4 years. The survival estimate will be biased high if patients were lost because they were beginning to fail, and it will be biased low if patients were lost because they were doing well. Both scenarios are plausible: desperate patients on advanced disease studies may go elsewhere if they are not doing well; patients on early stage studies who remain disease-free for many years may stop showing up for appointments.

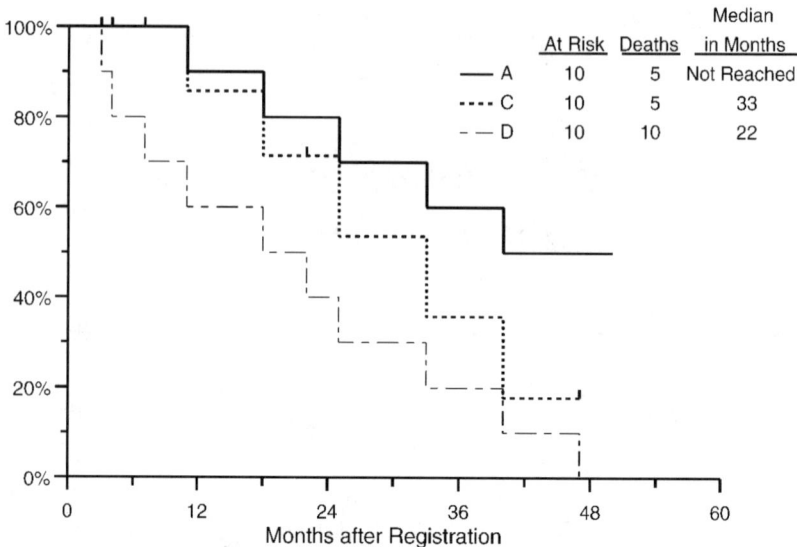

Figure 6.1. Potential bias in survival estimates where half of the patients sampled were lost to follow-up. Curve A indicates the estimate when the five patients lost to follow-up are assumed to be alive at the time of analysis. Curve C censors these five patients at the last contact date. Curve D assumes that the five patients died just after the last contact date.

Figures 6.2 through 6.4 illustrate with a real example how results change when the data are cleaned up. Southwest Oncology Group Study 7436 (Rivkin et al., 1989) compared CMFVP with L-PAM (L-Phenylalanine mustard, or melphalan) as adjuvant treatment in resectable node-positive breast cancer. Initially a significant difference was observed in postmenopausal patients, with logrank $p = 0.03$, as shown in Figure 6.2. After cleaning up the data with respect to eligibility and unrecorded events, this difference decreased, with the logrank p-value changing to 0.08 (Figure 6.3). After a request for updated follow-up, the difference decreased more, with a p-value of 0.17 (Figure 6.4). The example illustrates how uncorrected data can be misleading.

As a final example of how faulty data can bias results, consider the following scenario. A patient enters on study with a 2.0 cm lung lesion on computed tomography (CT) and a positive bone scan. At the first two assessments after entry the lung lesion is 0.5 cm; at the second a bone scan is also done, as required, and shows no change. At the third assessment the lesion is 1.5 cm. Using RECIST response criteria, the patient has a partial response (PR) starting at the first assessment, the response is confirmed at a second assessment, and

INTRODUCTION: WHY WORRY?

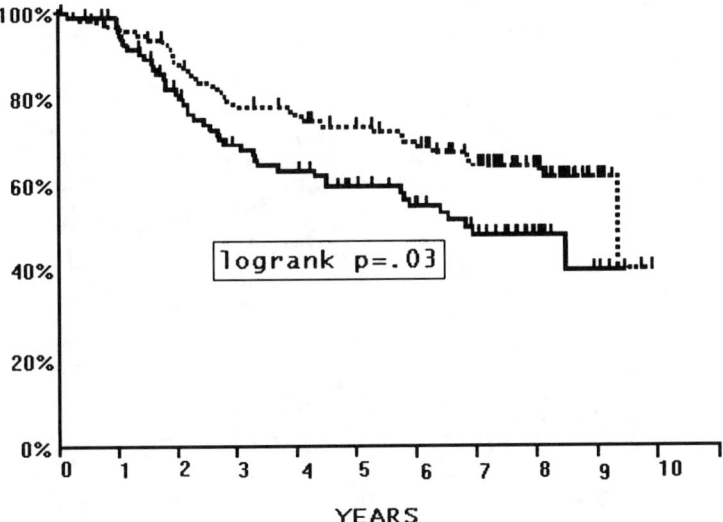

Figure 6.2. Survival distributions before data clean-up, and with follow-up overdue.

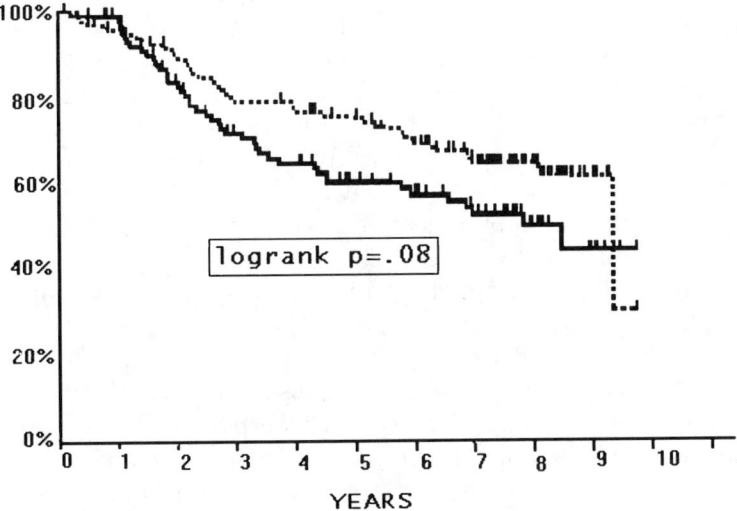

Figure 6.3. Survival distributions after data clean-up, and with follow-up overdue.

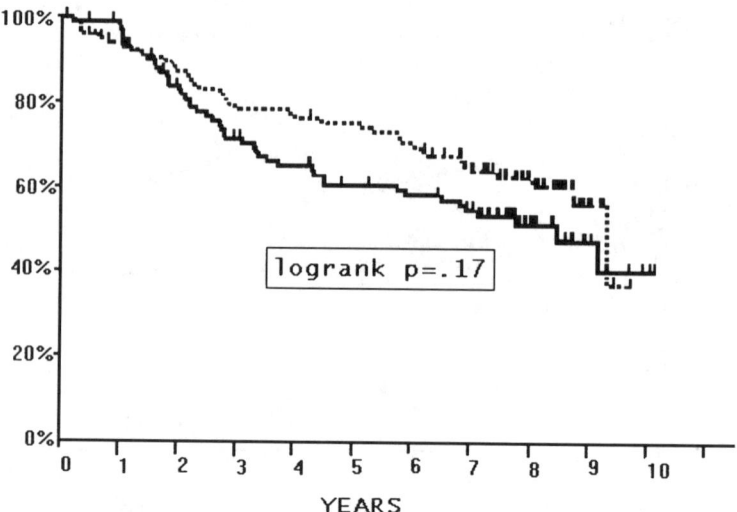

Figure 6.4. Survival distributions after data clean-up, and with follow-up updated.

progression of disease occurs at the time of the third assessment. (Note that while this 1.5 cm lesion is still smaller than the original 2.0 cm lesion, it represents a tripling over the minimum measurements at the second and third assessments, and is thus defined as a progression.) Table 6.1 shows what happens if tests are missed. If assessment 1 or 2 is missed or done differently, the response is either unconfirmed or missed altogether. If assessment 3 is missed, the time of progression is too late. If baseline measurements are missing, response is unknown and time of progression is difficult to assess. Worse, patients may remain on study long after they are no longer receiving benefit from the treatment.

The rest of the chapter describes some of the ways to maintain quality data: protocol development, standardized data items, data forms, protocol management, evaluation procedures, training, and data base management. Procedures are described from the point of view of a multi-institutional, multi-study organization, a setting in which it is most difficult to maintain consistency and quality. SWOG Study 8811 (Margolin et al., 1994), which is a Phase II study of 5-FU with continuous infusion high-dose folinic acid in advanced breast cancer, is used to illustrate. For this study, one of our investigators had interesting early data from her institution, which she presented at a meeting of the breast cancer working group at one of the semi-annual Group meetings. Preliminary interest was expressed by those

INTRODUCTION: WHY WORRY?

Table 6.1. Effect of missing assessments on response and progression determination.*

Baseline		Assessment				Outcome
		1	2	3	4	
Lung scan	2	.5	.5	1.5	(Pt off study due to progression)	PR starting at 1, confirmed at 2 Progression at 3 ('Truth' to the limits of the protocol requirements)
Bone scan	+	NR	S	NR		
Lung scan	M	.5	.5	1.5	(Pt off study due to progression)	Unknown response due to no baseline measuresssion Progression documented at 3 (at 1 if interpreted as new lesion)
Bone scan	+	NR	S	NR		
Lung scan	2	.5	.5	1.5	(Pt off study due to progression)	Unknown response due to no repeat bone scan, possible PR Progression documented at 3
Bone scan	+	NR	M	M		
Lung scan	2	.5	M	1.5	(Pt off study due to progression)	PR starting at 1, not confirmed Progression documented at 3
Bone scan	+	NR	S	NR		
Lung scan	2	M	M	1.5	2.2	PR starting at 3, not confirmed Progesssion documented at 4
Bone scan	+	NR	M	S	New sites	
Lung scan	2	M	.5	M	2.2	PR starting at 2, not confirmed Progression documented at 4
Bone scan	+	NR	S	NR	New sites	
Lung scan	2	M	M	M	2.2	???? No response, unknown if progression, patient continutued on treatment
Bone scan	· M	M	M	M	+	
Lung scan	2	1.5 on x-ray	1.5 on x-ray	2 on x-ray	2.2	Unknown response due to x-ray instead of scan, possibly stable Progression documented at 4
Bone scan	+	NR	S	NR	New sites	

*NR = not required; S = stable/no change; M = required but missing or not done; Pt = patient; PR = partial response.

attending the meeting, so a concept was written up by the investigator for circulation, review, and eventual approval.

6.2 Protocol development

A clearly written and well-justified study document is a critical early step in the conduct of good quality clinical trials. While there are many formats that produce successful protocols, it is important that the study document include explicit information on the topics presented below. All SWOG treatment protocols are written in the same format according to detailed protocol guidelines. Using a standard format is helpful in various ways. It allows for ease of reference by the institutions that have to use the protocol, for streamlining of production of the document, and for interpretation of the same items in the same way across protocols. It also allows for consistent inclusion of important aspects in the protocol, and for automatic clarification of common problems. During the process of developing the protocol, both the operations office and statistical center review the protocol carefully for consistency, clarity of instructions, correctness of procedures, and feasibility of the objectives. The statistical center, along with the study coordinator, also develops the design and statistical considerations for the study. The following is a general outline of SWOG treatment protocols.

6.2.1 Objectives

Section 1 of the protocol states the objectives for the trial. This section should include all primary and secondary objectives, and each should be explicitly defined. It is not sufficient, for example, to state that a goal is "to assess the use of adjuvant chemo-radiation in the treatment of gastric cancer." Instead, the primary goal for a Phase III trial should be stated as "to compare survival of gastric cancer patients treated with chemo-radiation following surgery to those treated with surgery alone." For study 8811, the primary objective was to assess response to 5-FU and folinic acid as treatment for advanced breast cancer to decide whether the regimen should be tested further. Secondary objectives also specified were to assess toxcities and survival for patients treated with this regimen.

6.2.2 Background

The background in Section 2 provides justification for addressing the objectives. The background in the protocol for SWOG 8811 included both biologic rationale and clinical observations. Biologically, it was hypothesized that folinic acid enhanced the activity of 5-FU by potentiating the inhibition of thymidylate synthetase. If true, then addition of folinic acid to 5-FU would be expected to improve the anti-tumor effect of 5-FU. The clinical observations supporting study of the regimen included an estimated response probability of 0.17 in a group of heavily pretreated patients, most of whom had previously failed on standard 5-FU therapy. The background also included information on response to standard therapy, which was necessary to justify the assumptions used in developing the statistical considerations.

6.2.3 Drug information

Section 3 has drug information. The section is standardized so that all protocols with the same agent have consistent information provided. Sections on new routes or agents are written up by the first investigator to use them in a study; they are then standardized for use in future protocols. Chemistry, toxicology, and pharmaceutical data are described in this section and the supplier is specified. Having standardized drug descriptions aids in efficient production of the protocol and avoids conflicting information across protocols.

6.2.4 Stage definitions

Applicable disease-specific stage definitions are provided in Section 4, and should be standard if at all possible. There are standard definitions for most cancers (typically based on the American Joint Commission on Cancer's staging definitions (Fleming et al., 1997)). This section may not be applicable for other diseases.

6.2.5 Eligibility criteria

Detailed eligibility criteria are listed in Section 5. Criteria typically cover disease characteristics, prior treatment, and patient characteristics. In addition, several standard sections covering regulatory requirements are automatically included in every protocol. These criteria should describe the patients to whom the results of the trial are to be generalized, and should be limited to only those requirements that are absolutely necessary. For SWOG 8811, disease requirements included adenocarcinoma of the breast, and bidimensionally measurable metastatic or recurrent disease. For prior treatment requirements, patients must have had no prior chemotherapy for metastatic disease or only one prior chemotherapy for metastatic disease. Required patient characteristics included pretreatment WBC above 4000, platelets above 150 000, creatinine and bilirubin less than $1.5\times$ upper limit of normal (ULN), and patients had to be ambulatory. The standard regulatory requirements concerned pregnancy (which was not allowed), Institutional Review Board approval (which had to be current), and informed consent (which had to be signed by the patient prior to registration). Careful attention to the eligibility sections when the protocol is developed saves a lot of trouble later. If the criteria are unclear, then there will not be a clearly defined patient population that can be precisely described in the manuscript. There will be misunderstandings by the participating institutions, resulting in too many ineligible patients being registered. There will be protocol revisions to be written and circulated. A clear and precise eligibility section is particularly important when there is a policy not to allow exceptions to the criteria — which there should be if the study is to be credible. For instance, if WBC above 4000 is required, then a patient with a WBC of 4000 cannot be accepted (what about 3999? Or 3998?). Criteria that are not meant to be enforced should not be in the eligibility section of the protocol.

6.2.6   *Stratification factors and subsets*

Stratification factors and subsets are in Section 6. Stratification factors are used in the study design to allocate patients to treatment on randomized studies (see Chapter 3 for a discussion of stratification factors). Subsets are those factors for which separate accrual goals and separate analyses are specified. Most Phase II studies do not have stratification factors or subsets. In SWOG 8811, however, there was interest in answering questions in two separate types of patients, so there was one subset factor. Patients were accrued separately into two groups: one with no prior chemotherapy for advanced disease and one with one prior chemotherapy.

6.2.7 Treatment plan

Section 7 begins with a subsection on Good Medical Practices, in which registration guidelines requiring medical judgement are listed. This section might include adequate renal function and general good health, for example. Guidelines for WBC or other lab results could be included here if absolute cutoffs are not necessary for safety, thereby avoiding the problem noted above of having to exclude all patients with values on the boundary. Items in this subsection do not affect eligibility, but generally require discussion with the Study Coordinator before a patient not meeting the guidelines is registered. The remainder of Section 7 contains a detailed treatment plan, including a table of dose level, route of administration, days of treatment, retreatment interval, and the order of the different agents. A sample treatment table is included at the end of this chapter. Section 7 of the protocol also specifies any restrictions on ancillary treatment. Typically, concurrent cancer treatment is not allowed so that outcomes can be attributed to the treatment under study. There may also be supportive care treatments that are preferred (e.g., a particular antiemetic regimen) or contraindicated (e.g., no corticosteroids), or guidelines for use of growth factors or antibiotics. The section also provides a list of acceptable reasons for removal of a patient from treatment.

6.2.8 Treatment modification

Section 8 gives detailed instructions for treatment modification if the patient experiences excessive toxicity. The section includes the phone number of the study coordinator and a backup clinician for institutions to contact with any questions concerning problems with treatment. These questions should not be left to a clinical research associate at the institution or to the statistical center personnel — it is inappropriate for them to give medical advice, even if what seems to be the same question is raised over and over. It is important that the treatment and dose modification sections be clear, not only for the safety of the patients, but also for consistency. If instructions are not clear, patients will be treated in a variety of different ways. For instance, suppose the protocol says "decrease dose by 25% after a 1 week delay if the patient experiences grade 3 vomiting." Does this mean to decrease by 25% of the starting dose or of the previous dose? If it means the starting dose and the patient experiences grade 3 vomiting a second time, does the patient stay at 75% starting dose, or is dose reduced by another 25% of starting dose? Should the dose be escalated back to starting dose if the patient recovers? What if the patient is still vomiting after 1 week? Obscure instructions will add variability to the study and may compromise its interpretation.

6.2.9 Study calendar

The study calendar is in Section 9. It specifies all baseline tests and the schedule for all follow-up tests that are required for eligibility, disease assessment, and toxicity assessment. It also specifies the follow-up schedule after a patient goes off treatment. The calendar helps ensure that patients are uniformly and correctly assessed. Check to be sure the baseline requirements include everything needed to determine eligibility and the follow-up requirements include everything needed to assess toxicity and disease. Omit any test not required. For instance, alkaline phosphatase might be fairly routine, but if not necessary for an adequate assessment, leave it to the discretion of the individual investigators. Also be sure to qualify requirements as appropriate. For instance, compliance with an unqualified requirement for a pregnancy test or for monthly CT scans is likely to be poor. Parts of the SWOG 8811 calendar are shown at the end of this chapter.

6.2.10 Endpoint definitions

Section 10 gives endpoint definitions, generally including response, performance status, survival, and progression-free survival or time to treatment failure. SWOG uses endpoint definitions that are consistent across protocols. For instance, all studies have the same definition of survival and performance status, and all solid tumor studies have the same definition of response. Clear definitions are needed so that endpoints are interpreted the same way at each institution. (Some of the difficulties in defining endpoints are discussed in Chapter 3.) Errors are avoided if the definitions are detailed and if the same definitions are always used. If there is inconsistency, it becomes difficult for institutions to keep track of and apply many different definitions across many different protocols. It also becomes difficult to interpret manuscripts when the same endpoint (nominally) always means something different.

6.2.11 Statistical considerations

Statistical considerations are included in Section 11. How these are produced is covered in Chapters 2 through 4. In general, this section includes accrual estimates, sample size with justification, study duration, and a specification of the types of interim and final analyses to be performed. With respect to study quality, the point to make is that what is written in the statistical considerations should be consistent with the rest of the protocol, particularly with respect to the objectives and the background.

6.2.12 Discipline review

Section 12 covers discipline review. Special reviews of pathology, radiotherapy, and surgery are done when quality control of these is important on a study. For example, radiotherapy typically should be reviewed if the procedures are nonstandard and an important part of protocol treatment. Surgery should be reviewed under the same circumstances, or if it is part of disease assessment, such as confirming a pathologic complete response. Reviews are probably too expensive to justify if the procedures are routine. For instance, SWOG does not review mastectomies done prior to registration on adjuvant breast cancer studies. Reviews were done at one time, but 287 reviews resulted in only one patient found to be ineligible solely as a consequence of surgical review; it was judged not worth the effort to continue routine review. On the other hand, surgical review of second-look surgeries has been important in ovarian cancer studies, and surgeons have a very active role in the gynecology committee.

Pathology should be reviewed if there is moderate difficulty in making a pathologic diagnosis. If there is little difficulty, the effort it takes to review slides is greater than the gain. If there is a great deal of difficulty, it is also probably not worth it, unless one of the specific aims of the study is to study pathology. For instance, SWOG has studies in non-small-cell lung cancer, but we generally do not try to separate out subtypes, as there is too little agreement among pathologists for this to be useful in the analysis of treatment effect.

For all of the disciplines, standard submission procedures should be used whenever possible. Limiting the number of routines the institutions have to follow results in fewer mistakes.

6.2.13 Registration instructions

Registration instructions are included in Section 13. In addition to the phone number to call or Web site to access and the hours patients can be registered, this section reminds institutions of registration policies. Registrations after treatment start are not allowed, registrations cannot be canceled after they are completed, and the planned treatment start date must be within 1 working day of registration for most studies (within a week for surgery or RT studies where scheduling cannot be accomplished within a day).

The first two policies are in place to minimize biases that can occur when there are options to include or exclude patients as a function of how well they are doing or as a function of which arm was assigned. If patients who have already started treatment can be registered, only those who do not quit or fail right away will be entered, making the treatment look better than it is. If cancellations are allowed, then it is possible that patients will be followed on study only when they are randomized to the arm they wanted anyway, which defeats the purpose of randomization. A trial (not in SWOG) of surgery vs. RT in prostate cancer had to be abandoned for just this reason. Each patient received the assigned treatment only if it was one the clinician wanted, and otherwise was omitted from the registration list — so patients received exactly the same treatments they would have without randomization, thereby reducing the trial to an observational study.

The third policy is enforced to minimize the number of patients who do not receive treatment. If long delays between registration and treatment start are allowed, some patients will deteriorate and no longer be candidates for treatment, some will die, and others will change their minds and refuse assigned treatment. Since *all* eligible patients who are registered on study must be used in the analysis of the study (see Chapter 7), it is best to have as few of these cases as possible.

6.2.14 Data submission instructions

Section 14 has data submission instructions. It includes the time limits for submission and instructions for submission over the Web (if applicable). For submission by mail, addresses and the number of copies of forms and materials that have to be sent are specified. As with most of our procedures, there are standards for location, timing, and number of forms that are generally applied. For adequate monitoring, time limits for data submission after registration, discontinuation of treatment, progression of disease, and death are short (14 days from event for most).

6.2.15 Special instructions

Any special instructions are included in Section 15. These might include sample submission instructions for biologic studies, or instruction on how to administer questionnaires for quality of life endpoints. Included are phone numbers for questions.

6.2.16 Regulatory requirements

Section 16 has regulatory requirements, including instructions for reporting adverse drug reactions, and an outline of informed consent requirements.

6.2.17 Bibliography

The bibliography is in Section 17.

6.2.18 Forms

Forms to be used in the study are included in Section 18. Forms are discussed below.

6.2.19 Appendix

The Appendix indicates toxicity criteria to be used. Standard toxicity definitions (Common Toxicity Criteria, see Section 3.2) are used across all disease sites and modalities. These definitions help institutions not have to guess what mild, moderate, and severe mean, and using the same definitions for all group protocols helps improve accuracy of grading and consistency of interpretation. The Common Toxicity Criteria are updated as new side effects to new agents become common.

6.2.20 Additional comments on SWOG study 8811

There were several issues we resolved during the review process for SWOG protocol 8811. One issue already mentioned was how to incorporate the extent of prior treatment into the study design — it was decided that patients with prior and no prior treatment for advanced disease were sufficiently different with respect to response to treatment that efficacy of the regimen should be studied separately in each subset. It was also decided that two-stage designs were appropriate for each subset. Endpoint issues were also resolved. Complete response was identified as the most meaningful endpoint for patients with no prior treatment for metastatic disease, while partial response was the best that could be anticipated for patients with prior treatment. In addition, response duration was omitted as an endpoint, because too few responses were anticipated to be able to estimate duration reliably.

Another issue that had to be resolved before the protocol document was complete was the definition of prior and no prior chemotherapy for advanced disease when the patient had prior adjuvant chemotherapy. For instance, patients who develop metastases while taking adjuvant chemotherapy have already demonstrated resistance of metastatic disease to chemotherapy, so probably should be categorized with the patients with one prior chemotherapy for metastatic disease instead of with those with no prior chemotherapy. It was decided that patients who relapsed within 1 year of completion of adjuvant therapy would be grouped with those who had failed one regimen for advanced disease, while those who failed more than 1 year after completion would not.

Issues of clarity and safety were also settled during the protocol review process. For instance, the planned starting dose of 5-FU was decreased from 400 to 370 milligrams per square meter of body surface area due to toxicity noted in additional pilot data. Another change was that eligibility was reworded to clarify that biopsies of metastases were not required. Also, requirements were reviewed with the result that repeat pulmonary function tests were deleted from the study calendar and diarrhea was added to the flow sheet as a toxicity to be monitored.

6.3 Data collection

The development and conduct of a clinical trial are expensive propositions, not only in dollars, but in terms of patient resources and researcher time. It is tempting to collect as much data as possible in hopes of maximizing the returns on any trial. Unfortunately, this strategy is likely to backfire. Anyone who has participated in a survey is familiar with the change from initial enthusiasm to tedium and impatience that accompanies the progression through completion of a lengthy questionnaire. There is a similar effect in data collection for clinical research. The quality of what is collected is inversely related to the quantity of information requested. A researcher will be more likely to take care to provide accurate information on five items, but is less likely to take the same care with a list of 50 data items. As a result, a manuscript based on a small number of carefully reported variables will be limited, but correct, whereas the second senario yields a manuscript that will be extensive, but less accurate, or possibly not worth writing at all. Even when the quantity of data is limited, care must be taken to insure that data are well defined, and reporting carefully controlled.

To achieve the goal of maximizing the accuracy of information reported on a trial, collection should be limited to those data crucial to the main goals of the trial. As data collection plans are developed, proposed variables should be included if they fall into one of the following categories:

1. Needed to support a specific aim of the study
2. Required to properly stratify a patient
3. Recognized as prognostic variables necessary for analysis
4. Required to document patient eligibility
5. Required to guarantee patient safety
6. Mandated for reporting purposes (e.g., race, method of payment are variables required by the National Cancer Institute).

Collection of any variables that do not fall into one of the above categories should be severely limited.

In the following sections we outline data collection strategies followed by the Southwest Oncology Group. While many of the discussions are specific to cancer research in a cooperative group, the principles remain the same in any clinical research setting.

6.3.1 Basic data items

A key way the Southwest Oncology Group has standardized study conduct has been to define a fixed set of data items used for all treatment studies. This has been very important for data management and quality control. It allows for uniform training of data coordinators and study coordinators, for consistency of interpretation of variables across all disease sites, and for extensive logic checks to be developed for application to all studies.

Our set of standard variables falls into four groups: eligibility, evaluability, treatment summary, and outcome summary. Various considerations went into the development of the set. We weighed the cost of collecting an item of information against its usefulness. For instance, collecting quality of life information is very expensive (Moinpour, 1996) and compliance is often poor; thus quality of life is not part of our standard outcome data set. Another example is calculation of dose received. This is also very time consuming and, particularly in the case of oral drugs, inaccurate. Furthermore, analysis by dose received is fatally flawed (see Chapter 8), so the primary use for the effort is a single line in a manuscript giving a (poor) estimate of how much of the planned drug the patients received. There are some studies where this may be sufficiently important (studies designed to investigate dose-intensity questions) to make received dose calculations a priority, but not enough studies to make this part of our standard data set. Our basic treatment items consist of start and stop dates and treatment status (which indicates whether or not the patient is on protocol treatment, and if not, the reason why not). We also code a crude summary of the amount of treatment received (none, minimal, or > minimal; for example, in SWOG 8811 minimal was defined as one course of treatment), and we also code whether or not there was a major deviation. Major deviations are reserved for gross treatment violations, such as no treatment given or the wrong treatment arm given or a major dosing error.

Another principle we followed in developing the basic data set was not to mix up different concepts, or to have items where more than one answer would apply. For instance, a previous version of Southwest Oncology Group evaluation variables included an item that combined eligibility, evaluability, major treatment deviations, and reason off treatment; the choices were: (1) Ineligible, (2) Fully evaluable, (3) Partially evaluable due to refusal, (4) Partially evaluable due to toxicity, (5) Partially evaluable due to early death, (6) Partially evaluable due to other reasons, (7) Lost to follow-up, (8) Not evaluable due to major violation, (9) Not evaluable due to insufficient information, (10) Not evaluable due to other reasons.

Since only one could be chosen, even though several could apply, the variable was inadequate for summarizing basic information needed for manuscripts. For instance, it could not be assumed that the number of patients lost to follow-up was the same as the number of patients coded "7."

In addition to cost and logic, a third consideration in defining the standard data set was to minimize what we asked for, as discussed above. This principle was implemented in two ways. The standard data set includes key variables that are collected on all patients, regardless of disease type. Additionally, each disease committee identified a limited standard set of basic data that are collected for all studies of a specific disease and stage type. Thus, for example, all studies of patients with metastatic colorectal cancer will collect a small basic set of variables that defines the sites and characteristics of the disease. In addition to guaranteeing that the most important variables are collected, this ensures consistent coding of variables across studies. Study-specific items may need to be added, but are also kept to a minimum.

The proper balance on detail can be difficult to judge. For instance, evaluability can be particularly difficult to define. All patients entered on a study are evaluable to some extent, but the extent can vary considerably — a simple yes–no or even yes–partial no does not cover enough of the possibilities. We decided to record information on baseline disease status (measurable disease, evaluable disease, nonevaluable disease, no evidence of disease, or incomplete assessment of baseline status). For evaluability after the patient is on study we have one item that indicates whether or not the patient was assessed for toxicity and, if so, the date of last toxicity assessment, plus items that indicate whether the patient had disease assessment adequate for determining response and time to progression. These are all coded, regardless of the eligibility of the patient — which brings us to the next example. The most basic eligibility variable would be a simple yes or no, but it may be worthwhile to keep some additional detail to be able to assess where problems are and address them. If patients are being found ineligible based on discipline review only, then perhaps educational sessions on what constitutes proper surgery or on how to interpret histologic criteria might be in order. If patients are being found ineligible because of inadequate documentation, then perhaps submission procedures need to be tightened. If ineligibility occurs because investigators ignore the criteria, then perhaps the investigators should be replaced.

A fourth consideration in defining our standard data items was completeness. Response is an example – the set "CR, PR, stable, increasing disease" is incomplete because too often tumor assessments are insufficient to determine response. When that happens, we use one of the following: "early death" is coded if the patient dies before disease can be assessed and death cannot be assumed due to disease, "unconfirmed response" is coded if there is only one assessment documenting response, and "no assessment" is coded if assessments are missing and there is insufficient information to determine best response.

Although the primary point of this section is the importance of standardization when many studies are being done by many institutions, the considerations for developing a standard data set are the same for the single institution/single study setting as well. Cost/benefit of items, separate items for different concepts, number of items limited to a number that can be collected accurately, and logical completeness will still be key.

6.3.2 Data forms

To maintain forms standards, new forms to be used in the Southwest Oncology Group go through a review before implementation. A draft form is produced at the statistical center based on content proposed by the study coordinator and others who will be responsible for the conduct of the study, including the study statistician and the disease committee chair. The draft is reviewed and must be approved by these same people, plus a protocol review committee that consists of data coordinators and statisticians, plus data base staff. If the forms are a significant departure from those to which institutions are accustomed, we also ask for comments from clinical research associates at the institutions. This process can be time consuming, but it is worthwhile to fix as many problems as possible before the forms are actually used in practice.

There are some very basic considerations that should be addressed when designing a form. For paper forms, if the margins are too close to the edge, then part of the form will be lost when copied; this is a particular problem for forms entered via optical scanners. If patient identifiers are not included on the second page of a form, then second pages cannot be processed when (inevitably) they get separated from the first page. If there is no space for notes on the form, explanations will be written on arbitrary and unidentifiable bits of paper. For electronic forms, if the form is on more than one screen, submission instructions or parts of the form can be missed so automatic warning messages ("you are about to exit without submitting..." or "part II has not been filled out...") need to be incorporated. For both types of forms, if they are too complicated or hard to read, parts will not be filled out. If there are too many "if xx, go to yy," then parts that should not be filled out will be. If definitions and instructions are not included on the form, the form will be filled out — inaccurately — from memory. On the other hand, it is not possible to include every possible clarification directly on a form, so guidelines addressing common problems and questions are necessary if forms are to be filled out consistently.

With respect to form content, most of the same considerations that go into developing a standardized data set go into the development of every form: standardizing where possible, weighing collection effort against usefulness (in this case the consideration is for collection effort at the institutions as opposed to effort in abstracting the standard data set from submitted information), restricting items on the form to ones that will be used (plus checking that no items that will be used are inadvertently left off), and making sure there are no logical difficulties in filling out the form.

Many of the basic data items discussed above have been abstracted from study-specific flow sheets. Flow sheets include, for multiple time points, spaces for the doses of each agent administered, for results of physical examination and of all required tests, for lesion measurements, for potential toxicities noted in the protocol, and a section for notes. Flow sheets are often used for patient care as well as for the research record. Even when not used for patient care, this amount of detail is often considered necessary for adequate safety monitoring by the study coordinator, particularly if new regimens are involved. An example of a flow sheet is included in Section 6.9. Although such forms have been very useful in collecting a lot of information efficiently, they are not particularly compatible with electronic form submission, which requires more explicit structure. For electronic submission, separate forms for disease assessments by evaluation cycle and for treatment and toxicity information by treatment cycle are necessary. An example of a treatment and toxicity form is included in Section 6.9.

For large studies, detailed treatment, toxicity, and outcome information may be beyond the limit of what can be collected accurately. If the treatment regimens being used are not new, a one-time form with simple treatment and toxicity summary information plus follow-up forms asking for relapse and survival updates may be sufficient. An example of a follow-up form is also included in Section 6.9.

Other forms used for a particular study are dictated in part by the type of disease being studied. As much as possible we limit study-specific data collection. It is inefficient to design a whole new set of forms every time a study opens. Ways in which we have standardized include standard headings and formats, standard disease-specific prestudies and baseline forms, and standard wording for identical items across prestudies, such as performance status. We also have a number of standard forms used for all studies as needed. The notice of death and off-treatment notice are common to all treatment studies; the same specimen submission form is used for all protocols requiring submission of pathology materials.

The forms set for SWOG 8811 included a study-specific flow sheet, the standard off-treatment notice and notice of death, and standard advanced breast cancer prestudy and baseline tumor assessment forms.

The advanced breast cancer prestudy form has basic baseline patient characteristics such as performance status and menopausal status. The disease history information is limited to receptor status and dates of diagnosis and first relapse. Current sites of disease are summarized as are the extent of surgery, radiotherapy, chemotherapy, and hormonal therapy received by the patient prior to registration on study. All items are needed for checking eligibility, for baseline information on which to base outcome evaluation, or later for analysis. A previous version of the prestudy asked for much more information, such as family history of breast cancer. This is an example of how asking for a lot of information just in case it might some day be interesting to examine was a waste of time. When the form was developed, there was little appreciation of how difficult family history information is to collect. In retrospect it is not surprising the data were so often incorrect or omitted that the information was unusable.

The former breast cancer prestudy also provides examples of potential logical difficulties on forms. Covering all the possibilities of missing information is a particular problem, e.g., it is not sufficient to ask only for "number of positive nodes," there also has to be a way to indicate "nodes not examined," "node positive, but number unknown," etc. At the other end of the logical completeness spectrum, it is probably not a good idea to go beyond all of the logical possibilities. The former prestudy, for instance, asked whether the patient's paternal and maternal relatives had breast cancer; unfortunately, paternal mother was included on the list. It never did become clear what either the question or the answers to it meant.

The baseline disease assessment form provides examples both for standardization and for the importance of asking specifically for information needed. The form is used for all solid tumor sites. Lesions are listed along with the method of assessment and the lesion size (measurements for measurable lesions to be followed, description of extent otherwise). Having all baseline disease sites and methods of assessment recorded is necessary to assess response. Before introduction of the baseline forms, baseline information was haphazardly recorded on the first flow sheet. It was then often unclear which lesions were being described on subsequent forms, and therefore it was often difficult to assess response.

A sample Notice of Death form is included in Section 6.9. This form, used for all studies, records date of death, causes of death (cancer, toxicity, other), and the sources of death information.

6.4 Protocol management and evaluation

6.4.1 Registration

Registration of patients onto a study is the first step in study management. Key to this process is consideration of patient eligibility. The Southwest Oncology Group utilizes an eligibility checklist (an example is in Section 6.9) that consists of the eligibility criteria specified in the protocol. This can be either a separate document or incorporated as part of the eligibility section of the protocol. All criteria must be verified for the patient to be eligible. The checklist may be submitted as part of the initial forms set after registration, or if a preliminary review is needed, prior to registration. For SWOG studies, there are also certain standard items of information collected at registration for patients on all studies, such as social security number, race, age, sex, method of payment and zipcode; these can be incorporated into the eligibility checklist or collected separately on a registration form. Institutions fill out the checklist and registration form before registering a patient. Fewer ineligible patients are registered when institutions are required to do a careful check to answer all questions before entering the patient on trial.

The Group's registration policies mentioned above are enforced at the time of registration; no exceptions are allowed. If an institution tries to register more than 1 working day prior to the planned treatment start, they are asked to register later. Patients are not removed from the data base if an institution tries to call back and say they made a mistake. If an eligibility criterion is not met, the registration is refused. We have found that if any exceptions are ever made, we wind up arguing endlessly about what should and should not be exceptions. Better to mishandle the rare case that should have been an exception than waste vast amounts of time trying to avoid mishandling the rest.

After the registration is complete, it is helpful to send a confirmation of registration to the institution. This confirmation reiterates the treatment assignment and reminds the clinical research associate which initial materials are due and when. Immediate confirmations should result in no forgotten patients, better compliance with the initial forms set submission, and quick correction if the wrong treatment arm was given mistakenly.

6.4.2 Data flow

Data flow is another important part of study management. Particularly in a setting with dozens of studies and hundreds of institutions, one must be ever vigilant against chaos.

In our Group, institutions submit copies of required forms to the statistical center by mail (still true for most studies) or by fax or Web (already implemented for large prevention studies due to the volume of forms). When these arrive, they are sorted by study and date stamped (so timeliness of form submission can be monitored) and are then entered into the data base. How much is immediately entered by data entry personnel for mail or immediately committed without review to the data base for electronic submission depends on the form — all of the information in the prestudies is entered, for instance, but for forms that require a lot of interpretation, such as the flow sheets or treatment and toxicity forms, only the last contact date is entered for mail forms or committed without review for electronic forms. Mailed forms are then sent to a data coordinator, who keeps them until it is time to evaluate, summarize, and enter the patient data. Information from electronic forms not yet reviewed can either be stored in holding files or can be flagged as pending until reviewed and verified by a data coordinator. After evaluation and entry of the basic data set into the data base, paper forms are filed in the patient chart (in SWOG, paper charts for old studies, electronic images for recent studies). Electronically submitted forms are automatically stored in an electronic chart. (Two filing hints for paper charts: (1) If there are thousands of charts to maintain, filing by terminal instead of leading digit of the patient number keeps them spread around the chart room instead of accumulating in one spot at a time. (2) When patients can be on multiple studies, there are fewer problems if all of the information on a patient is kept in the same chart instead of in several charts by study. This avoids problems such as having conflicting follow-up information on the same patient depending on which study chart is reviewed.) For studies requiring chart review by the study coordinator (all but the large prevention studies), copies of the charts are sent after evaluation and entry.

Submitted information that is not on forms, such as radiotherapy films and pathology material, are sent by the institution directly to the reviewer, with a form sent to the statistical center documenting the submission. For some protocols materials are sent to the statistical center first, which then forwards the material for review. Routing through the statistical center is considered when it is too difficult to track where materials are if they are sent elsewhere first.

One way we encourage timely submission of forms and materials from the institutions is through our Expectation report. This is a monthly report sent to institutions detailing forms and follow-up that will be due soon or that are overdue. The general requirements for data submission include: the initial forms set to be sent within 2 weeks of registration, pathology materials to be sent within 30 days, and RT materials within 30 days of completion of RT. Flow sheets or treatment and toxicity forms generally must be submitted every 3 months while the patient is on treatment, and follow-up forms every 6 months after off treatment. Notices of events (discontinuation of treatment, recurrence, second primary, death) are due within 2 or 4 weeks of the event. Long-term survivors are followed yearly. The Group has policies that cover institutions out of compliance with forms submission. If the initial forms set is overdue by more than 30 days for 10% or more patients at an institution, or if follow-up is behind (no last contact date for more than 7 months for patients on treatment, or more than 14 months for patients off treatment) on more than 20% of patients, the institution is given 3 months to get caught up. If the deadline is not met, registration privileges are suspended until the institution is in compliance. The threat of suspension has been a good deterrent, so has not often been necessary — but has been effective when imposed. Group institutions are continuing to improve and are currently running at about 6% overdue on initial forms sets and 13% overdue on follow-up.

6.4.3   Evaluation of data

Evaluation of the patient data is probably the most important aspect of study management. Data coordinators in the statistical center evaluate the patient chart first; this evaluation is then sent to the study coordinator for review and correction. Usually the data coordinators and study coordinators reach agreement on the evaluations. For the occasional cases where they do not, the disease committee chair decides what is correct. At the initial evaluation eligibility and stratification factors are checked against the prestudy, eligibility is checked against the first flow sheet and the pathology and operative reports, and the initial dose calculation is checked. At evaluations triggered by patient events, treatment and outcome information is abstracted. Clarification is often requested concerning missing information, causes of adverse reactions, and reasons for noncompliance. Study coordinators and data coordinators both look out for excess toxicity and misinterpretations of protocol. If problems are identified, the study coordinator submits any necessary changes or clarifications to the protocol to the operations office for distribution to the institutions.

We think this double review process works quite well. Review by data coordinators at the statistical center is important for consistency across studies within disease sites and for keeping study evaluations up to date. However, the data coordinators do not have medical expertise, so it is also important to have the study coordinator herself review the data, and not assign this task to anyone else. Clinical judgment is required for many aspects of evaluation, such as for adverse drug reaction reporting, for interpretation of pathology reports, for making judgments about circumstances not covered in response and toxicity definitions, in monitoring for excess toxicities and in recognition of clinical patterns of toxicity or response. For studies with nonstandard endpoints (such as imaging studies or secondary noncancer endpoints) additional endpoint reviews by an expert panel may also be important.

We generate a variety of reports to help in the evaluation process. Lists of which patients are due for evaluation are generated periodically. Typical times for evaluation include when the patient goes off treatment, when the patient progresses, and when the patient dies. Patient information on Phase II studies is evaluated more often because of the need for closer monitoring. Other types of reports consist of data consistency checks that are generated periodically by the study. An example of what is included in these reports might be a list of patients who went off study due to progression of disease, but do not have progression dates. Reports of possible Adverse Drug Reactions that have not yet been reported to NCI are also generated for review by the operations office and study coordinator to determine if action is necessary (if so, the institution is notified).

In addition to reports, standard data summary tables are generated at least every 6 months. The tables are used for the semi-annual report of studies produced for each Group meeting and for study monitoring. Note that it is possible to have standard summary tables only because we have a standard data set. Without standards the study monitoring process would be vastly more time consuming, requiring extensive programming efforts to create customized summaries for every study.

Some of the standard tables from SWOG 8811 are included in Section 6.10. The registration, eligibility, and evaluability table reports on the number of patients registered, those found to be ineligible, and those whose data can be evaluated for various endpoints. On SWOG 8811 there was one ineligible patient (no metastatic or locally recurrent disease). Since measurable disease was required, the baseline disease status in the table is measurable for all eligible patients. The table indicates that all patients were evaluated for toxicity, but assessment for response was not as good — 13 patients had disease assessments that were inadequate for the determination of response. This includes the types of patients mentioned previously — ones with unconfirmed responses, no assessments, and ones who died of other causes before response was determined.

The toxicity table gives the maximum grade of specific toxicities (there are about 300, most of which will not occur on a specific protocol) experienced by patients on treatment. On SWOG 8811 the most commonly experienced toxicities were leukopenia, granulocytopenia, thrombocytopenia, diarrhea, mucositis, nausea, and vomiting as expected. The fact that there are no grade 5 toxicities means that no patients died of treatment-related causes.

Response tables and survival curves are not routinely presented in the report of studies until the study is complete (per our data monitoring policy discussed in Chapter 5), but are generated for interim review by the monitoring committee (Phase II studies are monitored by a less formal committee consisting of the study coordinator, study statistician, and disease committee chair). The SWOG 8811 table indicates one CR and one PR in the group with prior treatment for metastatic disease, and four CRs in the no prior treatment group. The table also indicates there were four patients on the study with unconfirmed responses, eight more with inadequate disease assessment without suggestion of response, and one patient who died early. Median survival and progression-free survival on this study were 16 and 6 months, respectively (not shown).

Tables not included in Section 6.10 are a patient characteristic table, which includes characteristics collected on all patients (sex, age, race, ethnicity) plus the study-specific factors identified in the protocol (prior treatment groups in this case), a treatment summary table that indicates how many patients are off treatment (all off for this study), reasons off treatment (5 due to receiving maximum planned treatment, 37 due to progression, 2 due to death, 4 due to toxicity, 9 for other reasons), and number of major deviations (none).

6.4.4 Publication

The final step in the management and evaluation of a study is publication of the results. This involves a final cleanup of the data to resolve any outstanding evaluation questions and to bring everything up to date. The primary study analysis is dictated by the objectives and the design of the study; see Chapters 3, 4, and 7. After the statistician analyzes the study, the study coordinator drafts a manuscript. When both the study coordinator and statistician (who are first and second authors of the paper) are satisfied with a draft, it is circulated to other authors for review and approval.

6.4.5 Resolution of problems: Examples from SWOG·8811

We conclude the section on protocol management and evaluation with a discussion of a few of the problems that had to be resolved on SWOG 8811 during the course of the study. One problem concerned the definition of measurable disease. We were still working on our standard definitions at the time this protocol was opened. One of the issues we were considering was the problem of palpable disease. Is this measurable or not? It must be possible to reliably measure a lesion to considerate it measurable. The problem with palpable disease is measurement error — size estimates based on palpation have been shown to be highly variable. For instance, a 1×1 cm lesion needs to shrink only to 0.7×0.7 cm to be a PR; a change of this size cannot be reliably distinguished by palpation. For SWOG 8811 it was decided to define all palpable disease as nonmeasurable. Since then the new RECIST criteria have defined a palpable lesion as measurable only if it measures > 2 cm.

The problem of bone lesions was equally troublesome. Eventually all bone disease was termed nonmeasurable but evaluable, and it was specified that increased uptake on bone scans did not constitute evidence of progression (unless new sites appeared).

Other issues that had to be resolved on SWOG 8811 included disagreement on several responses. One case initially coded as a PR by the study coordinator was changed after discussion to unconfirmed response. In this case the confirmatory scan was done only 2 weeks after the first. The time cutoff we use for confirmation (3 weeks) is arbitrary, but necessary if confirmed response is to have a standard definition. In this particular case, the repeat scan had been done due to increasing symptoms in the patient, so treating this patient as a nonresponder was probably the correct decision in any case.

In a second problem case, the statistical center initially classified a case as having inadequate disease assessment; after clarification by the study coordinator that a poorly visible mediastinal node could not be reliably assessed and should be considered nonevaluable, this was changed to a PR.

One final case was changed from PR to not assessed. In this case the only evidence of PR was based on MRI scans after a baseline CT. Since the evidence was not based on the same tests as baseline, it could not be used to document a partial response.

SWOG 8811 also provides an example of how studies are amended after the first evaluations are done. The study coordinator in this study observed excess toxicity on the initial protocol chemotherapy doses. The toxicities were not so severe that the initial dose had to be reduced again, but it was decided to amend the protocol by adding another dose reduction, so that patients could be kept on some level of treatment for a longer period of time.

The final issue that had to be resolved for SWOG 8811 was the conclusion in the manuscript. There were a few responses in patients on study, so the regimen did have some activity. However, neither group met the design criteria for sufficient activity to be of interest, so in the end we agreed to a fairly negative summary and conclusion.

6.5 Quality assurance audits

A statistical center can ensure only that the data base is internally consistent. Without copies of the primary patient records, we cannot be sure that what we receive matches what happens at the clinics. External audits done by clinicians are necessary to ensure this aspect of quality. Our Group recommends institutions be audited at least every 3 years (more often if problems are discovered). Charts reviewed should include a representative sample of patients entered on study by the institution, plus any specific charts identified by the statistical center or study coordinators as problem cases. How many charts are reviewed is, unfortunately, more a function of how much money is available than how many should be reviewed, but do note that a review of less than 10% will not be credible. In addition to chart review, compliance with regulatory requirements (e.g., drug logs) needs to be reviewed.

Review is not sufficient of course. Standards must be established and corrective measures applied when institutions are out of compliance. Measures might include scheduling another audit in 6 months, recommendations for new procedures, or suspension of registration privileges until improvement is documented.

Detection of fraud requires extreme measures: expulsion of all involved, audit of all records from the institution, omission of all falsified data from analysis. Someone careful who is determined to falsify data is extremely difficult to detect, however. Even if auditors were to assume dishonesty, there would be time for only a superficial search for duplicate records. It is unlikely anything would be found, and the ill will generated by the assumption would be highly counterproductive to a cooperative effort. Fraud is more likely to be detected within the institution by someone whose job could be in jeopardy, so it is reasonable to establish procedures for anonymous reporting of suspected fraud. Not to minimize the seriousness of the offense — fraud is intolerable — but at least in a setting of multiple institutions and investigators the effects on a study of falsified information from a single source are diluted and should result in relatively small biases.

6.6 Training

Another important aspect of data management and quality control is training. Standardization of definitions and procedures allows development of standard training courses as well. In SWOG, training courses are presented to all new data coordinators, statisticians, clinical research associates, and study coordinators.

Data coordinator and statistician training occurs at the statistical center. The courses cover such things as the goals and history of the Group, computer training, explanations of SWOG structures and procedures, and a detailed review of SWOG standards.

Institutional clinical research associates and study coordinators are trained at the group meetings. Topics covered for clinical research associates include how to fill out the forms, methods for tracking down patients who are lost to follow-up, toxicity reporting, elements of informed consent, how to register patients, and how to order investigational drugs. Study coordinators are told in detail what their responsibilities will be and what policies with which they are expected to comply; they are also initiated into the mysteries of protocol development and response assessment. For both clinical research associates and study coordinators, hands on exercises are useful in illustrating the points made in the lectures.

Training courses are a good introduction but cannot possibly cover everything — thus, we maintain extensive documentation detailing responsibilities, procedures, standards, etc. for data coordinators, clinical research associates, and study coordinators. Writing documentation is an onerous task, but dealing with the data messes that occur without documentation is even worse.

6.7 Data base management

The field of data base management is a highly specialized one with a large body of literature and a language all its own. We will only touch on some of the more important aspects, focusing on computerized data base management for organizations carrying out multiple clinical trials, whether in single institutions or in cooperative groups. A good review of this field is given by McFadden et al., 1995.

6.7.1 Data base structures

The software used by most trial organizations today is one of several commercially available relational data base management systems. The relational model can be thought of simply as organizing data into tables that can be linked to other tables by certain key variables. For example, the SWOG data base has a table for data unique to a patient (patient identifier, sex, date of birth, race, vital status, last contact date, etc.) and other tables for data unique to a patient on a given study, such as the toxicity table (patient identifier, study number, types and degrees of toxicities) and the evaluation table (patient identifier, study number, eligibility, time to progression, etc.). Data from the patient table can be linked to these other tables through the patient identifier. This kind of structure is highly flexible (tables can be added as needed) and very intuitive; there is a close correspondence between many of the tables and the data collection forms (for instance, tables corresponding to prestudy forms). Retrieval of data for analysis is a matter of specifying and linking the relevant tables (forms). The relational model is thus particularly suited to statistical analysis, as opposed to hierarchical data bases. Hierarchical structure consists of a pyramid of record types, where each record type is owned by the record type next up in the hierarchy. For instance, if the basic unit (highest record type) is the patient, the first record type might be characteristics of the patient that do not change (date of birth, sex, date and type of diagnosis, etc.), the next might be visit basics (date of visit, BSA, etc.), the next level outcomes from the visit (lab values, agents and doses administered, etc.) Hierarchical data bases that are patient oriented are more suited to retrieving data on individual patients (e.g., for clinical use) than for retrieving data for analysis. For instance, accessing a toxicity table for analysis is much more straightforward than identifying all visits for which patients were on a particular study and summarizing toxicities from those visits. A hierarchical structure with study as the basic unit is better but not ideal when patients can be on multiple studies (then information that does not change for a patient must be repeated for each study) or when the same forms are used for multiple studies (then the same table cannot be used for all occurrences of the same form). For more information about the advantages of the relational model for clinical trials organizations, see Blumenstein (1989).

The standards described in the preceding sections of this chapter for common definitions of data items find their expression in the data base. This standardization also facilitates the development of *edit checks*, which are programmed rules added to the data base management system to make sure individual data items are within specified ranges or take values from the right set of codes, and to make sure items have the proper relationships (date of progression is later than date of registration on study, for example). Edit checks can be implemented at data entry (within a form) or when data are submitted to the data base (to cross-check against other forms). In either case the programming job is made easier by the fact that basic patient items are standardized across all studies; some other items are standard within a disease type, etc.

6.7.2   Data collection, transmission, and entry

A dream of many of those involved in the conduct of clinical trials is that the day will come when all the data needed to analyze a study have already been captured in the hospital information system or computerized medical record and merely need to be transmitted to a research data base and summarized. That day is a long way off. If everyone agreed to use compatible hardware and software the technological hurdles would not be particularly hard to overcome, but the universal experience to date is that data collected for one purpose (such as patient care) are not suitable for another (such as clinical research). The requisite data are not available, are not coded appropriately, or are not of sufficient quality. Thus, research data must be culled by skilled clinical research associates from several sources, some computerized and some not, and put into shape for transmission to the central statistical center.

Organizations differ as to whether the CRAs enter data directly into a computer system or onto forms for transmission to the statistical center. An argument for the former is the belief that those closest to the source of the data have the best chance of making sure that data entry is done correctly. In practice this argument has the most validity when the data are of use at the clinical site and when entry occurs at the same time the data are generated. With multi-center cancer clinical trials this is rarely the case, because the trial organization is just a small part of the cancer practice at the site and is often just one of many such organizations, all with different data requirements. What often happens instead with remote data entry is that forms are filled out at the site, then entered into the computer later as a separate step, also at the site. Because of the relatively low volume of data entry from a given site, this means that the task of data entry is done by people with many other things to do instead of by people at the statistical center for whom data entry is the primary job. Both timeliness and quality suffer as a result. Also, a great deal of effort is involved in setting up data entry procedures at multiple sites and maintaining the necessary hardware and software, so many cancer clinical trial groups still ask that CRAs fill out paper forms for transmission to the statistical center, where they are entered into the central data base (often with duplicate entry as a verification step). The transmission is most often done by mail, but lately the use of facsimile (fax) transmission followed by supervised optical character recognition (OCR) has been growing because of better timeliness and lower data entry personnel requirements. On the other hand, entry at the site does mean that basic edit checks can be done immediately and the form can be refused until obvious problems are resolved, such as missing items or out-of-range values. This saves time in the data query and resolution process, which can be excessively time consuming when handled by mail. Other advantages are automatic resolution of expectations; no mail delays; and computer access by clinical research associates to previous submissions, facilitating forms management at the institution. Furthermore, managing Web entry through a dedicated central server represents a significant improvement in resource needs over older distributed data entry procedures. Instead of installing and maintaining entry programs at every participating institution (or requiring dedicated programming staff at each institution), statistical center staff can do all programming maintenance at the statistical center. Help (by telephone or email) for configuring local PCs for internet access to the programs is needed, so extra resources are still required compared to mailing, but the extra resources are becoming affordable. SWOG has implemented fax and OCR for its first prostate cancer prevention trial and a combination of Web and fax-OCR submission for its second prostate cancer prevention trial. Paper forms mailed to the statistical center for data entry are still the standard method for therapeutic trials, although this is changing.

Our paper systems have a proven quality and were the only practical alternative in the statistical center until recently, particularly considering the wide range of technical capabilities — from highly sophisticated to nonexistent — at the participating institutions. Change is now becoming feasible as institutional capabilities expand and comercial products, such as those that allow for both fax-OCR and Web submission, improve.

6.8 Conclusion

To those coordinating a study: be as clear as you possibly can, about absolutely everything you can think of, to absolutely everyone involved. Then you will have something useful at the end of the study in addition to a beautiful initial concept. To those participating on a study: every mistake made in following the protocol or recording information on the data forms jeopardizes the credibility of the trial. Be compulsive!

6.9 Appendix: Examples

6.9.1 Treatment table for 8811

Agent	Starting dose	Route	Days	ReRx interval	Notes
Folinic acid	500 mg/m^2 per day	IV continuous infusion	5 1/2 days, starting day 0	4 weeks	Start infusion 24 hrs before day 1 5-FU
5-FU	370 mg/m^2 per day	IV bolus	1,2,3,4,5	4 weeks	

6.9.2 Sample study calendar

Required study	Pre-study	Day 15	29	43	57	71	85	99	113	*
PHYSICAL:										
H & P	x		x		x		x		x	
Toxicity assessment	x	x	x	x	x	x	x	x	x	
Tumor assessment	x		x		x		x		x	
LABORATORY:										
CBC, platelets	x	x	x	x	x	x	x	x	x	
Serum creatinine	x		x		x		x		x	
Bilirubin	x		x		x		x		x	
SGOT	x		x		x		x		x	
X-RAYS & SCANS:										
Chest x-ray	x		x		x		x		x	
Scans for tumor assessment	x				x				x	

* Continue according to the same schedule until patient is off treatment. After discontinuation of treatment, schedule follow-up visits at least every 6 months.

6.9.3 Sample flow sheet

SWOG 8811						
Date year:____ m/d	/	/	/	/	/	Pt #_____Reg dt_/_/_
Treatment						Pt initials_____
BSA						Investigator_____
Folinic Acid						Institution_____
5-FU						**Progress notes** (date each)
Laboratory						
Hgb						
Platelets/μl						
WBC/μl						
granulocytes						
lymphocytes						
Serum creat. IULN____						
Bilirubin IULN____						
SGOT IULN____						
Calcium						
Physical						
Temperature						
Weight (kg)						
Hemorrhage/infection	/	/	/	/	/	
Performance status						
X-rays and scans						
Chest x-ray						
Bone scan						
Other scans						
Lesions						
#1						
#2						
#3						
#4						
List other lesions in notes						
Toxicity (record grade)						
Nausea/vomiting						
Stomatitis/mucositis		*				
Diarrhea						
Alopecia						
Other, specify						

APPENDIX: EXAMPLES

6.9.4 Sample treatment and toxicity form for a single agent treatment given every 4 weeks for 1 day

SOUTHWEST ONCOLOGY GROUP
TOXICITY AND DOSAGE FORM

SWOG Patient ID [ ][ ][ ][ ]   SWOG Study No. [S][ ][ ][ ][ ]
Patient Initials _____ (L, F M)
Institution _____ Physician _____

Instructions: Complete after every course of treatment, just prior to initiation of next course; and at time of discontinuation of treatment, after resolution of all toxicities of the final course. All dates are **MONTH, DAY, YEAR**. Place an [X] in appropriate boxes. Circle **AMENDED** items in red.

PATIENT STATUS
Date of Last Contact or Death: [ ][ ] / [ ][ ] / [ ][ ][ ][ ]
Vital Status: ☐ Alive ☐ Dead *(submit Notice of Death)*

TREATMENT STATUS
Course number: [ ][ ]   Dose of agent A administered this course: [ ][ ].[ ] mg/m^2
Date administered: [ ][ ] / [ ][ ] / [ ][ ][ ][ ]

Were there any omissions, additions, or modifications to treatment since the last form?
☐ No   ☐ Yes, type and reason:

Is the patient still on protocol treatment? ☐ Yes   ☐ No *(Submit Off Treatment Notice)*

TOXICITIES EXPERIENCED THIS COURSE
(From the date of administration noted above to just before administration of next course.)
Date of toxicity assessment: [ ][ ] / [ ][ ] / [ ][ ][ ][ ]   Use CTC 2.0 definitions.

Grade	Toxicity	Grade	Toxicity	Grade	Toxicity
☐	Edema	☐	Neutropenia	☐	Nausea
☐	Headache	☐	Leukopenia	☐	Vomiting
☐	Fatigue	☐	Thrombocytopenia	☐	Diarrhea
☐	Fever	☐	SGOT	☐	Stomatitis
☐	Chills	☐	Bilirubin	☐	Other: _____
☐	Myalgia	☐	Alkaline Phosphatase	☐	Other: _____
☐	Dyspnea	☐	Creatinine	☐	Other: _____

Notes:

6.9.5 Sample follow-up form

SOUTHWEST ONCOLOGY GROUP
FOLLOW-UP FORM

SWOG Patient ID ☐☐☐☐☐   SWOG Study No. [S]☐☐☐☐

Patient Initials _____ (L, F M)

Institution _____   Physician _____

Instructions: Please submit at each follow-up after completion of treatment until recurrence, at time of recurrence, and at protocol-specified intervals after recurrence. All dates are **MONTH, DAY, YEAR**. Answer all questions and explain any blank fields or blank dates in the **Notes** section. Place an [X] in appropriate boxes. Circle AMENDED items in red.

VITAL STATUS
Vital Status: ☐ Alive   ☐ Dead   Date of last contact or death: ☐☐ / ☐☐ / ☐☐☐☐
If vital status is Dead, complete and submit Notice of Death form.

DISEASE FOLLOW-UP STATUS
Has the patient had a documented clinical assessment for this cancer since submission of the previous follow-up form?
☐ No   ☐ Yes   If Yes, Date of Last Clinical Assessment: ☐☐ / ☐☐ / ☐☐☐☐

NOTICE OF FIRST RELAPSE OR PROGRESSION
Has the patient developed a first relapse or progression that has not been previously reported?
☐ No   ☐ Yes   If Yes, Date of Relapse or Progression: ☐☐ / ☐☐ / ☐☐☐☐

Site(s) of Relapse or Progression: _____

NOTICE OF NEW PRIMARY
Has a new primary cancer or myelodysplastic syndrome (MDS) been diagnosed that has not been previously reported?
☐ No   ☐ Yes   If Yes, Date of Diagnosis: ☐☐ / ☐☐ / ☐☐☐☐

New Primary Site: _____

NON-PROTOCOL TREATMENT
Has the patient received any non-protocol cancer therapy (prior to progression/relapse) not previously reported?
☐ No   ☐ Yes   If Yes, Date of First Non-Protocol Therapy: ☐☐ / ☐☐ / ☐☐☐☐

Agents: _____

LONG-TERM TOXICITY
Has the patient experienced (prior to treatment for progression or relapse or a second primary, and prior to non-protocol treatment) any severe (grade ≥ 3) long-term toxicity that has not been previously reported?
☐ No   ☐ Yes   If Yes, Toxicities and Grades: _____

Notes:

APPENDIX: EXAMPLES

6.9.6 *Sample notice of death*

SOUTHWEST ONCOLOGY GROUP
NOTICE OF DEATH

SWOG Patient ID [ ][ ][ ][ ][ ] Most Recent SWOG Study No. [S][ ][ ][ ][ ]

Patient Initials _____ (L, F M)

Institution _____ Physician _____

Instructions: Answer all questions and explain any blank fields or blank dates in the **Notes** section. Place an [X] in appropriate boxes. Circle AMENDED items in red.

Date of Death: [ ][ ] / [ ][ ] / [ ][ ][ ][ ]   (month / day / year)

CAUSES OF DEATH

Any cancer (select one):
☐ No ☐ Primary Cause ☐ Contributory ☐ Possible ☐ Unknown

If cancer was the primary cause or if cancer possibly or definitely contributed to death, and the patient had had multiple tumor types, specify those which were causes of death:

☐ Cancer of most recent SWOG study, specify cancer: _____
☐ Cancer of other SWOG study, specify cancer: _____
☐ Other cancer, specify: _____

Toxicity from disease-related treatment (select one):
☐ No ☐ Primary Cause ☐ Contributory ☐ Possible ☐ Unknown

If Primary Cause, Contributory or Possible, specify treatment and toxicity:

[   ]

Non-cancer and non-treatment related causes (select one):
☐ No ☐ Primary Cause ☐ Contributory ☐ Possible ☐ Unknown

If Primary Cause, Contributory or Possible, specify:

[   ]

Death information obtained from (select all that apply):
☐ Autopsy report
☐ Medical record / Death certificate
☐ Physician
☐ Relative or friend
☐ Other, specify: _____

Notes:

[   ]

6.9.7 Sample checklist

SWOG-8811 Phase II trial of 5-fluorouracil and high dose folinic acid as first or second line therapy for advanced breast cancer.

SWOG Patient ID		Pt. initials	
Caller's ID		Pt. date of birth	
Investigator ID		Pt. sex	
Institution ID		Pt. race/ethnicity	/
Payment method		Pt. SSN	
IRB approval date		Pt. zip code	
Date informed consent signed		Projected treatment start date	

Each of the items in the following section must be verified for the patient to be considered eligible for registration. The checklist should be filled out entirely before registration.

Verify each item:
___ 1. Patients must have a histologic diagnosis of adenocarcinoma of the breast.
___ 2. Patients must have incurable metastatic or locally recurrent disease.
___ 3. Patients must have sites of measurable disease.
___ 4. All measurable lesions must have been assessed within 28 days prior to registration. All nonmeasurable disease must have been assessed within 42 days prior to registration.
Date measurable disease assessed_____
Date nonmeasurable disease assessed_____
___ 5. Patients must not have received more than one prior chemotherapy for advanced disease. (If the patient relapsed within 12 months of adjuvant chemotherapy, count this as one chemotherapy for advanced disease.)
___ 6. If the patient has received prior RT, it must have been completed at least 2 weeks prior to registration.
Date prior RT completed_____ (Indicate NA if no prior RT).
___ 7. If the patient has received chemotherapy, it must have been completed at least 3 weeks prior to registration.
Date last chemotherapy_____ (Indicate NA if no prior chemo)
___ 8. Patients must not have had previous treatment with 5-FU plus leukovorin as a modulator of antimetabolite activity (Note: Prior 5-FU is acceptable. Prior leukovorin as protection against methotrexate is acceptable.
___ 9. Patients must have recovered from all toxicities of all prior treatment.

APPENDIX: EXAMPLES

___ 10. Patients must have performance status 0–2.
Performance status_____
___ 11. Patient must have WBC >4000, granulocytes >2000, platelets > 150,000 and hemoglobin > 10, obtained within 14 days prior to registration.
WBC_____Granulocytes_____ Platelets_____Hemoglobin_____
Date obtained_____
___ 12. Patients must have creatinine <1.5 × institutional upper limit of normal obtained within 14 days of registration.
Creatinine_____ IULN_____Date obtained_____
___ 13. Patients must have bilirubin <1.5 × institutional upper limit of normal obtained within 14 days of registration.
Bilirubin_____ IULN_____Date obtained_____
___ 14. Patients must not have had any prior malignancies other than non melanoma skin cancer, carcinoma in situ of the cervix, or cancer for which the patient has been disease free for 5 years.
___ 15. Patients must not be pregnant or nursing. Women of reproductive potential must agree to use an effective contrceptive method.

Stratification Factor (Response does not affect eligibility.)
Group:
___ A. Previous exposure to chemotherapy for metastatic disease, or relapse within 12 months of completing adjuvant chemotherapy.
___ B. No previous exposure to chemotherapy for metastatic disease AND if adjuvant chemotherapy was received, disease free for at least 12 months after completion.

6.9.8 Sample tables

SWOG 8811 registration, eligibility, and evaluability.

	Total	Prior Chemo. for Adv. Disease	No Prior Chemo. for Adv. Disease
Number registered	58	21	37
Ineligible	1	0	1
Eligible	57	21	36
Baseline disease status			
Measurable	57	21	36
Response assessment			
Adequate to determine response	44	16	28
Inadequate	13	5	8
Toxicity assessment			
Evaluable for toxicity	57	21	36
Not evaluable	0	0	0

SWOG-8811 Number of patients with a given type and degree of toxicity.

TOXICITY	unk	0	1	2	3	4	5
Abdominal pain	0	56	0	0	1	0	0
Allergy/rash	1	51	4	1	0	0	0
Alopecia	1	50	5	1	0	0	0
Anemia	0	46	3	4	3	1	0
Chills/fever	0	53	0	3	1	0	0
Diarrhea	0	21	14	15	6	1	0
Dizziness/hot flashes	0	55	2	0	0	0	0
DVT	0	56	0	0	1	0	0
Granulocytopenia	0	21	6	7	9	14	0
Headache	0	56	1	0	0	0	0
Ileus/constipation	0	54	3	0	0	0	0
Infections	0	54	0	2	0	1	0
Leukopenia	0	20	14	15	5	3	0
Lymphopenia	0	53	1	1	1	1	0
Stomatitis/mucositis	0	16	13	12	13	3	0
Nausea/vomiting	1	20	24	6	6	0	0
Thrombocytopenia	0	51	4	1	1	0	0
Weight loss	0	55	1	1	0	0	0
MAXIMUM GRADE ANY TOXICITY	1	3	9	8	20	16	0

SWOG 8811 Responses.

	Prior Chemo. for Adv. Disease		No Prior Chemo. for Adv. Disease	
Complete response	1	(5%)	4	(11%)
Partial response	1	(5%)	3	(8%)
Unconfirmed response	1	(5%)	3	(8%)
Stable	7	(33%)	12	(33%)
Assessment inadequate	4	(19%)	4	(11%)
Increasing disease	7	(33%)	9	(25%)
Early death	0	(0%)	1	(3%)
Total	21		36	

CHAPTER 7

Reporting of Results

Cave quid dicis, quando, et cui.

Reporting of the results from a clinical trial is one of the most anxiously awaited aspects of the clinical trials process. This reporting can take on many forms: reports to investigators during the conduct of the trial, interim outcome reports to the Data Monitoring Committee, abstracts submitted to scientific meetings, and finally, the published report in the medical literature. For any type of study report, it is important to recognize what type of information is appropriate to transmit, and how that information can be communicated in the most scientifically appropriate fashion. Recently, an international committee comprised of clinical trialists, statisticians, epidemiologists, and editors of biomedical journals reviewed the quality of reporting for randomized clinical trials. The result of this review led to two publications (Moher, Schultz, and Altman, 2001, Altman et al., 2001), under the title of CONSORT (Consolidated Standards of Reporting Trials). The CONSORT statement proposes a flow diagram for reporting trials, and a checklist of necessary items.

While there are still no absolute standards for the reporting of clinical trials, some basics regarding timing and content should be observed (see also, Simon and Wittes, 1985). For routine reports, accrual, ineligibility, major protocol deviations, and toxicity should be presented. Such reports are important for early identification of excess toxicity, ambiguities in the protocol, and other study management problems; this is discussed in Chapter 6. In this chapter we concentrate on interim (to the Data Monitoring Committee) and final reports on the major trial endpoints. Information in these reports should allow the reader to evaluate the trial: its design, conduct, data collection, analysis, and interpretation.

7.1 Timing of report

Once a trial has been opened, researchers turn their attention to the design of future trials, and are impatient for any clues that the current trial can provide for new study designs. Thus, almost from the beginning of patient accrual, there is pressure to report any data accumulated so far. As discussed in Chapter 5, a common problem in Phase III reporting has stemmed from a tendency to report primary outcome results while a trial is still accruing patients, or after study closure but before the data have "matured." Accrual may be affected and too many incorrect conclusions may be drawn when results are reported early. The use of monitoring committees and appropriate stopping rules minimizes such problems.

Early reporting causes similar problems in Phase II studies. Consider a trial designed to accrue 40 patients with advanced colorectal cancer. Of the first 25 patients accrued, 15 have gone off study and are evaluable for response, while the other 10 are either still on treatment, or have not had their records updated sufficiently to assess response. These 10 patients are not necessarily the last 10 to have registered — they might include patients who have been on therapy for a long time, patients who have poor compliance regarding return visits, or patients for whom required tests have been run, but have not yet been reported. Moreover, there may be a tendency for institutions to report the negative results first (less documentation is required). If this is the case, then the estimated response probability in the first evaluable 15 patients may be pessimistic as an estimate of the true response probability. The early pessimism may even result in changes in the types of patient registered to the study. For example, patients with less severe disease may now be put on other trials perceived to be more promising. This change in patient population could cause the registration of patients who are less likely to respond, resulting in a final response estimate that remains overly pessimistic. Thus, as for Phase III studies, care should be taken not to report results until the data are mature.

The definition of mature data is dependent upon the type of study being conducted, and should be specified prior to the opening of the trial. No matter the definition, however, the principle to be strictly enforced is that outcome information should not be reported until the study is closed to accrual, and the appropriate reporting time has been reached. This rule limits biases in the final outcome of the trial that can occur when early data are released.

7.1.1 Phase II trials

Typical Phase II trials have either response or survival at a specific time as the endpoint. For two-stage designs (commonly used for studies of investigational new drugs), reporting only occurs once permanent closure has taken place, and all registered patients were evaluated. Response is never reported at the conclusion of the first stage of accrual (unless the study closes after the first stage), for the reasons given above. Specific rules, which are established during the study planning phase, specify the results needed to continue to the second stage of accrual. When it is determined that accrual should continue, the actual number of observed responses is not reported; investigators are only informed that the minimum number of responses necessary for continuation has been observed and that the study will continue to completion. Once the study has closed and all patients have been evaluated for response, the final study report is prepared for presentation at professional meetings and for publication in the medical literature.

7.1.2 Phase III trials

Phase III trials typically last for many years, making the desire for early reporting even more acute. The literature is replete with examples of studies that reported early promising results, only to have those results negated once additional follow-up was available. SWOG 7924 (a study of radiotherapy vs. no radiotherapy after complete response to chemotherapy in patients with limited small-cell lung cancer) is an example. This was reported in ASCO abstracts as promising during accrual to the study (Kies et al., 1982) and positive after accrual (Mira, Kies, and Chen, 1984). The conclusion after the final analysis, however, was that there was no survival benefit due to radiotherapy (Kies et al., 1987). The timing of study reports should be defined in the study protocol, including the time of final analysis and times of interim analyses. At interim analysis times confidential outcome analyses are provided to the study's data monitoring committee (see Chapter 5). Only if this committee recommends early reporting (based on predefined guidelines) may the results of the study be released prior to the final analysis time defined in the protocol.

7.2 Required information

The amount of detail in a report will vary according to its purpose. Not everything needs to be included in a toxicity update to the data monitoring committee, whereas a manuscript should contain sufficient detail to allow informed judgment about whether, and if so, how, to use the regimens being discussed. In general, though, it will be important to include the following information.

7.2.1 Objectives and design

The aims of the trial should be stated in any report or manuscript (in the abstract and methods sections of a manuscript). Primary and secondary endpoints should be clearly defined. Response and toxicity, in particular, require definition as so many variations of these are in use. If an explanation is necessary, the relation of the endpoints to the objectives of the study should be stated.

The study design should be described, including whether the study is a Phase II or Phase III trial and if there are any predefined patient subsets with separate accrual goals. The target sample size should be given (for each subset if applicable), along with justification (precision of estimation, or level of test and power for a specified alternative). The interim analysis plan, if any, should be specified. For Phase III trials, some details of the randomization scheme should be given, including whether or not the randomization was balanced on stratification factors, and how that balance was achieved (see Chapter 3 for a discussion of randomization schemes).

7.2.2 Eligibility and treatment

A definition of the patient population under study is provided by a clear description of the eligibility criteria. Among the items that should be included are the site, histology, and stage of disease under study, any prior therapy restrictions, baseline laboratory values required for patient eligibility, and medical conditions contraindicating patient participation on the trial.

The details of the treatments should be defined (not just "5-FU therapy"), including dose, schedule, method of delivery, and required supportive therapy (e.g., hydration, growth factors). In the final manuscript dose modification plans should also be included.

REQUIRED INFORMATION 169

7.2.3 Results

The results section should include the timing of the report, i.e., whether it is the planned final analysis, a planned interim analysis to the DMC, or, if neither of these, justification for the early report. The results section should also include the time interval over which patients were accrued, the total number of patients registered in that period, the number of patients ineligible and reasons for ineligibility. If any patients are excluded from analyses, the reasons for the exclusions should be given (there should be very few of these, see below for guidelines).

Since eligibility criteria allow for a variety of patients to be entered on trial, a summary of the basic characteristics of patients actually accrued is necessary to indicate the risk status of the final sample. Examples of variables to include are patient demographics (age, sex, race, ethnicity), stratification factors, and other important descriptive factors (e.g., performance status, extent of disease, number of prior treatment regimens). For randomized trials, a statement on how well balanced the treatment arms are with respect to basic characteristics should also be included.

The text should also contain a summary of the treatment experience. This summary should include a report on the number of patients who completed therapy as planned, and the numbers and reasons for early termination of therapy. Reasons for early termination might include toxicity, death not due to disease, or patient refusal. For Phase III trials, if large numbers of patients have failed to complete therapy, some comparison between treatment arms with respect to patient compliance may be of interest. A summary of deviations to protocol specifications should also be included. Definitions of protocol deviation may vary and are rather subjective. Thus, a definition of what constitutes a deviation is appropriate in this summary.

The number of patients evaluated for toxicity, the number with adequate response and progression/relapse information, and an indication of maturity of follow-up should be provided. This last typically would include the number dead and the number lost to follow-up, plus minimum, maximum, and median follow-up time. However, there is some debate on how to calculate median follow-up time (Schemper and Smith, 1996). Among the ways to estimate this is to compute the median follow-up only for patients who remain alive (which we prefer), or compute the median of time from registration to last contact date (without regard to survival status). The manuscript should specify what statistic is being used. Some or all of survival, progression-free survival, response, and toxicity are generally primary and secondary outcomes in a trial; these should be summarized as discussed in the analysis section below. Exploratory results should be relegated to a separate section of the results and be accompanied by numerous statements minimizing the importance of anything observed.

7.3 Analyses

7.3.1 Exclusions, intent to treat

All patients entered onto the trial should be accounted for. In general, all eligible patients are included in any analyses from a study. This is the well-established intent-to-treat principle, which is the only method of analysis that eliminates selection bias. However, there may be some legitimate reasons for patient exclusions in certain analyses. For example, when estimating toxicity probabilities, it usually makes sense to exclude patients who were never treated. Keep in mind, though, that patient exclusions often can contribute to biased estimates of outcomes.

For Phase II trials with the goal of evaluating drug activity, all patients who receive drug should be included in the analyses. A bias in response probability estimates is caused when patients for whom response was not evaluable are excluded. Since the reasons for not being evaluable generally are indicative of treatment failure (death prior to formal tests of disease assessment, early progression, or early refusal of treatment), the result of excluding these patients from the analysis is that the response estimates are inflated. A recent American Society of Clinical Oncology abstract in the treatment of hepatocellular carcinoma with a thymidylate synthetase inhibitor reported an 8% response rate in 13 evaluable patients (Stuart et al., 1996). However, this study had enrolled 24 patients, 8 of whom had been judged to be inevaluable due to toxicity or rapid disease progression and 3 of whom were too early for evaluation. If one assumes that all 8 of the patients with toxicity or rapid progression failed to respond to therapy, then a revised response estimate becomes $1/21 = 0.05$, over a third less than the original estimate. Why is the original estimate in error? The goal of Phase II studies is to decide whether to continue study of the regimen. The decision is based on whether sufficient activity is observed in the type of patient defined by the eligibility criteria. The goal is not to estimate the response probability in the subgroup of patients who, after the fact, are known not to progress too fast on therapy, and not to develop early toxicities. (If this were the goal, then eligibility would have to include a requirement that patients be succeeding on the regimen for a specified time before registration is allowed.) The after-the-fact response probability might hold some interest, but it is useless for deciding whether a new patient should be treated with the regimen. We want the estimate that most nearly matches the prediction we can make for an individual patient prior to receiving drug, not the estimate we can give of what the chances are of response if they do not fail right away.

For Phase III trials, which by definition are comparative, the intent-to-treat principle states that all eligible patients are analyzed according to the arm to which they are randomized, even if the patient refuses therapy according to that arm, or even if their treatment involves a major deviation from protocol specifications. It is important to stress that eligibility is based on patient characteristics or tests done prior to registration. For example, a pathology specimen obtained prior to registration, but read as ineligible by the pathologist after the patient has been registered still means the patient is not eligible. The determination of ineligibility relates to the timing of patient information, not timing of the review.

The reason behind the intent-to-treat concept is to avoid the bias that can occur by arm-specific selective deviations or refusals. Reasons for treatment deviations cannot be assumed to be random. High-risk patients might be more likely than low-risk patients to refuse assignment to a less aggressive treatment arm, for instance, or very good-risk patients might decide toxicity is not worth whatever small benefit from treatment they might expect. Patient groups defined by initial treatment assignment are approximately comparable with respect to pretreatment characteristics because of randomization; systematically throwing some patients out of the study destroys that comparability. Note intent-to-treat does *not* mean that ineligible patients must be included in the analysis. It means that treatment received *after* randomization (or anything else that happens to the patient after randomization for that matter) cannot be used as a reason to exclude patients. No systematic bias should occur when patients on all treatment arms are omitted based on events or characteristics that occur or are collected prior to registration — randomization takes care of that. In fact, it is generally detrimental to leave ineligible patients in the primary analyses — it becomes impossible to characterize what type of patient the sample represents, and might mask whatever treatment effect there is.

7.3.2 Summary statistics: Estimates and variability of estimates

For Phase II trials, the primary outcome measure is usually response or survival. When it is response, the report should include the estimate of response probability (number of responses/number of eligible patients), as well as a survival curve (product-limit estimate, see Chapter 2). Survival should be included if response is the primary endpoint, since survival is always an important secondary endpoint. For Phase III trials, all major endpoints should be presented by treatment arm, along with estimates of medians and/or hazard ratio estimates for time-to-event endpoints. Estimates of differences adjusted for important prognostic factors are also often appropriate. When the proportional hazards model is correct, adjusting for important prognostic factors in a Cox model provides a better estimate of treatment effect (Anderson et al., 2002).

There is often a temptation to provide survival curves for responders vs. nonresponders. However, as discussed in Chapter 8, such comparisons are virtually meaningless. Duration of response out of context with the rest of the times to failure is not particularly useful either. Instead, a progression-free survival curve based on all patients on trial should be given. The durable responses will appear on these curves as late failures. The duration-of-response information is still there, while the additional failures provide information on what proportion of patients are early and late failures — thus you get a more complete picture of the results of the trial than an estimate based only on responders.

For both Phase II and Phase III studies toxicity summary information is important. More detailed summaries generally are required for Phase II studies, for which further characterization of toxicity of the regimen typically is a goal. An exhaustive list of toxicities observed on the study, including all degrees of toxicity, may be in order. For Phase III studies employing only well-characterized treatment agents, it may be sufficient to report the number of patients with high degrees of common toxicities, plus any unexpected toxicities of any degree that were observed.

For quality of life (QOL) endpoints, a description of the QOL instrument and its properties (reliability, validity, and sensitivity to change in patient status) should be provided, as should the timing of assessments and compliance with filling out the forms. A summary of QOL data is particularly challenging due to the fact that these data are often missing and that this pattern of missing data is not random, but related to the endpoint. Patients may not fill out forms due to factors related to poor quality of life (such as deterioration due to disease, excess toxicity, depression, or death) or due to factors related to good quality of life (such as going on vacation when the form is due).

In analyzing change in QOL from baseline to subsequent times, estimates are biased if either all patients at baseline are compared to all patients who fill out forms at each time, or if only patients with both baseline and all subsequent forms are used in the comparison. In the first case, if patients with seriously decreased quality of life at time T do not fill out forms, the average at time T is biased toward good QOL and any favorable difference between baseline and time T is an overestimate. In the second, differences between baseline and time T in the subset of patients who filled out all forms may not reflect differences in the whole group; in this case it may be less clear which way the bias goes, but typically this also overestimates any improvement.

An approach to examining QOL data that addresses some of the difficulties and allows for identification of bias involves summarizing according to the drop-out pattern and reason for drop-out. Averages for patients with only baseline and the first assessment are presented, along with averages for patients with only baseline plus the first and second assessments, and so on, which constitute a more comprehensive summary of the results than the simpler approaches often used. The averages can be restricted further according to reasons for drop-out. Such summaries often reveal worse QOL for early drop-outs, decreased QOL at the time of last completed assessment, and steeper decline when the reason for discontinuing QOL assessments is due to illness or death. All of these indicate drop-out is related to QOL. Figure 7.1, adapted from part of a figure in Moinpour et al. (2000), shows the result of such a strategy for a measure of symptom distress collected in SWOG 8905 (Leichman et al., 1995), a study of 5-FU in advanced colon cancer. The two dashed lines give the symptom distress score for patients who discontinued follow-up due to death or illness, with separate plots for patients who completed two or three QOL questionnaires. These two lines show higher baseline values (corresponding to worse symptom distress), and steeper slopes than the solid lines, which represent patients who dropped out after two or three visits for other reasons. Patients who completed follow-up (dotted plot) started with the lowest baseline values, and had the flattest slopes over time. Analysis methods using models that incorporate patterns of drop-out are becoming common. (See Troxel et al., 1998 and Hogan and Laird, 1997 for discussions of issues and methods.)

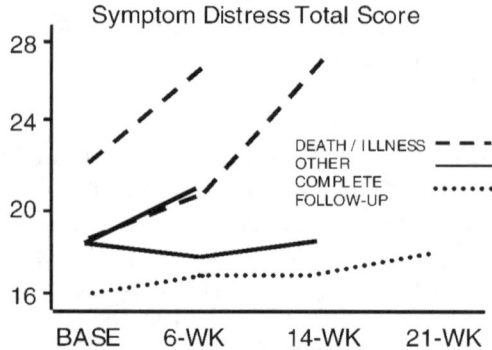

Figure 7.1. Example of biased follow-up due to nonrandomly missing QOL data.

Perhaps the most important summary information in a report is an indication of how reliable the results are. Generally this is done with confidence intervals (see Chapter 2) for the reported estimates. An estimated treatment hazard ratio of 1.9 with a confidence interval of 0.94 to 3.8, for instance, could be interpreted as exciting if the confidence interval was not reported. When the confidence interval is reported it becomes clear the result is highly unreliable (consistent with no difference at all as well as with an astonishing benefit) and worth at most guarded optimism, not excitement. While it is always important to report confidence intervals, it is absolutely critical to report them for interim reports lest early trends be overinterpreted. For these, the confidence intervals should not be the standard 95% intervals, but should reflect the early conservatism built into the design (see Chapter 5). If a test of level 0.01 is being done at an interim analysis, then a 99% confidence interval is more suitable than a 95% interval.

Estimation and confidence intervals when interim analyses are part of the design bring up a difficult statistical issue. If a study continues after the first interim analysis, then one decision has already been made that results are not consistent with very small response probabilities (Phase II) or that differences are not exceptionally large (Phase III). Incorporation of these observations into estimates at the next interim analysis time tends to increase the response estimate and shift up the confidence interval a bit (Phase II) or decrease the difference estimate and shift down the confidence interval a bit (Phase III). The statistical difficulty is that there is no unique or even standard way to do this. For example, Jennison and Turnbull (1983), Chang and O'Brien (1986), and Duffy and Santner (1987) propose three different ways to adjust confidence intervals to account for two-stage Phase II designs. The biggest differences in adjusted and unadjusted intervals generally occur when results at later analysis times become extreme (e.g., if there are no responses in the second stage of accrual in a Phase II study after several in the first stage, or if a very large difference is observed at the final analysis of a Phase III following only modest differences at earlier analyses). In some cases it might be worth adjusting, but in practice we expect that if conservative early stopping rules are used, then unadjusted intervals will present a reasonable impression of the results of the study (Green, 2001).

7.3.3 Interpretation of results

One-sided vs. two-sided tests

The choice of whether to perform a one-sided or two-sided test is determined during study development, and should be specified in the statistical considerations section of the protocol. The one-sided p-value for the test of the primary endpoint should be reported for a study designed with a one-sided hypothesis. The possible conclusions from such a study are "the experimental treatment has been shown to be better, use it" and "the experimental treatment has not been shown to be better, stick with the standard." (Also see Chapter 3). If the experimental arm appears worse than the control, this will mean the p-value is close to 1 rather than being close to 0. The possibility that the experimental arm is actually worse may be of some interest but does not represent one of the decisions used to plan the statistical error rates for the trial. In a multi-arm setting with an ordered hypothesis, think of one-sided as ordered instead and the same comments apply. Either conclude there is evidence for the hypothesized ordering or not; changing the ordering after the fact invalidates the design considerations.

A two-sided p-value should be reported for a study designed with a two-sided hypothesis. The possible conclusions for a two-arm trial are "arm A is better, use it," "arm B is better, use it," and "there is insufficient evidence to conclude either one is better, use either." The possible conclusions from a multi-arm trial are not so simply listed. If a global test (all arms equal vs. not all arms equal) is planned first, one possible conclusion is "there is insufficient evidence to conclude any of the arms are inferior or superior;" after this the possible outcomes will depend on the specific hypotheses stated in the protocol. (See Chapter 4.)

The primary test statistic reported for a Phase III trial should be either an unadjusted logrank test if simple randomization was used, or a stratified logrank or Cox model adjusting for the stratification factors if randomization followed a stratified scheme. Failure to adjust for variables used in the randomization results in conservative testing when the stratification factors have strong prognostic effects (Anderson et al., 2002).

For either one-sided or two-sided settings, the test statistic specified in the protocol's statistical considerations section should be the test used. For a two-arm trial this is often a logrank or stratified logrank test (see Chapter 2). When proportional hazards assumptions do not appear to be met after a study is complete, it is tempting to use a test other than the logrank test to improve power. However, using a second test, especially one based on looking at the data, means an extra opportunity for a false positive error, making the significance level specified in the design incorrect. To allow for two tests the study must be designed for two tests — with levels for each adjusted so that the overall false positive probability for the study (probability either test rejects when there are no differences) is the desired level α.

Positive, negative, and equivocal trials

Positive results on a Phase II or a two-arm Phase III study are relatively easy to define. If the protocol-specified hypothesis test of your protocol-specified primary endpoint is significant using protocol-specified levels, the result is positive. The definition of negative is not so easy. What distinguishes a negative trial from an equivocal trial is the extent of the confidence interval around the null hypothesis value (see Chapter 3). On a two-arm Phase III trial the null hypothesis generally is that the death hazard ratio equals 1. Thus for a trial in which the null hypothesis of treatment equality cannot be rejected, a confidence interval for the hazard ratio that contains only values close to 1 constitutes a negative trial; if some values are not close to 1, the trial is equivocal. One should never conclude there is no difference between treatment arms — the confidence interval never consists precisely of the value 1. Similarly, a Phase II trial is convincingly negative if all values in the confidence interval are close to p_o and equivocal if not.

What is "close" and what is "not close" to the null hypothesis are matters of clinical judgment, but for a well-designed trial with sensible alternatives, these can be interpreted as "less than the difference specified in the alternative hypothesis" and "greater than the difference specified in the alternative hypothesis," respectively. In this case, a confidence interval lying entirely below the alternative would constitute evidence of a negative result. If power for the alternative is high, failure to reject the null hypothesis will generally result in such confidence intervals (unless the p-value is close to α). Trials that are too small to have good power for reasonable alternatives, however, stand a good chance of being interpreted as equivocal if the null hypothesis is not rejected. For example, an adjuvant trial designed to have 80% power to detect a hazard ratio of 1.5 may well turn out not to reject the null hypothesis, but the confidence interval may contain hazard ratios on the order of 1.25, a difference many would argue is clinically important. Be very careful not to overinterpret trials of inadequate size that do not reject the null hypothesis.

A multi-arm trial is positive if a superior arm is identified according to the design criteria. It is negative if the differences among arms are not consistent with a moderate benefit due to any one of the arms over another. In practice, it is very hard to conclude that a multi-arm trial is anything but equivocal. Variability guarantees differences between the arms, and chances are some of these will be large enough not to exclude differences of interest unless the sample size is very large. Furthermore, even if a protocol-specified test statistic is significant, readers may not be persuaded that the hypothesized best arm truly is best unless stricter testing is also significant. For instance, suppose a test of equality against an ordered alternative, A < AB < ABC, rejects in favor of the alternative. According to the design, ABC should be concluded the best arm. If, however, ABC was only a little better than AB (and not significant in a pairwise comparison), there would be doubt as to whether adding C to the regimen was necessary.

Multiple endpoints

In general there should be only one primary endpoint for a trial, the one on which sample size and statistical error rates are based. However, there are usually several important secondary endpoints. Results for each endpoint should be presented separately, not combined into some arbitrary aggregate (see also, Chapter 3). If analyses of all endpoints lead to the same conclusion, there is no problem of interpretation. A positive result in the primary endpoint not accompanied by positive results in secondary endpoints is still positive, but may be viewed with less enthusiasm. For instance, a new agent found to have a modest survival advantage over a standard agent but with a serious toxicity increase or a decrease in quality of life will likely be concluded useful, but less useful than if there was no difference in toxicity or quality of life. On the other hand, if there is no significant difference in the primary endpoint, then results are still negative, but differences in secondary endpoints might be useful in making clinical decisions concerning what regimen to use.

7.3.4   Secondary analyses

Everything but the intent-to-treat analysis of all eligible patients with respect to the protocol-specified primary endpoint using the protocol-specified test is a secondary or exploratory analysis. In addition to protocol-specified secondary analyses, there are frequent requests for additional tests during the analysis phase of the trial. One of the most common such requests is to evaluate treatment results within subsets of patients (including stratification factors).

The most common mistake in the analysis of subsets is to perform a test of treatment effect separately within levels of the variable of interest. For example, if it is thought that treatment may vary by sex, the temptation is to produce (and test) a separate set of survival curves for men and women. This strategy yields tests that have poor power and inflated level (see Section 8.5). The safest strategy is to perform a test of interaction between treatment and the variable(s) of interest. A test of interaction tests whether the magnitude of the treatment effect (hazard ratio) differs between levels of the factor. A nonsignificant test of interaction suggests there is no evidence of differences in treatment effect within subsets, and further exploration should stop. (Note the cautious wording "no evidence of differences." As for any nonsignificant test with low power, interpretation of a nonsignificant result is not equivalent to proving no difference.)

For all but the primary endpoint, results of any exploratory analyses must be viewed and reported with caution. Although an occasional new insight is uncovered, data dredging leads to mainly incorrect conclusions (see Chapters 8 and 9). Care should be taken to report only strong statistical associations with plausible biological explanations, and even then the observations should be reported as exploratory, needing confirmation in other studies.

7.4 Conclusion

The introductory quote says "Be careful what you say, when, and to whom." Treatment and management decisions will be made based on what you report. Given the long history of premature enthusiasm and exaggerated claims for new treatments in cancer, there is reason to take every care that conclusions do not go beyond what your trial data support. Patients' lives may depend on it.

CHAPTER 8

Pitfalls

The crooks already know these tricks; honest men must learn them in self-defense.

–**Darrel Huff** (1954)

8.1 Introduction

The results of a well-designed and executed clinical trial should be evident from a few summary statistics — but stopping at those summaries in a manuscript is rare. It is reasonable to want to see if more can be learned from a long, expensive effort. The temptation to overinterpret secondary analyses can be irresistible. Although exploring data and analyzing different endpoints do sometimes lead to new insights, far too often they lead to implausible hypotheses and faulty conclusions. In this chapter we discuss problems with some common types of analyses that have been used to try to draw treatment conclusions beyond those supported by the study design. In Chapter 9 we discuss methods for exploratory data analysis.

8.2 Historical controls

As noted in Chapter 3, any nonrandomized choice of a control group will be systematically different from the experimental group in countless ways, some known, many unmeasurable. We know from numerous examples that there are historical trends in disease incidence and survival that are difficult to explain. For example, diphtheria is a heterogeneous disease caused by several bacteria that vary in deadliness. The bacteria were discovered in 1894 and antiserum was produced and made available in Europe in 1894–1895. Mortality due to diphtheria decreased at this time, but the decline had started *before* the introduction of antiserum. The prevalences of

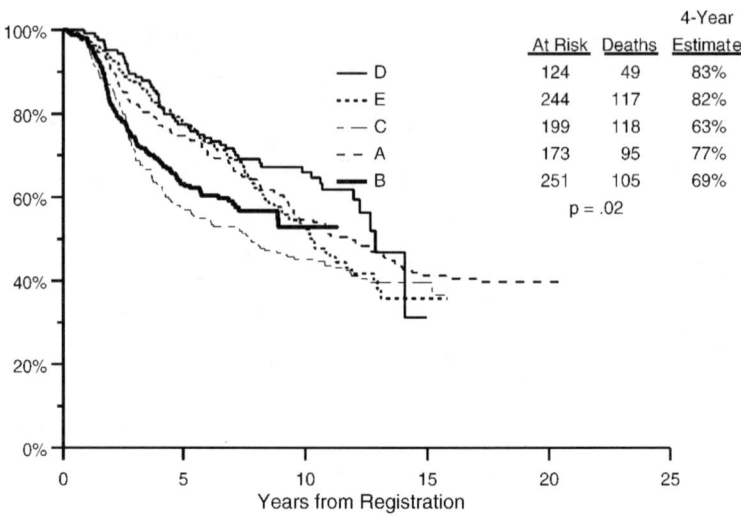

Figure 8.1. Survival distributions for CMFVP arms of five SWOG breast cancer trials.

the various types of bacteria were changing, making the contribution of treatment uncertain. Thirty years later it was still unknown whether treatment helped, as deaths in 1924 had risen to 1871 levels (Lancaster, 1994).

For a modern cancer example, Figure 8.1 shows the CMFVP (defined in Chapter 1) arms from five Southwest Oncology Group adjuvant breast cancer studies conducted in node-positive patients between 1975 and 1989 (Rivkin et al., 1989; Rivkin et al., 1993; Budd et al., 1995; Rivkin et al., 1994; Rivkin et al., 1996). Survival differs widely despite use of the same treatment in the same stage of disease in the same cooperative group. At the time of the first study, single agent LPAM was the standard adjuvant treatment. If the worst of the CMFVP arms had been compared to historical experience on LPAM, combination chemotherapy would have been concluded to be no better (Figure 8.2). Fortunately a randomized trial was done, and the appropriate comparison (arm A, Figure 8.3) demonstrated the superiority of CMFVP.

Some of the reasons for the differences between the CMFVP arms are clear — studies B and C consisted of estrogen receptor-negative patients (who generally have a less favorable prognosis), studies D and E required estrogen receptor-positive disease, and study A was a mixture. Unfortunately, identifying the biases is not always so easy. Between 1977 and 1989 the Southwest Oncology Group did a series of four Phase III trials with the same eligibility criteria in multiple

HISTORICAL CONTROLS

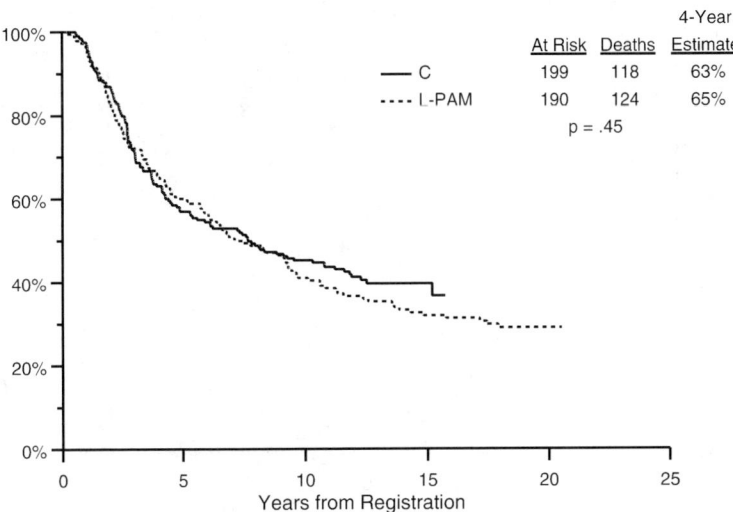

Figure 8.2. Survival distributions for worst arm of CMFVP vs. L-PAM based on five SWOG breast cancer trials.

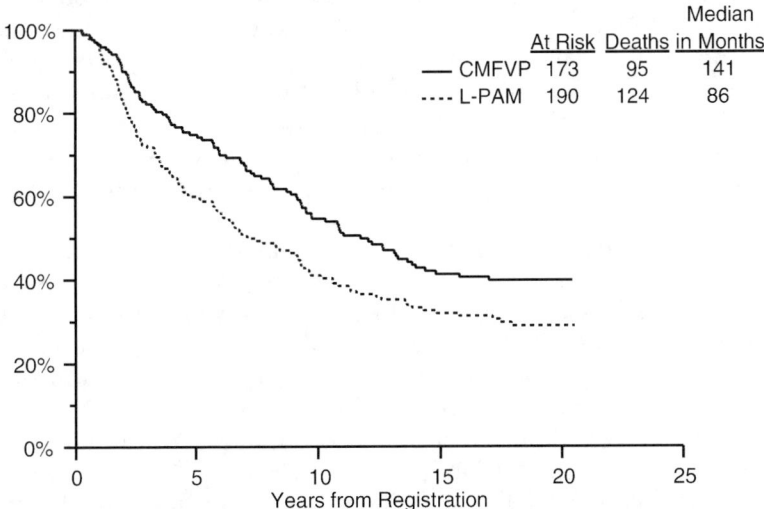

Figure 8.3. Survival distributions based on randomized comparison of CMFVP vs. L-PAM on SWOG breast cancer trial 7436.

myeloma (Salmon et al., 1983; Durie et al., 1986; Salmon et al., 1990; Salmon et al., 1994). Figure 8.4 shows survival on the four studies (arms combined). The estimates of the survival distributions of the four studies are nearly the same; it would appear that little progress was made in myeloma treatment during this time. Contrast this with

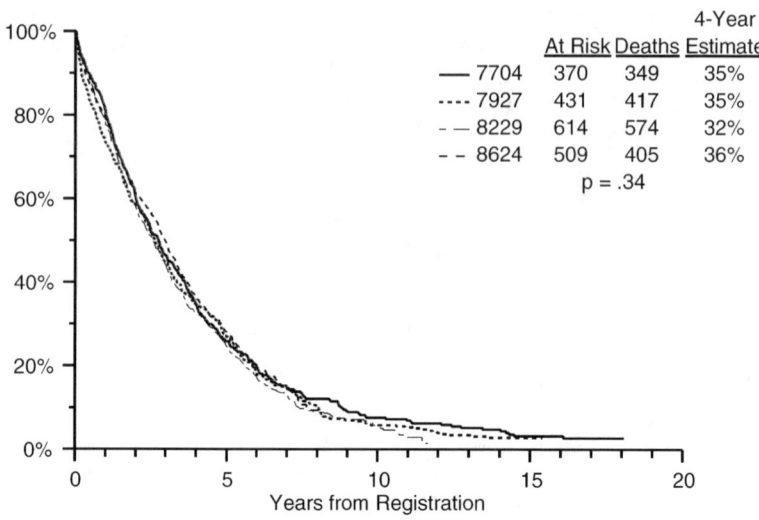

Figure 8.4. Survival distributions for four successive SWOG myeloma trials.

Figure 8.5, which shows survival on the arm common to each of the trials. Despite the same eligibility, the same treatment, and largely the same participating institutions, the survival curves on the four arms appear quite different — almost statistically significant at the conventional 0.05 level! If comparability cannot be counted on in this ideal setting, it certainly cannot be counted on when control groups are chosen arbitrarily from the literature or from convenient data bases.

The next examples illustrate the potential magnitude of selection bias in historical comparisons. Consider the results in Figure 8.6 from a myeloma pilot study of high-dose therapy with autologous bone marrow transplant (Barlogie et al., 1995). Viewed next to standard results in Figure 8.4, transplant results appear quite promising. Is this observation sufficient to declare transplant the new standard without doing a randomized trial of transplant vs. a standard chemotherapy control group? Would it be unethical to do a randomized trial of transplant vs. control? When the difference is this large it is tempting to conclude that results could not all be due to systematic biases. Figure 8.7 suggests otherwise, however. Major sources of bias in the historical comparison are the different eligibility criteria for the two types of trials. Potential transplant patients must be young and in good condition; criteria for standard therapy are not so strict. Figure 8.7 shows how results on one possible historical control arm (VAD, one of the arms of SWOG 8624, and the induction arm for the transplant protocol) look when restricted to patients under 70 years

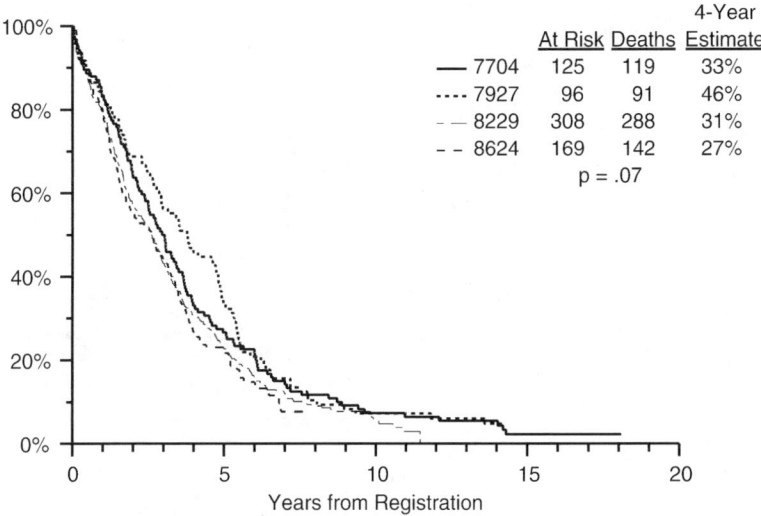

Figure 8.5. Survival distributions for common VMCP/VBAP arms of four successive SWOG myeloma trials.

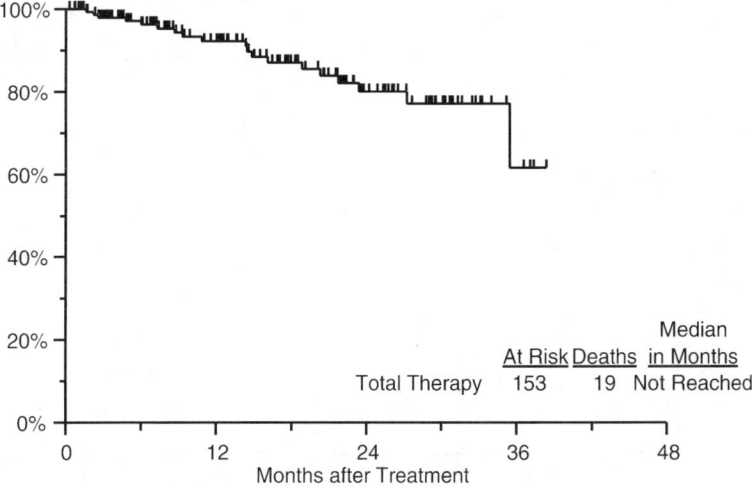

Figure 8.6. Survival distribution for pilot trial of high-dose therapy in myeloma.

of age with good renal function. Results look quite a bit better for standard therapy – and this is after adjustment for just two known factors. Unknown and unmeasurable selection factors may play an even larger role. A randomized trial coordinated by SWOG (trial 9321) to answer the question has completed accrual, with final analysis awaiting data maturity.

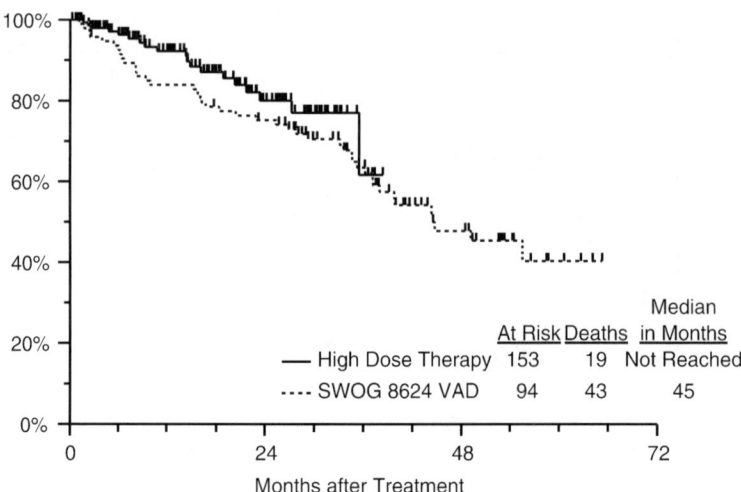

Figure 8.7. Survival distributions for historical comparison of high-dose therapy with standard therapy for myeloma, using only patients under 70 and with good renal function.

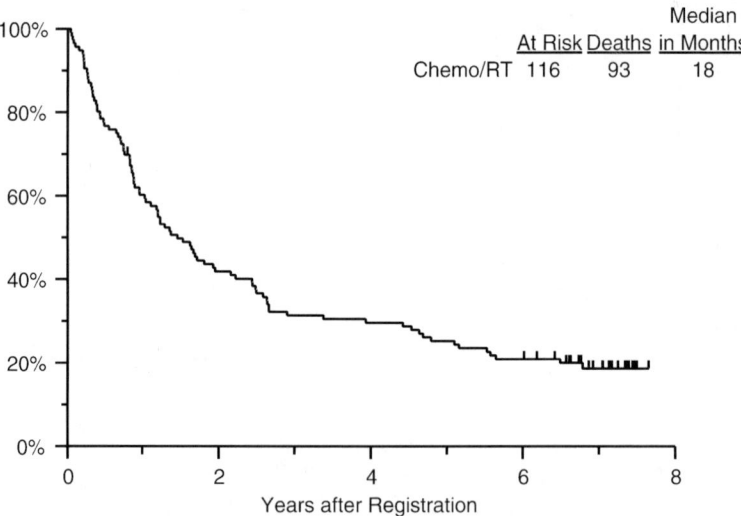

Figure 8.8. Survival distribution for all patients on SWOG lung cancer trial 8269.

Now consider the sequence of curves in Figures 8.8 to 8.10 from a pilot study in limited small-cell lung cancer (McCracken et al., 1990). The first figure shows survival for all patients on the study; median survival was 18 months. Transplant advocates claimed that

HISTORICAL CONTROLS 187

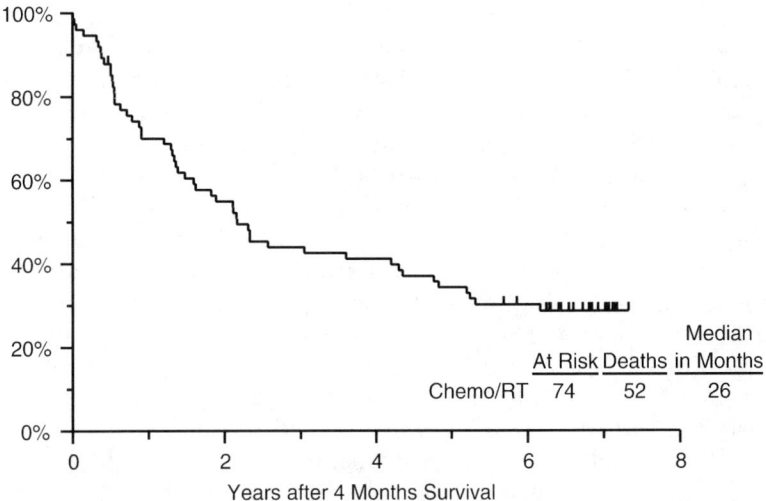

Figure 8.9. Survival distribution for patients on SWOG lung cancer trial 8269 with good performance status and survival beyond 4 months.

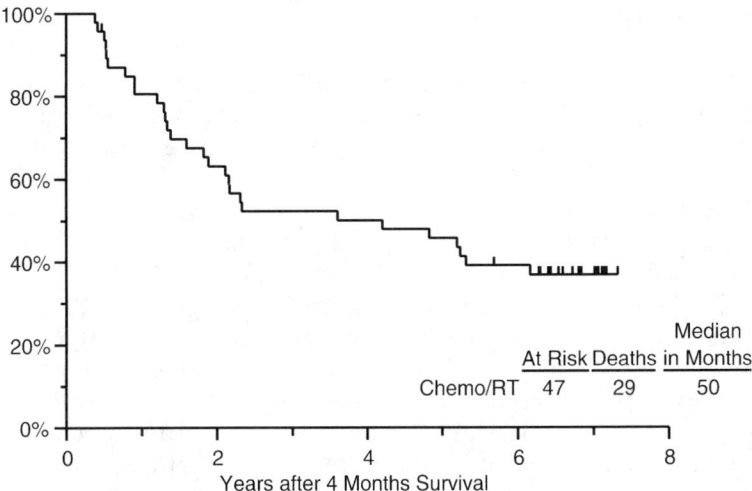

Figure 8.10. Survival distribution for patients on SWOG lung cancer trial 8269 with good performance status and disease in complete response at 4 months.

survival on high-dose therapy might be two to three times longer than on standard treatment. To get high-dose therapy plus transplant on most pilot studies, however, patients had to have been in good physical condition, and must have received and responded to induction treatment with conventional chemotherapy. Figure 8.9

shows survival on the SWOG pilot when restricted to patients with good performance status who survived 4 months. It is evident that these requirements select out a relatively good risk subset of patients; median survival for this subset is 26 months. (Note: we could make this look even better by including the 4 months the patients were being treated on induction.) Results improve even more (Figure 8.10) when patients are further restricted to those with disease in complete response at 4 months; we are now up to a median of 50 months, 2.7 times the median on standard treatment, right in the range of claimed benefit for high-dose therapy plus transplant. In this case further pilot studies are being done before a possible randomized trial of high-dose therapy.

From these examples it should be clear that randomized trials to test new cancer treatments are indeed ethical. In fact, it might be unethical to claim superiority without a randomized trial demonstrating efficacy, especially for such costly and toxic treatment as high-dose therapy.

8.3 Competing risks

Competing risks refers to the problem of analyzing multiple possible failure types. For instance, patients being followed for relapse do not necessarily do so before they die, so relapse and death from other causes are the competing failure types for a disease-free survival endpoint. If particular sites of relapse are also of interest (e.g., local vs. distant), then these are additional failure types. A common but misguided aim is to determine the effect of treatment on one endpoint (e.g., time to distant recurrence) after eliminating the risk of other endpoints (e.g., local recurrences and deaths due to other causes). Biology does not allow for elimination of outcomes without influence on other outcomes, and statistics cannot either. A typical approach to estimating the distribution of time to a specific type of failure is to censor the observation at the time of any other type of failure if it occurs first, and calculate the Kaplan-Meier estimator from the resulting data. If outcomes were independent (meaning the probability of one outcome is the same regardless of the occurrence of other outcomes) there would not be a major problem, but such independence is an unrealistic assumption. For instance, patients who have had a local relapse might then have a higher probability of distant relapse. Or, the same factors that result in a low probability of distant recurrence might influence the probability of death due to other causes as well. Sensitivity to chemotherapy might result in a higher probability of toxic death but a lower probability of distant recurrence. Alternatively, a poor immune system might result in a higher probability of both death and distant recurrence. Figure 6.1, repeated as Figure 8.11, which illustrates the potential bias when patients are lost to follow-up, applies here as well. Assume the loss to follow-up is due to the occurrence of a secondary endpoint. If patients who experience the secondary endpoint never experience the primary one (extreme case of chemosensitivity), the top curve would apply. If patients who experience the secondary endpoint always experience the primary one immediately afterward (extreme case of poor immune system), the bottom curve would apply. Censoring (middle curve) can result in bias in either direction. Endless combinations of relationships among endpoints can yield the same results. There is no way to tell which combination is correct without more complete information on all endpoints. There is no easy way to interpret such estimators.

Another approach sometimes taken is to follow patients for all types of endpoints until death or last known follow-up time. This approach is a slight improvement in that fewer endpoints have to be assumed independent. It does require that follow-up for all endpoints continues uniformly until death, which we often find not to be the case. Once a patient has metastatic disease, efforts to screen for —

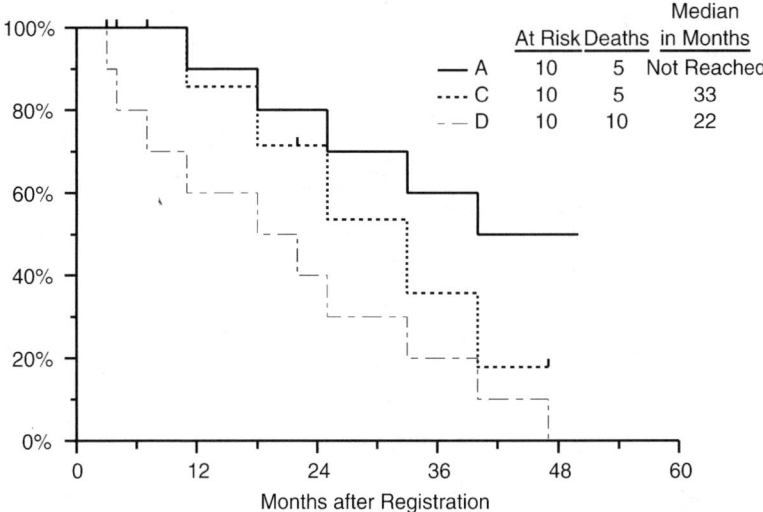

Figure 8.11. Potential bias due to competing risks. Curve A assumes failure types are related, and the second failure type never occurs. Curve C assumes failure types are unrelated. Curve D assumes failures are related, and the second failure always occurs.

or at least to report — new local sites, new primaries, and other diseases are reduced.

The approach to estimation in the competing risks setting with perhaps the most support from statisticians is to decompose overall time to first failure into cause-specific first failure components. In this approach, no unrealistic assumptions are made to estimate a distribution in the absence of competing causes of failure. Instead, a subdistribution function in the presence of all other failure types is estimated. This is also called (among other names) a *cumulative incidence* curve, although this term has also been used for other purposes. In this context, the cumulative incidence curve estimates, at each time t, the probability of failing due to a specific cause by time t in the presence of competing failure types. Here is an example to illustrate. Suppose all 20 patients on a study of treatment Q have failed at the following times for the following reasons.

Patient ID	Time to First Failure	Failure Type
1	1	Death
2	11	Death
3	2	Distant
4	12	Distant
5	3	Death
6	13	Local
7	4	Local
8	14	Death
9	5	Distant
10	15	Distant
11	6	Distant
12	16	Local
13	7	Distant
14	17	Death
15	8	Distant
16	18	Local
17	9	Death
18	19	Distant
19	10	Distant
20	20	Death

Figure 8.12 shows overall failure and cumulative incidences of the three failure types. For instance, the probability of failure at time 10 or before is estimated by the number of failures by time 10 over the total number on study, or 10/20. The probability of failure type *local*

COMPETING RISKS

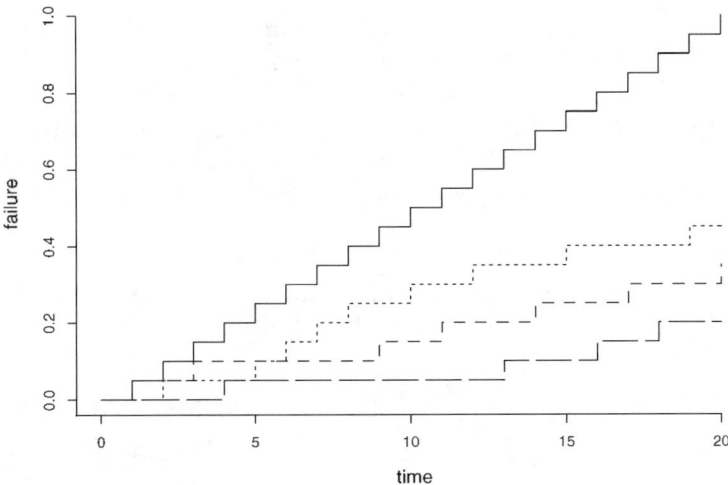

Figure 8.12. Overall failure (solid line) and cumulative incidences of three failure types, local recurrence (long dashed line), distant recurrence (dotted line), deaths (short dashed line).

at time 10 or before is estimated as 1/20; the estimated probability of type *distant* is 6/20; the estimated probability of type *death* is 3/20. Since overall failure consists of the three types, the overall probability is the sum of the probabilities of the three types.

With censored data the estimates are more complicated (Kalbfleisch and Prentice, 1980), but the idea of estimating the components of overall failure is the same. Gooley et al. (1999) have a nice description of the difference between the cumulative incidence and Kaplan-Meier (censored) approach. In Chapter 2 the Kaplan-Meier (K-M) estimator was described as a product

$$\left(\frac{n_1 - 1}{n_1}\right)\left(\frac{n_2 - 1}{n_2}\right)\ldots\left(\frac{n_i - 1}{n_i}\right),$$

where $n_1 \ldots n_i$ are the numbers of patients remaining at risk just before failure times $1 \ldots i$. Another way to describe the K-M estimator is to note that if there are N patients and no censoring, there is a drop of size 1/N at each time of failure. If there is censoring, then for the first patient censored, the assumption is made that failure for this patient should be just like failures for all other patients remaining alive at this time, so the K-M estimator divides the 1/N drop for this patient among everyone left alive. For the next censored patient, 1/N plus whatever was allocated from the previous censored patient is divided among everyone left alive at this time, and so on.

For censorship due to the patient still being alive without failure, this is not unreasonable. With competing risks, however, the allocation generally does not make sense — death without relapse cannot be followed by a relapse. Rather than allocate the 1/N for a death without relapse to subsequent relapses (the K-M approach), the cumulative incidence approach recognizes that no relapse is possible and nothing is allocated.

There are methods for analyzing the cumulative incidence (Gray, 1988), but these methods should be interpreted carefully. Consider a second set of 20 patients treated with agent X:

Patient ID	Time to First Failure	Failure Type
a	1	Death
b	11	Death
c	2	Death
d	12	Distant
e	3	Death
f	13	Death
g	4	Death
h	14	Death
i	5	Death
j	15	Distant
k	6	Death
l	16	Death
m	7	Death
n	17	Death
o	8	Death
p	18	Death
q	9	Death
r	19	Distant
s	10	Distant
t	20	Death

Figures 8.13–8.15 show the comparisons of cumulative incidence for local and distant recurrence and of death between the two data sets. Agent X appears to prevent local recurrence and to reduce distant recurrence. However, agent Q appears to reduce death. Is Q better? Or does Q cause recurrences so we do not see the deaths? The overall failure rate (time to local recurrence, distant recurrence, or death) is identical. A better endpoint for the choice of treatment would seem to be time to death (not recorded here for all patients).

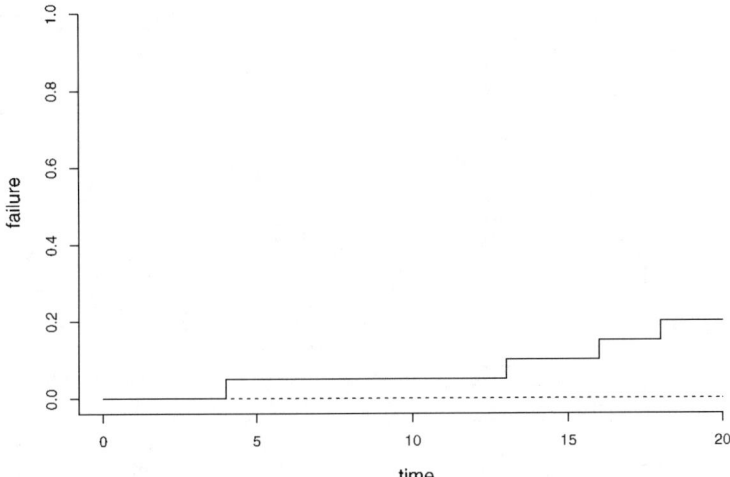

Figure 8.13. Cumulative incidence of local recurrence in two data sets, Q (solid line) and X (dotted line).

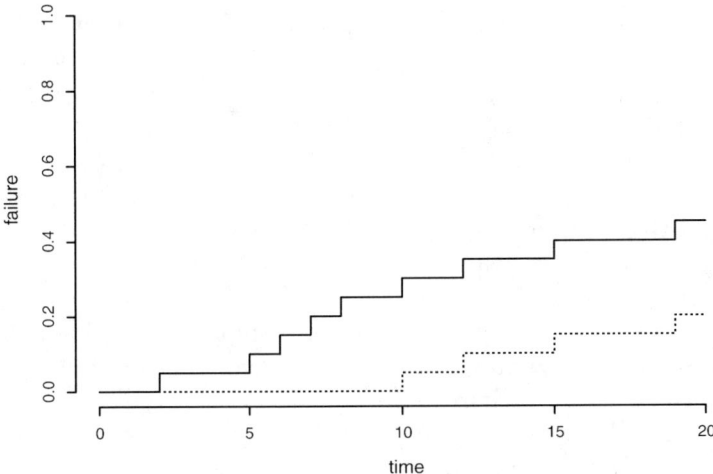

Figure 8.14. Cumulative incidence of distant recurrence in two data sets, Q (solid line) and X (dotted line).

Another approach to analysis (Prentice et al., 1978) is to compare cause-specific hazards (also called subhazards). A cause-specific hazard at time t is the rate of failure due to a specific cause given the patient is failure free at time t. The sum of all the cause-specific hazards is the overall failure hazard (defined in Chapter 2). Just as for the overall hazard, differences in cause-specific hazards between

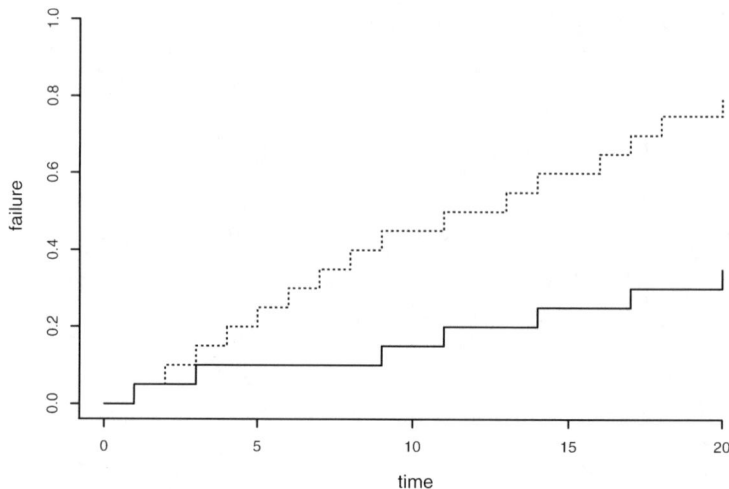

Figure 8.15. Cumulative incidence of death in two data sets, Q (solid line) and X (dotted line).

two arms can be tested using a proportional hazards model (also defined in Chapter 2).

For this type of analysis, probabilities of cause-specific failure are not being compared, but rather the relative rate of failure. The two approaches are not equivalent. For instance, suppose the relapse hazard is the same on two arms, but the death hazard is higher on arm two. Comparing relapse probabilities will result in the conclusion that there are fewer relapses on arm two. Since patients are dying faster on arm two, fewer are at risk for relapse so fewer relapses are seen. Comparing relapse hazards using a proportional hazards model, on the other hand, will result in a conclusion of no difference between the arms with respect to relapse. Roughly speaking, the computation looks at the number of patients at risk on each arm at the time of a failure and assigns a score depending on whether or not the failure came from the more likely arm. If relapse rates are equal, a relapse is more likely on the arm with more patients remaining at risk. As long as about the right number of patients relapse on each arm (conditional on the number at risk at each time of relapse), the comparison will not indicate that there is a difference.

As for analysis of cumulative incidence, analysis of cause-specific hazards must also be interpreted cautiously. A smaller hazard on one arm with respect to one failure type does not mean there might not be a larger hazard with respect to another type.

8.4 Outcome by outcome analyses

Another faulty analysis strategy involves correlating two time-dependent outcomes and trying to draw causal conclusions from the result. For instance, it is commonly thought that certain treatments are ineffective unless sufficient myelosuppression is achieved. (Presumably if blood cells, with their high turnover rate, are being killed, then so are cancer cells.) How would you prove this? A naive approach would be to look at minimum WBC achieved while on treatment vs. survival time. Inevitably, low counts can be shown to be associated with longer survival. A little thought should reveal that the patients with the maximum number of shopping trips achieved in a week while on treatment live longer, too, as do the ones who experience the most rainy days, the highest vitamin A levels, or the most mosquito bites in a month. Patients have to be alive for a measured variable to be observed; the longer a patient is alive the more often that variable is observed; the more often it is observed, the higher the maximum and the lower the minimum of the observations.

8.4.1 Survival by response comparisons

Perhaps the longest-standing misuse of statistics in oncology is the practice of comparing survival of responders to that of non-responders. The belief appears to be that if responders live longer than non-responders, then the treatment must be effective.

It should not be surprising that patients who respond live longer than ones who do not — patients have to live long enough to get a response, and those who die before evaluation of response are automatically classified as non-responders. Suppose, for example, that everyone treated for 6 months gets a response at that time, and that response and survival are unrelated. In this case the responder vs. non-responder comparison is equivalent to comparing patients who are alive at 6 months vs. ones who are not. People alive at 6 months do indeed survive longer than those who die before 6 months, but this observation has nothing to tell us about the effectiveness of treatment.

The comparison of responders to non-responders is completely analogous to the first published analysis of the potential benefit of heart transplantation (Clark et al., 1971), which compared the survival of those patients healthy enough to survive the waiting period for a donor heart, to that of patients who died before a new heart arrived. Most oncologists immediately recognize the latter as a fallacy, but the former persists. The fallacy has been given a mathematical formalization by Liu, Voelkel, Crowley et al. (1993).

A better method of comparing responders with nonresponders is the landmark method (Anderson, Cain, and Gelber, 1983). In this approach, response status is determined among living patients at a particular time (the landmark) after start of treatment. Then survival times subsequent to that time are compared. This eliminates the biases introduced by (1) defining early death as nonresponse and (2) by including the time before response as part of the survival time for responders (lead time bias). The cost of reducing the bias is loss of information from early deaths and classification of some late responders as nonresponders. Even though less biased than the simple comparison, the landmark method does not allow for a biologic interpretation of results. Responders might not live longer because they have achieved a response, but rather response might be a marker identifying patients who would have lived longer anyway — statistically there is no way to tell the difference. Still, it might be of clinical interest to know that among patients alive at 3 months, those who respond will generally live longer/the same/shorter than those who have not responded.

A related common, but misguided, analysis involves comparing treatments with respect to survival of responders or to duration of response. The reasoning behind such analyses seems to be that patients who do not respond to treatment receive minimal benefit from treatment, so responders are the primary group of interest. SWOG 8616 (Antman et al., 1993) provides a good example of the difficulties with this type of analysis. In this study, patients with advanced soft-tissue sarcoma were randomized to receive either Adriamycin plus DTIC (AD) or these same two agents plus Ifosfamide and Mesna (MAID). Response, time to failure, and survival were all endpoints of the study. In the next three paragraphs we demonstrate that AD is superior, that MAID is superior, and that AD and MAID are equivalent.

Figure 8.16 shows that survival of responders on AD is somewhat better than survival of responders on MAID. Under the assumption that patients who do not respond to treatment do not benefit from treatment, then the superior results of responders on AD suggest the superiority of AD.

Figure 8.17 shows that responders live longer than nonresponders on the study as a whole. The number of responders on MAID was 55/170 while the number on AD was 29/170. Clearly, since responders live longer and there were more responders on MAID, then MAID has been demonstrated to be superior.

OUTCOME BY OUTCOME ANALYSES

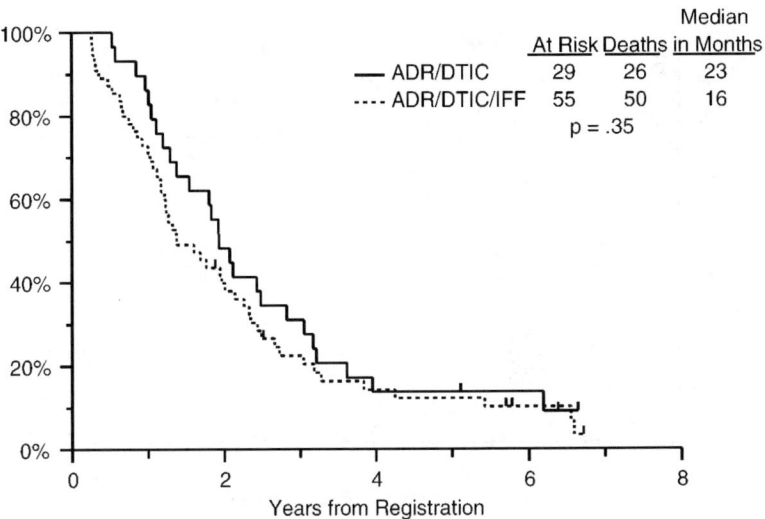

Figure 8.16. Survival distributions by treatment arm for responding patients on SWOG sarcoma trial 8616.

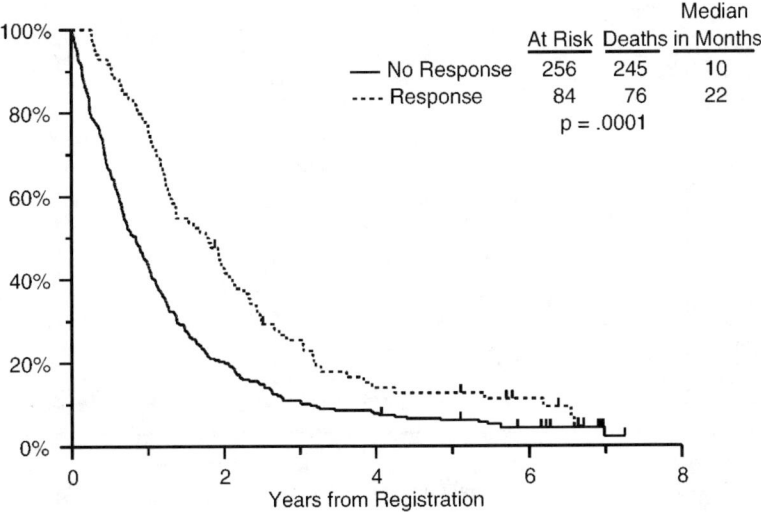

Figure 8.17. Survival distributions for responders vs. non-responders on SWOG sarcoma trial 8616.

Time to failure and survival curves for AD vs. MAID are shown in Figures 8.18 and 8.19. The time to failure estimate is a little better on MAID, while survival is a little better on AD. Neither difference is significant. Neither regimen is shown to be preferable.

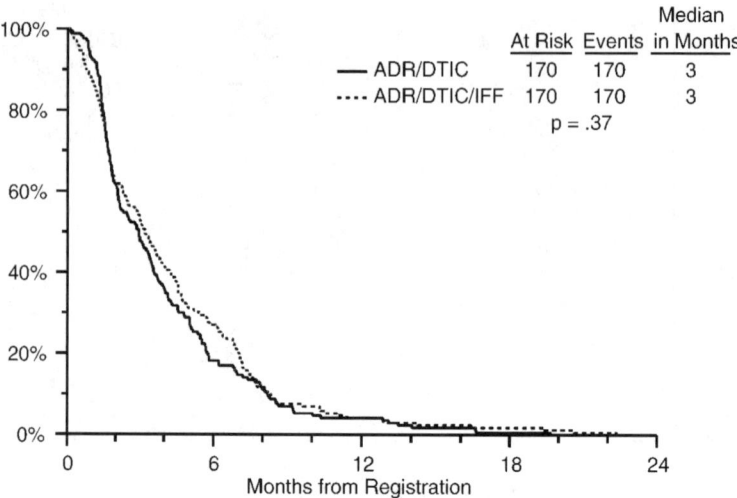

Figure 8.18. Time to treatment failure distributions by treatment arm for SWOG sarcoma trial 8616.

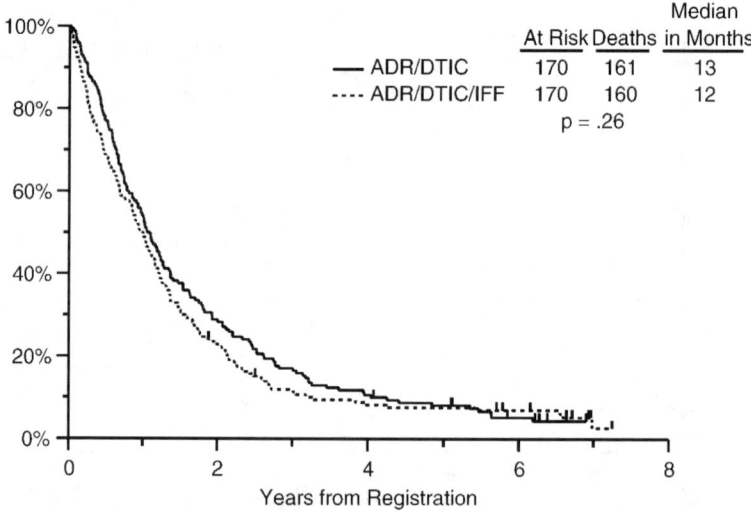

Figure 8.19. Survival distributions by treatment arm for SWOG sarcoma trial 8616.

Which regimen should be recommended? MAID does result in more responses, although the ones gained over AD appear to be short (considering Figure 8.16). If the value of fleeting tumor shrinkage in the absence of survival benefit outweighs the substantial excess toxicity and cost due to Ifosfamide, then MAID should be recommended.

If not, then AD would appear to be the better choice. Either way, it would have been a mistake to base a decision on Figure 8.16 or 8.17; these confuse the interpretation of treatment differences more than they clarify.

8.4.2 Dose intensity analyses

The latest variation on the theme of outcome by outcome analysis we have encountered is the analysis of survival according to planned or received total dose or dose intensity of treatment. These analyses usually are performed to show that more is better without the hassle of a clinical trial comparing doses. Famous examples are due to Hryniuk and Levine (1986), who observed a positive association of planned dose intensity with outcome in a collection of adjuvant studies in breast cancer, and Bonadonna and Valagussa (1981), who purport to demonstrate that high doses of received adjuvant chemotherapy are associated with improved survival, also in breast cancer.

Our own results with CMFVP noted above illustrate the difficulty in interpreting correlations of study outcomes with study characteristics such as planned dose intensity. Hryniuk and Levine hypothesized the importance of dose intensity based on (among other analyses) a plot of 3-year disease-free survival vs. a weighted sum of the weekly doses of certain agents in the prescribed regimens of 27 arms from 17 adjuvant breast cancer studies. The apparent association was striking: disease-free survivals were 50 to 57% for regimens of 0 intensity (no treatment); 53 to 69% for intensities 0.1 to 0.5; 64 to 86% for intensities 0.5 to 1.0. One of the problems with the analysis is that the studies compared may have differed with respect to factors not analyzed in the paper. As demonstrated by our series of CMFVP arms, factors other than dose may have major influences on outcome. Despite a planned intensity of 1.0 for our CMFVP regimen, 3-year disease-free survivals on the five studies range from 58 to 73%, covering the middle 2/3 of survivals reported in the Hryniuk and Levine table. The arms in the table below 58% were all no treatment and single agent LPAM arms; the ones above 73% had planned intensities no greater than ours (lowest 0.71). It is not necessary to invoke intensity to explain the results of the table. A close look suggests an alternative explanation: no treatment or single-agent LPAM is insufficient (50 to 63%), and CMF-based regimens (64 to 86%) are better than LF-based regimens (60 to 69%). Henderson, Hayes, and

Gelman (1988) discuss additional problems with the assumptions in the paper, such as the implied assumption that there were no time trends in breast cancer results (the more intense regimens were generally on studies conducted later in time).

Now consider the Bonadonna and Valagussa approach to showing high doses are beneficial, that of comparing patients who received higher doses on a trial with those who received lower doses. It should by now come as no surprise that analysis by dose received is as severely biased as the other outcome by outcome analyses in this chapter. Studies can be conducted in ways that prove high doses, low doses, or intermediate doses are superior.

An example that illustrates the point clearly is taken from the cardiovascular literature (Coronary Drug Research Project Group, 1980). The Coronary Drug Project was a randomized double-blind, placebo-controlled, five-arm trial of cholesterol-lowering agents. The 5-year mortality for 1103 men on one of the agents, clofibrate, was 20% vs. 21% in 2789 men on placebo, a disappointing result. A ray of hope might have been seen in the fact that clofibrate adherers had a substantially lower 5-year mortality than did poor adherers (15% for those who received $\geq 80\%$ of protocol prescription vs. 25% for those who received $<80\%$). Perhaps at least the compliant patients benefitted from treatment. Alas, no. Compliance was even more strongly related to mortality in the placebo group: 15% mortality for $\geq 80\%$ vs. 28% for $<80\%$. Evidently compliance functioned as a measure of good health.

Redmond, Fisher, and Wieand (1983) have an excellent cancer example. Doses received were collected for both arms of an adjuvant breast cancer trial of LPAM vs. placebo. In the first comparison, the total received dose divided by the total planned dose was calculated for each patient and the following levels compared: level I $\geq 85\%$, level II 65 to 84%, level III $<65\%$. Overall 5-year disease-free survival on the LPAM arm was 51%. The results for the three levels were 69, 67, and 26%, respectively, apparently a nice dose response. Disease-free survival in the placebo group was 46%, however. If we conclude that doses over 65% are beneficial, then must we also conclude that receiving $<65\%$ is harmful, since placebo was better than level III?

Most of the bias in this analysis comes from the fact that patients discontinued treatment if relapse occurred before the completion of the planned therapy, and therefore could not have had the highest doses. In effect, early failures were required to have low doses. This is seen clearly when the same analysis is done for placebo patients — an even better dose response is observed! Five-year disease-free survivals for patients who took $\geq 85\%$, 65 to 84%, and $<65\%$ of placebo were

69, 43, 12%. Patients did not fail because their received dose was low, but received a low dose because they failed.

No method eliminates all the biases. The next comparison in the Redmond paper shows how another approach fails. To reduce the bias in the first method, it might seem logical to calculate instead the total dose received divided by the dose planned prior to the time of failure. Unfortunately, this is not much better — the bias switches the other way. Patients who fail late are more likely to have received low protocol doses, since they have had more time to experience toxicity requiring dose reductions, or to become noncompliant. For LPAM, 5-year disease-free survivals by level I, II, and III defined this way are 47, 59, 55%; for placebo they are 47, 43, and 60%.

The third method discussed is a landmark method, similar to that described for response in section 8.2. The landmark chosen was 2 years (the length of prescribed treatment) and survival after 2 years among those who had not yet failed was compared as a function of dose received. Although the differences were not significant, middle doses were the winners for this analysis. The first 2 years of information were a lot to ignore, however, so one final method was used, a time-dependent Cox model (Cox, 1972). This can be thought of as a way to switch to a new landmark at each failure time. While quite sophisticated statistically, this final method still has problems: the placebo dose was again significantly associated with survival.

Dose analysis problems start the instant one tries to define received dose intensity. The amount of drug administered per unit time is a common definition of intensity, but it is not complete unless a single agent is administered at the same dose at the same unit interval for the same number of intervals in every patient. If there are multiple agents, a method must be devised for combining agents into a single intensity measure; the possibilities for weighting schemes are infinite. If doses are modified over time, then there is no single amount per unit time; some sort of average must be devised. If treatment is given according to an interval other than the unit interval, then again there is no single "amount per unit time". If treatment duration is variable, then "amount per unit time" is a function not only of unit doses, but also of how many units. Should per unit time be calculated during the time the patient received treatment, during the time the patient was supposed to receive treatment, or during some fixed interval?

Southwest Oncology Group study 7827 again provides an example. As noted in Chapter 3, this trial compared 1 year vs. 2 years of SWOG standard CMFVP in node-positive receptor-negative breast cancer patients. The regimen consisted of daily administration of cyclophosphamide (ctx), weekly administration of methotrexate (mtx) and 5-fluorouracil (5-FU), plus short-term vincristine (vcr) and prednisone. How should intensity be summarized?

First consider how to define interval intensity. Summaries per week are more common than per day, but note that in choosing a weekly interval the assumption is being made that daily doses of cyclophosphamide are equivalent to the same total dose given weekly. Then consider how to combine weekly doses into a single measure. Weighting according to the content of the Cooper, Holland, and Glidewell (1979) CMF regimen is typical, i.e., ctx/560+mtx/17+ 5−FU/294. Note this weighting makes the assumption that 1 mg/m^2 of single agent mtx, 33 of ctx, and 17 of 5-FU are all interchangeable, and that vcr and prednisone contribute nothing to intensity. If we want to add contributions for vcr and prednisone, how to do so is problematic since these agents are not given for as long as the others. Should the 10 weeks of vcr be averaged over the year treatment is given? Should the intensity measure be changed after 10 weeks?

A large number of fairly arbitrary assumptions and decisions have to be made to define interval intensity. Another set of assumptions and decisions has to be made to combine all the intervals for a patient into a single measure. Is a simple average of unit intensities over the course of treatment a sufficient summary? If so, then the assumption is being made that 6 months of 95% doses followed by 6 months of 5% is equivalent to the reverse. If a patient on the 1-year arm and the 2-year arm have identical doses for the first year, should the intensity summary be the same? If yes, then the assumption has to be made that doses in the second year contribute nothing to intensity. If no, and weekly intensities are averaged over the planned course of treatment, then if the patient on the 2-year arm quits after 1 year (recall from Chapter 3 that compliance with 2 years was poor) intensity will be half the intensity of the 1-year patient despite identical treatment.

Better statistical methods will never yield results that answer the question of whether more myelosuppressive, more responsive, or more intense regimens are more effective. Many factors associated with survival are also associated with other outcomes. For instance, in the SWOG study just discussed, we found menopausal status and age to be associated with dose. (Premenopausal patients received the highest doses, post 60 and older the lowest, and post less than 60 middle range doses.) It might be possible to adjust for the few factors we know about, but most factors are unmeasured or unknown or both. Part or all of any association (or lack of association) of survival with attained dose or any other outcome may well be explained by these other factors.

Considering all the biases in analyzing survival by dose, and the fact that intensity cannot even be defined sensibly, we hope you are persuaded that dose intensity analyses have no useful scientific interpretation. The way to answer questions about dose intensity is through randomized trials!

8.5 Subset analyses

The temptation to go beyond a simple treatment comparison of the primary endpoint is almost irresistible. If the study is negative overall, it would be nice if there were some subset of patients (women, good performance status, young, etc.) for which a benefit associated with the new treatment could be shown. Similarly, if in the overall comparison there is an advantage for the new treatment over the standard, it is of interest to find subsets for which the advantage is greater, and some for which it is not beneficial at all. The problem with such good intentions is that most such subset analyses arrive at incorrect conclusions.

In 1989 the North Central Cancer Treatment Group and the Mayo Clinic published a study that demonstrated a survival advantage for the combination of 5-FU and levamisole over observation after surgery for patients with Dukes' C colon cancer (Laurie et al., 1989). The authors then looked at subsets of patients to see whether some groups benefited from therapy more than others. They found that adjuvant therapy was most effective for females, and for younger patients. A large confirmatory trial was undertaken, involving several groups, with the Southwest Oncology Group as the statistical center. The overall result was consistent with the earlier trial: patients with Dukes' C colon cancer treated with 5-FU plus levamisole after surgery had a better survival outcome than did patients on observation (Moertel et al., 1990). However, when we looked at the same subsets as in the NCCTG/Mayo study, we found that adjuvant therapy was most effective for males, and for older patients: the exact opposite! Figure 8.20 illustrates the results for males.

We recently reviewed eight trials testing the efficacy of infusion of 5-FU into the portal vein following surgery for colorectal cancer (Crowley, 1994). Three trials were reported as positive for portal vein infusion therapy, five as negative. Among the positive trials, therapy was found to be more effective in Dukes' C patients in one trial and in Dukes B in another. A formal statistical test of whether

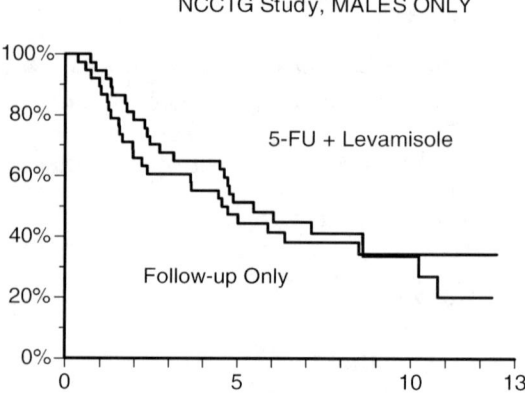

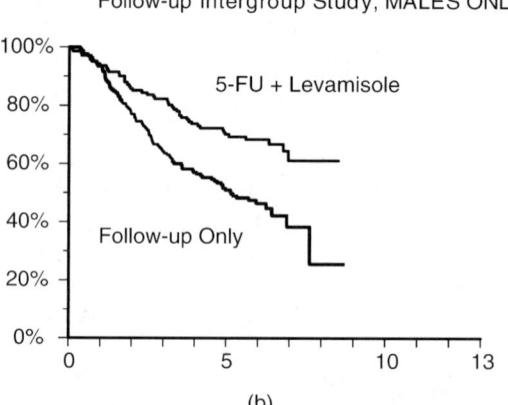

Figure 8.20. Subset analysis of males from: (a) original study; and (b) confirmatory study.

treatment results varied by subset was negative in the third trial. Among the negative trials, positive subsets were found for Dukes' C patients in one, for all those surviving 6 months in another, and for Dukes' C patients surviving 3 years in a third. No subset differences were found in the other two trials. The overall benefit of portal vein infusion is in doubt (and is the subject of a published meta-analysis — see Chapter 9); the subset analyses are clearly noise.

Why do such subset analyses so often go wrong? Most cancer clinical trials are designed with sample sizes just large enough to have reasonable power to detect a clinically interesting treatment difference for the primary comparison of interest. In some cases the power is not even sufficient for this main outcome. Thus, a particular subset, with around half (or less) of the patients, will have even lower power. As a result, a given subset analysis will have a high false negative rate (low power); many real differences will go undetected. In particular, this means that for a study with an overall positive treatment result, there is a strong likelihood that there will be a nonsignificant result within some subsets. This could have detrimental implications for patient treatment. Would one want to make a treatment decision that differed from the overall study conclusions for a patient from a specific subset, based on a test with low power?

As an example, consider SWOG 9008, a recently reported trial in gastric cancer (Macdonald et al., 2001) that established the benefit of using chemoradiation after gastric resection compared to no additional treatment. Among the many variables for which subset analyses were requested, there was interest in whether tumors of the gastro-esophageal (GE) junction behaved differently from tumors of other sites. A test of interaction between site and treatment was not significant (see Section 7.3.4). Despite this, queries continued regarding treatment effects within the subset of patients with GE junction tumors. However, of the 553 eligible patients on this trial, only 20% had tumors of the GE junction. We determined that based on these numbers, the power to detect the study-specific hazard ratio in this subset was approximately 40%. Would we want to publish a result that had such a poor chance of demonstrating the clinical result? Based on the nonsignificant interaction, and such low power, we did not pursue further exploration in this subset.

Fleming (1995) performed a simulation study to assess the reliability of subset analyses when the overall treatment effect was positive. This simulation, based on data from a double-blind, placebo-controlled trial of dornase alfa in 968 patients with cystic fibrosis, estimated false-negative rates when only three covariates were the subject of subset analyses. The covariates were age (categorized into three levels, representing 50%, 20%, and 30% of the population, respectively); sex (50%, 50%), and baseline forced vital capacity (FVC) (40%, 30%, 30%). The simulation assumed that the overall treatment effect was constant across all subsets of patients, and 1000 trials were generated, randomly assigning patients to different covariate levels for each trial. In 67% of the trials, the treatment was estimated to be of no benefit, or even harmful in at least one level of one of the three covariates. This false-negative rate would have been even higher if the number of subsets tested had been increased.

Subset analyses suffer from more than low power. When the overall test of treatment does not conclude a benefit of one treatment over the other, subset analyses are viewed as a way to save something from the trial, or at the very least, make the manuscript more interesting. Once one starts down the road of doing subset analyses, it is very difficult to stop. After looking within races, sexes, stages, performance status categories, histologies, tumor grades, *ad infinitum*, something is bound to show up as being statistically significant just by chance (this is the multiple comparison problem considered in the context of multi-arm trials in Chapter 4, interim analyses in Chapter 5, and exploratory analyses in Chapter 9). Multiple subset analyses are subject to a high false-positive rate; many of the differences detected are not really there.

The combined problems of poor power for real differences, and high false-positive rates mean that almost all subset analyses are wrong. Thus, all subset analyses must be confirmed in subsequent trials before they can be believed.

What can be done to minimize the difficulties inherent in subset analyses, given the imperative to explore data for clues? First, understand that if results in a given subset are important and likely to be different, separate trials should be designed, or a given trial should be designed with adequate power for that subset analysis, including proper attention to the multiple comparison problem. Second, understand that stratification for the purpose of balance at randomization (Chapter 3) does not justify subset analyses by stratification factors. Such analyses are still subject to a high false-negative rate due to inadequate sample size, and a high false-positive rate unless each comparison is done at a very low significance level or using a model that first allows for a formal statistical test of whether treatment differences vary by subset. Third, be aware that subset analyses are exploratory and hypothesis generating, and thus not to be given nearly the same credibility as the overall treatment comparison. Any presentation or publication of results (Chapter 7) should make clear which results can be taken as definitive and which as exploratory. As a rule, the overall treatment comparison of the primary endpoint is definitive (in a well-designed trial), the rest is speculative.

8.6 Surrogate endpoints

Survival is the preferred primary endpoint in cancer clinical trials, being both objective and of obvious validity. In certain adjuvant trials (in breast cancer, for example) it is not practical to insist on survival as the primary endpoint, because not enough events will be observed in a realistic time-frame; thus disease-free survival is used instead. It could be said in such cases that disease-free survival, which is known sooner but is somewhat subjective and does not perfectly reflect long-term outcome, is used as a replacement or surrogate for survival (which is usually an important secondary endpoint). A more common use of the term surrogate endpoint is for very short-term outcomes such as tumor response, tumor markers in cancer prevention trials, and CD4 count in AIDS trials. The motivation for the use of such surrogate endpoints is obvious: we would like to be able to make decisions about treatment efficacy with smaller sample sizes and without having to wait for the real endpoint to occur.

A few examples should suffice to give pause about the use of surrogate endpoints. We have already seen in the sarcoma trial of AD vs. MAID that a higher tumor response rate does not necessarily translate into better survival (Section 8.4.1). The same phenomenon occurred with 5-FU and leucovorin in advanced colon cancer. A review of several trials (Advanced Colorectal Meta-Analysis Project, 1992) indicated that response was strikingly improved with the combination ($p < 0.0001$) but that there was no effect on survival ($p = 0.57$). The opposite can also happen. Gil Deza et al. (1996) reported a survival advantage for vinorelbine and cisplatin over vinorelbine alone in patients with advanced non-small cell lung cancer ($p = 0.02$) but no response advantage ($p = 0.97$).

In the Cardiac Arrythmia Suppression Trial (Echt et al., 1991) in patients having a recent myocardial infarction, encainide and flecainide were compared to placebo for survival post MI. These agents reduce ventricular arrhythmias, which are a risk factor for subsequent sudden death. Many argued that a placebo-controlled trial was not only unnecessary but unethical, since an effect on the surrogate endpoint of ventricular arrhythmias had already been established. The trial was done anyway, and with over 1500 randomized patients the startling result was that the drugs more than doubled the death rate relative to placebo (the rate was more than tripled for causes to due arrhythmias).

From the field of AIDS research, a trial conducted in the United States by the Aids Clinical Trials Group (Volberding et al., 1990) testing the effect of zidovudine for slowing disease progression in asymptomatic HIV-infected people was stopped early for positive results based on interim analysis of this surrogate endpoint (progression). A later trial done in Europe (Concorde Coordinating Committee, 1994) found that with longer follow-up the effect on the surrogate was lost, and no effect on survival was found. (See DeMets et al.,

(1995) for a discussion of the first trial from the point of view of the data monitoring committee.)

Prentice (1989) has given mathematical conditions that would permit the use of surrogate endpoints. To guarantee that the inference from the surrogate is the same as would be obtained from the primary endpoint, it is necessary to assume that all the information on treatment differences is contained in the surrogate, clearly an impossible case. There were suggestions to model the association of the surrogate with the primary endpoint as you go along and to use the information gained to strengthen inferences on the primary endpoint. It turns out that the information gained is highly dependent on being able to model the relationships correctly. Even the enthusiasts of this approach agree that it does not help unless there is a very high correlation between the primary and surrogate endpoints. Hsieh, Crowley, and Tormey (1983) investigate various realistic models of the relationship between disease progression and death, and find that incorporating progression into the analysis of survival adds little strength to the inference, even when the correct model is assumed.

The inescapable conclusion is that trials must be designed to detect differences in real clinical endpoints of interest. Surrogates are most useful in the context of Phase II trials to screen agents for further randomized testing of effects on primary endpoints.

CHAPTER 9

Exploratory Analyses

> *In real life research is dependent on the human capacity for making predictions that are wrong and on the even more human gift for bouncing back to try again.*
>
> –**Lewis Thomas** (1983)

9.1 Introduction

Cancer clinical trials should be designed primarily to get precise answers to important questions about the efficacy of treatment. However, there is considerable interest in also trying to learn something about the underlying biology of the disease during the course of a trial or a series of trials. Data are collected on patient demographics, tumor characteristics, and various other host factors in an attempt to understand which variables are useful in predicting patient outcome, both for use in subsequent trials and in explaining the results of a given trial. As opposed to the definitive treatment comparison, these statistical analyses are exploratory, serving to generate and not prove hypotheses. The general kinds of questions addressed include the following: What are the important prognostic factors? How can they be used in the design of future trials? Are there identifiable subsets of patients who do so well that there is little room for improvements in treatment? Are there subsets of patients who do so poorly that much more aggressive strategies should be devised?

We illustrate some aspects of these exploratory analyses using data from two Southwest Oncology Group trials of multiple myeloma with survival as the outcome of interest (SWOG 8229, Salmon et al., 1990; SWOG 8624, Salmon et al., 1994), but the issues are of course more general. More detailed analyses of these data are given in Crowley et al., 1995 and Crowley et al., 1997).

9.2 Some background and notation

Patients with multiple myeloma have a predominant clone of affected plasma cells and thus a compromised immune system. They are thus subject to various infections, and also often have kidney trouble and bone lesions and fractures. The introduction of therapy with melphalan and prednisone in the 1950s increased the median survival for patients with this disease from less than 1 year to 30–36 months. The course of the disease is extremely variable but most patients eventually die of myeloma or its complications. Consequently, there is an interest in understanding which factors at diagnosis predict survival, and in developing staging systems that could be used in stratification or in defining subsets for differing therapeutic interventions.

SWOG 8229 was designed to test whether two four-drug combinations (vincristine, melphalan, cyclophosphamide, prednisone; vincristine, BCNU, Adriamycin) should be given in rapid succession or in a more slowly alternating fashion. There was evidence that cancer cells resistant to one combination would be susceptible to treatment with the other, and some theory (the Goldie-Coldman hypothesis, Goldie 1982) that such noncross-resistant regimens should be given as close in time as possible for maximum effect. We randomized 614 patients to the two regimens and found virtually no difference in survival (Figure 9.1). SWOG 8624 compared one of the arms from SWOG 8229 with two other regimens containing more steroids, with modest differences in favor of the latter two arms.

The staging system currently in common use is due to Durie and Salmon (1975) and is based on a quantification of the number of tumor cells (stages I-III) and a classification of kidney function (A, B). This system was used to stratify the patients in SWOG 8229 (I-II vs. IIIA vs. IIIB, Figure 9.2). Besides Durie-Salmon stages, information routinely collected on the myeloma prestudy form includes albumin, creatinine, age, race, myeloma subtype (light- and heavy-chain proteins involved), and serum β_2 microglobulin (sb2m), a prognostic factor first identified in the 1980s (Norfolk et al., 1980; Battaille et al., 1983) which rises with either increasing tumor burden or decreased kidney function. We wanted to know if these variables predicted survival and if we could derive a more predictive and reproducible staging system than the Durie-Salmon.

Statistically, these questions can be addressed within the framework of Cox (or proportional hazards), and regression, introduced in Chapter 2. (Analogously, other measured variables not subject to censoring can be explored using ordinary multiple linear regression or

SOME BACKGROUND AND NOTATION

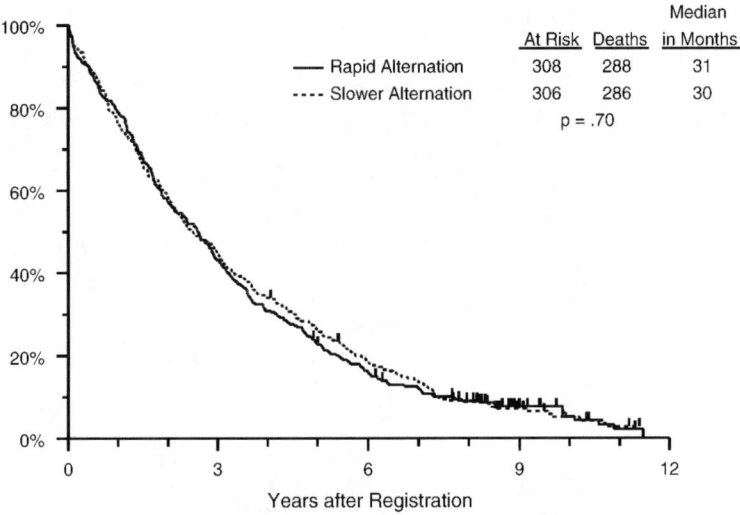

Figure 9.1. Survival distributions by treatment in SWOG myeloma trial 8229.

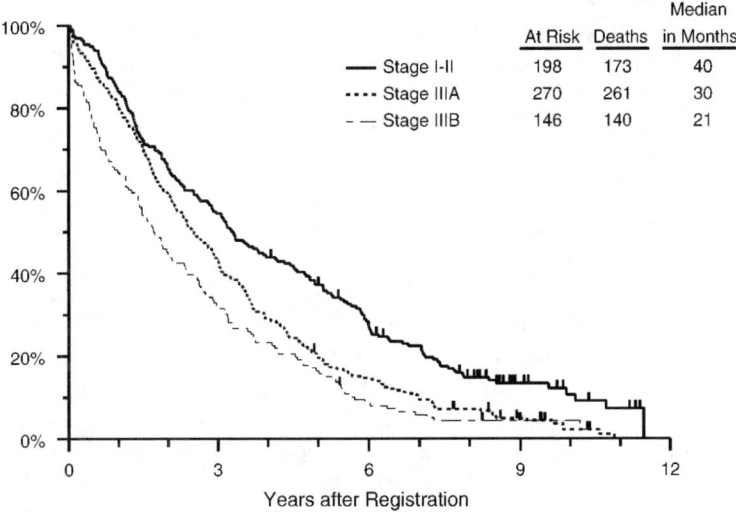

Figure 9.2. Survival distributions by Durie-Salmon stage in SWOG myeloma trial 8229.

any of its generalizations, and dichotomized categorical variables can be explored using a model relating probabilities to covariates, such as logistic regression (see, for instance, Farewell and Matthews, 1996).) Since the methods are exploratory, there is more of an emphasis on looking at data graphically to find relationships, but some aspects of formal hypothesis testing and estimation are usually employed (subject to caveats regarding multiple comparisons and post-hoc fallacies). With survival analysis the fact that some survival times may be censored makes the graphical aspects all the more challenging.

Recall from Chapter 2 that the proportional hazards model characterizes a patient's hazard or risk of dying as a function of time and measured variables of interest. Thus the model states that a patient with covariates x (x_1 = age, x_2 = stage, x_3 = sb2m, etc.) has hazard function

$$\lambda(t, x) = \lambda_0(t) \exp\left(\sum_i \beta_i x_i\right),$$

or in logarithmic form

$$\ln \lambda(t, x) = \ln \lambda_0(t) + \left(\sum_i \beta_i x_i\right). \tag{9.1}$$

The underlying or baseline hazard $\lambda_0(t)$ is not of interest so much as whether a particular covariate x_i should be in the model (statistically, whether we can reject the hypothesis that β_i is 0); and in how the model might be used to make predictions or derive patient groupings (which involves estimating β).

9.3 Identification of prognostic factors

In principle the answer to the question of whether, say, sb2m is an important prognostic factor can be answered very simply by the statistician: fit a Cox model and test whether the coefficient associated with sb2m is 0 or not (the test statistic is a generalization of the logrank test). In practice, there are a host of difficulties and complications that the user of such models needs to appreciate. First, there is the issue of the scale of measurement. A covariate like sb2m is continuous. Should it be used as a continuous variable in the regression modeling, or dichotomized or otherwise turned into a categorical variable? If continuous, should it be in the original scale or some other scale (e.g., logarithmic)? If categorical, how are the cutpoints of the categories to be chosen? Second, is it of primary interest to see if sb2m is prognostic at all (in a univariate model, with no other variables present), or prognostic even in the presence of other variables (in a model with multiple other variables, i.e., a multivariate model). If the latter, how is this multivariate model developed, from the literature or the data at hand? If from the data, there is the question of the scale of measurement for each of the other variables, the question of whether derived variables are considered (e.g., products of two variables), and the question of how a final model is chosen from among countless possibilities even given answers to the other questions (step-down, step-up, stepwise, all subset selection, etc. (see Draper and Smith (1968) for a general discussion of these methods, and also Section 9.3.2 below). We address each of these areas in turn.

9.3.1 Scale of measurement

As usual, there are trade-offs regarding the choice of a scale of measurement for a putative prognostic factor. The simplest choice for a continuous covariate is to use the measurements as recorded and ask whether the coefficient is significant in a Cox regression model. This is also the most powerful, in the sense of detecting an effect if there really is one, provided the assumed model is correct. However, there is little likelihood that any regression model is exactly correct, and it is well known that a few extreme values of the covariate can greatly affect the results of a regression analysis. Transformations of the covariate (e.g., by taking logs) can reduce the dependence on extreme values, but the choice of a particular transformation can be problematic. Covariates can be categorized to create two or more groups, but the choice of boundaries for the groupings can be difficult (possibilities include using previously published values, using the median or other percentiles of the observed covariate distribution, or using data-driven cutpoints). We illustrate these choices using sb2m as a potential predictor of survival in our sample of myeloma patients treated on SWOG 8229.

The covariate sb2m was recorded for 548 of the 614 eligible patients on study. For various reasons, it is typical to have some missing values of a covariate. Such missing data can jeopardize an analysis of prognostic factors, especially if the reasons for missing data are related to the variables under study. The best approach is to minimize this problem through protocol requirements (sb2m was not an eligibility criterion for 8229); a distant second best is to investigate whether the other covariates and the outcome of interest vary depending on whether data are missing on a particular covariate. Figure 9.3 shows that the patients with and without available sb2m measurements have roughly comparable survival, a reassuring but not conclusive observation.

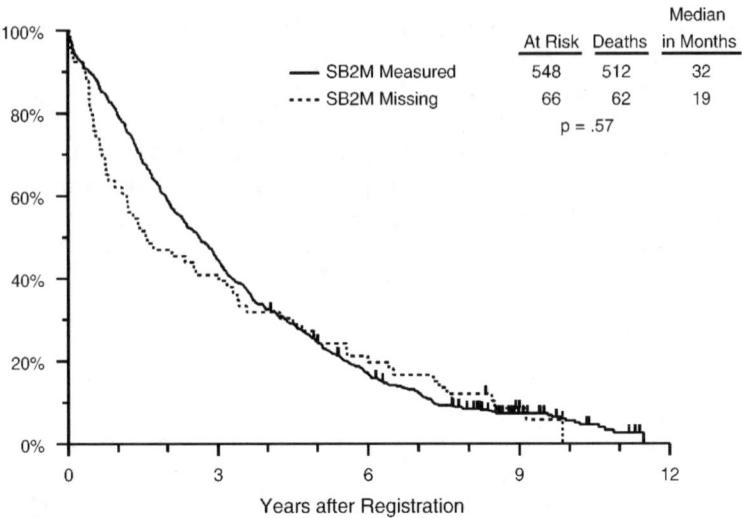

Figure 9.3. Survival distributions by presence of sb2m in SWOG myeloma trial 8229.

The result of fitting a Cox model with the single covariate sb2m as measured gives a χ^2 of 38.11 ($p < 0.0001$) and an estimated β coefficient of 0.035, meaning that an increase in one unit of sb2m is associated with an estimated increase of $\exp(0.035) = 1.035$ in the risk of dying per day (survival was measured in days). But is this real or artifactual? Figure 9.4a shows the distribution of sb2m values, which as is typical for laboratory measurements is highly skewed, with a few large values that have a great deal of influence on the fit of the Cox regression model. Figure 9.4b shows that the distribution of the log of sb2m has fewer extreme values. Fitting log sb2m in a Cox model gives a χ^2 of 36.45 ($p < 0.0001$) and an estimated coefficient of 0.360, which means an estimated increase in risk of dying of $\exp(0.360) = 1.434$ for a unit increase in log sb2m. But which model is better? Statistical techniques now exist for estimating the regression relationship (the summation in Equation (9.1)) without assuming it has the linear form $\sum \beta_i x_i$ (Tibshirani and Hastie, 1987; Gentleman and Crowley, 1991a). One such fit is shown in Figure 9.4a for sb2m, suggesting a highly nonlinear relationship. A similar fit for log sb2m is given in Figure 9.4b; the latter relationship is more nearly linear, indicating that using $x = \log$ sb2m in the Cox model with the linear form $\sum \beta_i x_i$ is more appropriate than using $x =$ sb2m without such a transformation.

It would seem wise in any case to step back from fitting a regression model and take a look at the data. When plotting survival

IDENTIFICATION OF PROGNOSTIC FACTORS

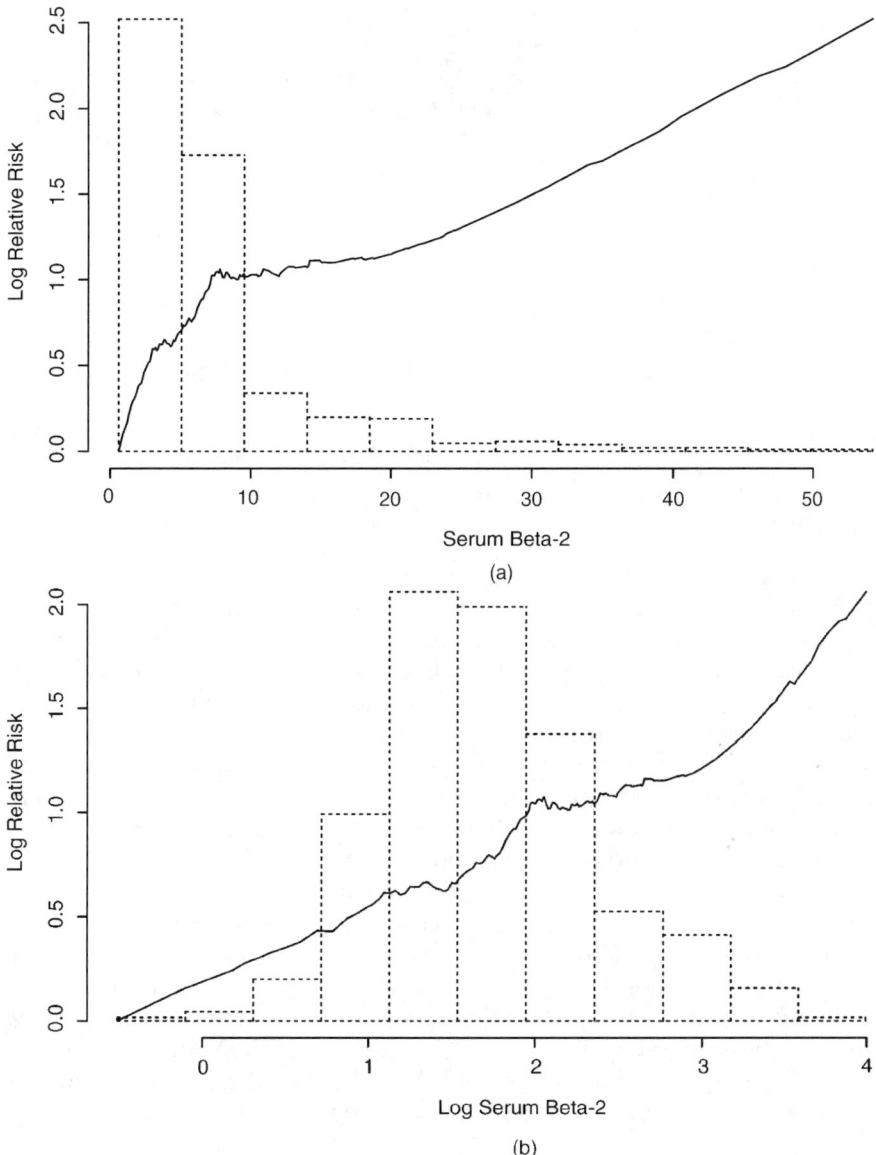

Figure 9.4. Local full likelihood estimate of the log relative risk for: (a) sb2m; (b) log sb2m. Histograms of (a) sb2m and (b) log sb2m are also shown.

data, however, the censored data points can distort the message that complete data would provide. Figure 9.5 is a scatterplot of survival and log sb2m with censored observations plotted with open circles, uncensored ones with closed circles. It is difficult to discern trends

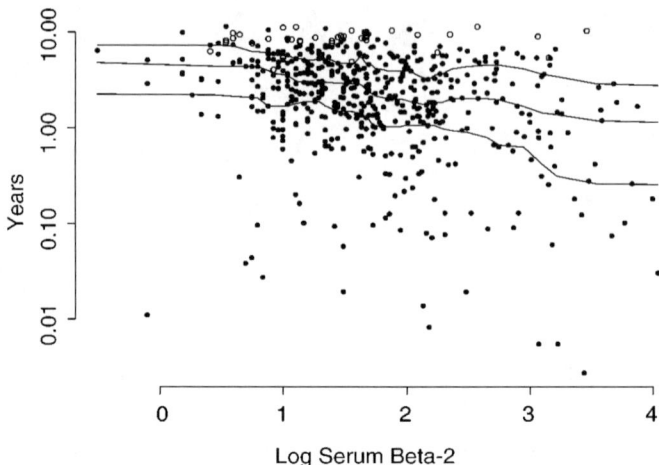

Figure 9.5. Scatterplot of survival vs. log sb2m with smoothed quartile estimators.

in the scatter plot by itself, because of the censoring and because of the inherent variability of the data. Merely superimposing a straight line fit would not be appropriate because some of the data are censored. However, one can use recently developed techniques to fit a curve through the center of the data, where for a given value of log sb2m those patients with nearby covariate values are grouped and the median survival or other percentiles of the distribution are calculated (Gentleman and Crowley, 1991b). Figure 9.5 shows these running quantile plots for the median and the 75th and 25th percentiles, indicating a decrease in survival with increasing values of log sb2m. An even simpler approach would be to categorize sb2m into a few groups (three or more are recommended, depending on how much data one has) and plot survival curves for each group. An example is given in Figure 9.6 (the choice of cutpoints is arbitrary, but could be based on having enough data in each group if an indication of trend is all that is desired). It would seem from these various analyses that sb2m is indeed an important prognostic factor.

9.3.2 Choice of model

Once we have established that a covariate such as sb2m does have some use in predicting the survival of myeloma patients, the next question is: Does sb2m have prognostic value added to what is already known about the covariates that predict survival? If there is already

IDENTIFICATION OF PROGNOSTIC FACTORS

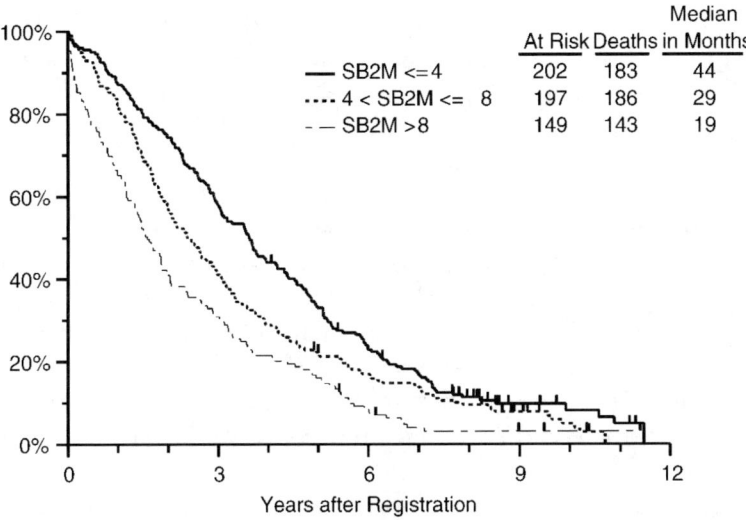

Figure 9.6. Survival distributions by values of sb2m in SWOG myeloma trial 8229.

an agreed upon regression equation, this question is only slightly more complicated than the question of whether sb2m has any prognostic value (the problem is that graphs that take into account other factors are harder to draw than those involving a single covariate). One merely has to decide on an appropriate scale of measurement, then add sb2m to an agreed upon model containing the known factors and test the hypothesis that the β coefficient associated with sb2m is 0. However, it is fair to say that no situation exists in cancer research where there is agreement on which prognostic factors are important, much less on the form of the model containing those factors. One is thus left with having to decide the scale of measurement for each known factor and whether derived variables such as products are to be included in a model before even addressing the question of the added value of sb2m. Often the situation is even more complicated than that, the question being not "does this covariate add information" but rather, which of dozens of candidate variables are "the" important prognostic factors (and which is the most important, which is next, etc.).

An extensive statistical literature on fitting such regression models is available, especially but not exclusively in the context of uncensored data. Excellent recent reviews of regression methods with censored data are given in Schumacher et al., 2001; Ulm et al., 2001; Thall and Estey, 2001; and Sasieni and Winnett, 2001. At least as many strategies exist as there are statisticians. One can step up in the sense that all variables (and derived variables such as products? products of three or more variables? different scales for each variable?) are considered by themselves one by one, in univariate models, and the most statistically significant is chosen in the first step. The remaining variables are then considered as to whether they add to the first, etc. Or, one can step down, first fitting a model with all possible variables and then seeing which can be eliminated as least significant. (This approach is rarely possible due to the large number of candidate variables and the fact that few patients will have complete data on all of them.) Or, one can adopt a stepwise strategy, stepping up but seeing at each step if any previously included variable can now be excluded. Yet another approach is to select the best from all possible models, something conceivable only in statistical textbooks.

A related technique to Cox regression modeling is the use of neural networks (or neural nets), which are really no more than complicated regression models hidden behind the language of artificial intelligence. An example using the data from SWOG myeloma study 8229 is given by Faraggi, LeBlanc, and Crowley, 2001. The results are not much different from the use of Cox regression, provided one keeps the neural net to a manageable number of parameters, and includes product terms (also called interactions) in the Cox model. The disadvantage of neural nets is that the results are difficult to interpret in terms of the effects of the original variables.

Apart from all the more subjective modeling decisions, there is the fact that a multitude of formal statistical tests are being done. This multiple comparison issue was also raised in Chapters 4 and 5, but it is an even more severe problem in the present context. (Should each test be done at the 5% level? The 0.5% level? Is there a level for each test that is small enough to protect against making false positive statements?) This is not science, and perhaps not art. Many of us have heard confident proclamations that such and so variable is important in multivariate analysis; perhaps now you can appreciate the fact that this translates to "my statistician and I think we have something here." In the case of sb2m, we think we have something. It has been found to be important by others. It is important in our data in univariate analyses using various scales of measurement. It is the first variable entered in the stepwise modeling we have done. And, "it is statistically significant in a multivariate analysis, after adjusting for other known prognostic factors ($p < 0.001$)."

9.4 Forming prognostic groups

Given an agreed upon Cox regression model (!) one can make predictions about the survival of patients with given prognostic factors. While it should be clear that this cannot be done with any precision, one might use a Cox regression model to group patients into broad prognostic categories or stages (based on deciles, quartiles, etc. of patient values of the regression function βx, or by assigning patients into categories based on how many of the good or bad values of prognostic variables they had). While such staging schemes have proven useful, they are difficult to interpret. A more direct technique called recursive partitioning or regression trees may have some advantages in this regard.

Recursive partitioning can be described as follows. Each candidate prognostic variable is used to divide the patients into two groups, based on all possible cutpoints for that variable. The best (over all variables and all cutpoints) such split is found, where "best" might be defined as maximizing the logrank statistic between the two groups (Ciampi et al., 1986; Segal, 1988). This rule is then applied to each of the resulting two groups, and then recursively to the data until there are a large number of groups, each containing only a small number of patients. Next, there are rules that allow one to combine groups and choose the best staging system. There are several potential advantages to this approach to forming prognostic groups. One is that the scale of measurement is not an issue, except that a monotonic relationship must be assumed between covariates and survival (e.g., survival tends to go down as sb2m goes up). Another is that the resulting groups are easily described (a good prognosis group being those with low sb2m and high albumin, for example). In addition, there are built-in mechanisms (sample re-use, such as cross-validation, Breiman et al., 1984) that try to minimize the extent to which one is fooled by making multiple comparisons. However, there are still difficulties, among them that use of another statistic besides the logrank test results in different groupings and that the precise split points for a given set of data are unlikely to be duplicated in the next.

Figure 9.7 is a plot of the value of the logrank statistic as a function of the value of the covariate for several covariates in the SWOG 8229 data set. The best split into two groups based on the logrank statistic is for the covariate sb2m, at a value of 5.4 nanograms per milliliter. The Chi-squared statistic for this split is 38 ($p < 0.0001$) but this needs to be adjusted because it is the maximum logrank

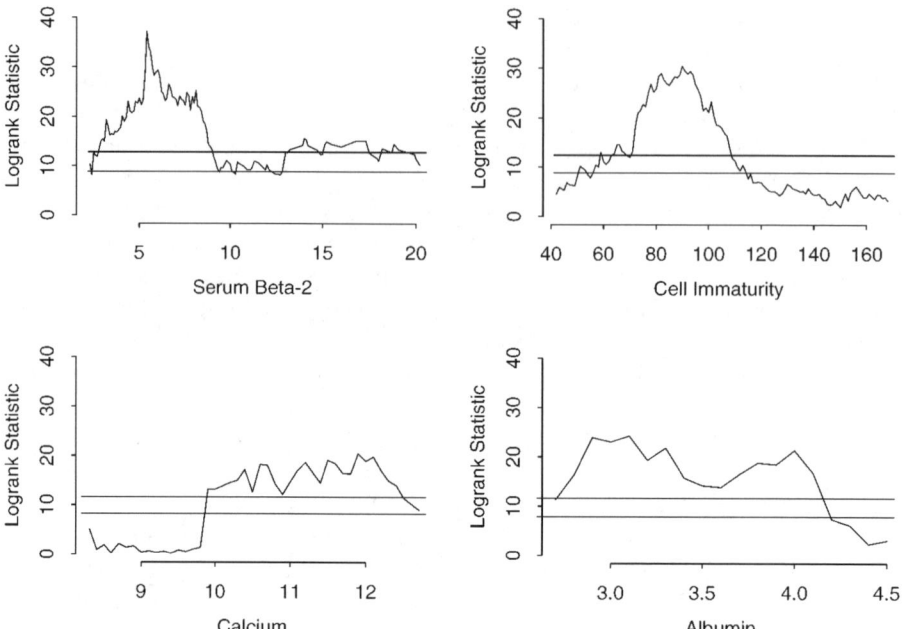

Figure 9.7. The logrank statistic as a function of several covariates in the SWOG myeloma trial 8229 data set. Values above the horizontal lines are significant at the 1 and 5% levels adjusted for multiple comparisons.

statistic over all possible cutpoints. The p-value adjusted for multiple comparisons is still highly significant (see LeBlanc and Crowley, 1993, for a discussion of the details of the adjustment procedure).

A regression tree based on our recursive partitioning algorithm (LeBlanc and Crowley, 1992) using all candidate variables is given in Figure 9.8. The value of the variable for each split is given along with the logrank test statistic in χ^2 form and the p-value adjusted for multiple comparisons. The median survival in years and the sample sizes for the final groupings are also displayed. Thus the first split in the tree is based on sb2m at a value of 5.4, with a χ^2 of 35.93 and an adjusted p-value listed as 0 ($p < 0.001$), resulting in two groups. The group with low sb2m is split on the variable calcium, at a value of 10.6, and so on. Finally, groups with similar survival can be combined giving a proposed staging system with three stages as shown in Figure 9.9 that can be contrasted with the Durie-Salmon system (Figure 9.2). The best prognostic group in Figure 9.9 consists of younger patients with low sb2m, low calcium, and high albumin. The worst group has high sb2m and high age, or high sb2m, low age, and high creatinine. The rest of the patients form the intermediate

FORMING PROGNOSTIC GROUPS

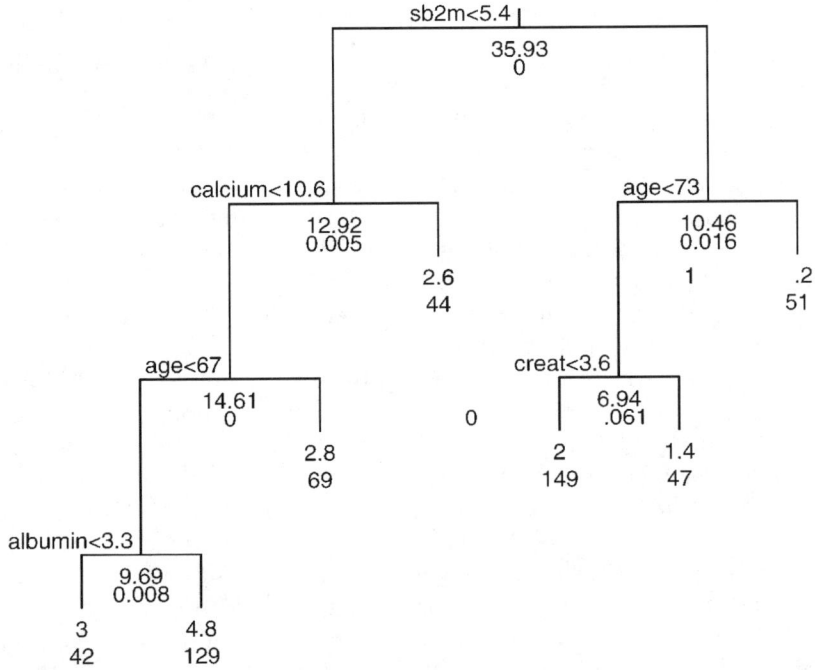

Figure 9.8. A regression tree based on a recursive partitioning analysis of the SWOG myeloma 8229 data set. Numbers beneath the variable names are the χ^2 value of the logrank test and the adjusted p-value. Median survival in years and sample size are also given for the final groups.

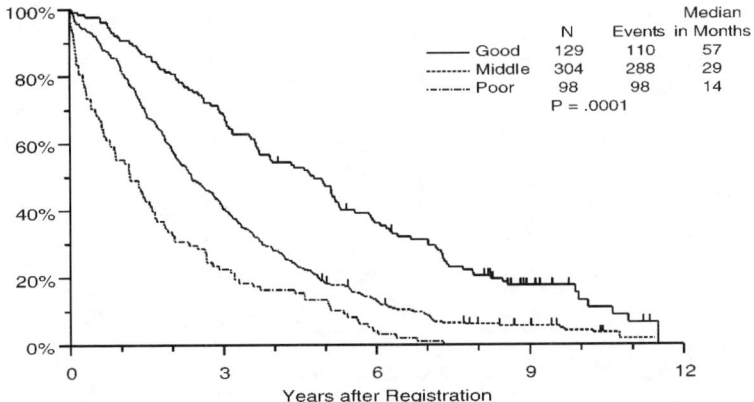

Figure 9.9. Prognostic groups from a recursive partitioning analysis of the SWOG myeloma trial 8229 data set.

group. Because this entire process has been exploratory in nature, this new proposed staging system needs to be validated in independent data sets before it can be regarded as reliable and useful, and that effort has been completed (Crowley et al., 1997) using validation data from the subsequent myeloma trial, SWOG 8624 (Salmon et al., 1994). As shown in Figure 9.10, the staging system does appear to generalize beyond the data from which it was derived. An even simpler system based just on sb2m and albumin has also been proposed recently (Jacobson et al., 2001).

A related statistical technique to recursive partitioning is called peeling. Here the idea is to find one group of patients with a particularly poor (or good) prognosis, but with enough patients for the grouping to be useful. An example using the myeloma data is given in LeBlanc, Jacobson, and Crowley, 2002. The goal was to identify a group with a median survival of 18 months or less, thinking that such a group would be a good candidate for more intensive therapy. The algorithm based on SWOG 8229 identified those with sb2m ≥ 10.1, constituting 17% of the sample, and a second group with $10.1 > \text{sb2m} \geq 4.7$, albumin <3.7 and age ≥ 68, which added another 10%. The 2 groups together had a median survival of 18 months. In contrast, from the regression tree in Figure 9.8, one could identify those with sb2m ≥ 5.4 and age ≥ 73, along with those with sb2m ≥ 5.4, age <73 and creatinine ≥ 3.6, constituting 19% of the sample with a median survival of 17 months. Figure 9.11 shows the results of these two approaches for finding a poor prognosis subset applied to the data from SWOG 8229. Applying these groups to the validation data from

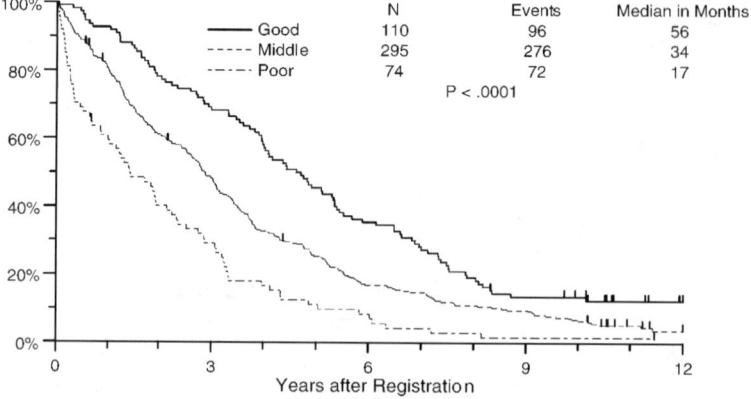

Figure 9.10. Validation of the prognostic groups derived from the SWOG myeloma trial 8229 data set using data from the subsequent myeloma trials, SWOG 8624.

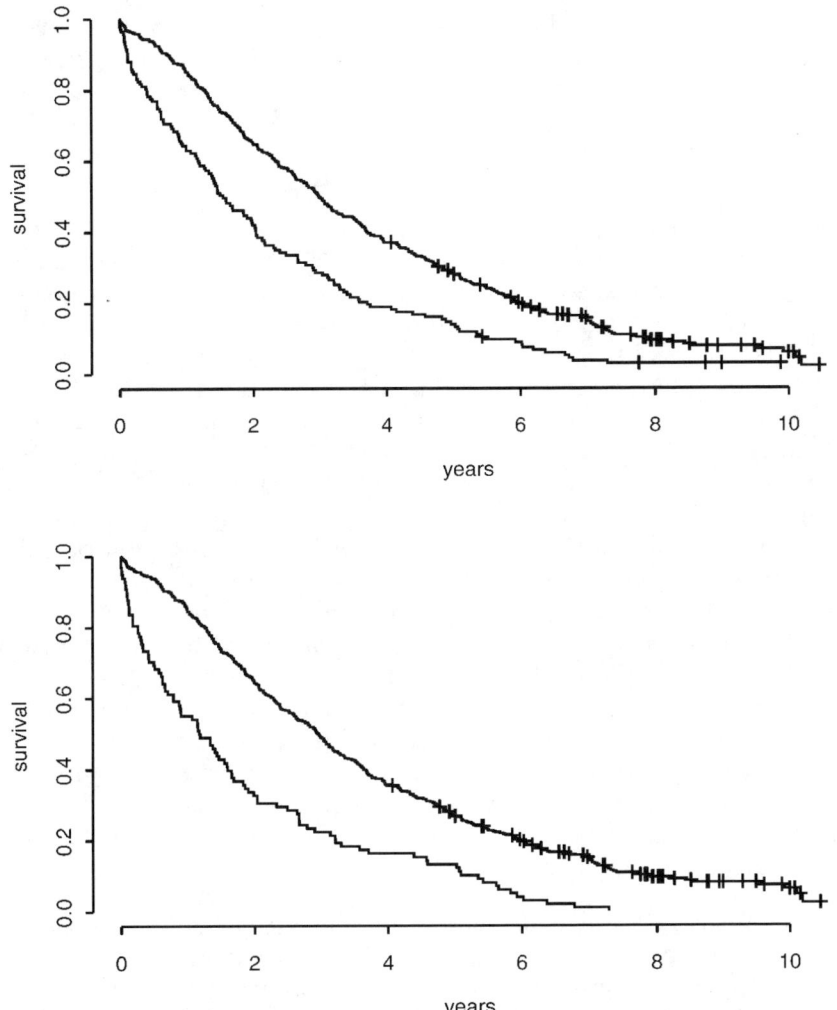

Figure 9.11. Survival curves for poor prognostic groups vs. the remaining patients, based on data from myeloma trial 8229. The top panel is based on peeling, and has 27% of the patients in the poor prognosis group. The bottom panel is based on regression trees, and has 19% of the patients in the poor prognosis group.

SWOG 8624 yielded very similar survival results, with 27% of the sample in the poor prognosis group using peeling, and 15% from the regression tree approach. Again, the results generalize beyond the data from which they were derived. Note that the peeling algorithm generates a larger subset of poor prognosis patients and so might be more useful clinically than regression trees for the purpose of isolating a single prognosis group from the rest of the patients.

9.5 Analysis of microarray data

The past decade has witnessed an explosion of knowledge about the human genome and the genes that play a role in the development and progression of cancer. The coming decade holds the promise of moving that knowledge from the bench to the bedside.

A key to this revolution was the development of the microarray chip, a technology which permits the researcher to study literally thousands of genes in a single assay. There are several approaches to developing these chips, but the basics are that known genes or key parts of genes (sequences of nucleotides) are fixed on a small slide, and a sample from a subject is prepared in such a way that the genes existing in the sample will attach to the genes on the slide. The output for each gene is compared to either an internal or external control and is expressed as either a categorical (gene present or not) or a measured variable (usually a ratio or a log ratio of experimental to control, quantifying the degree of over or under expression). The chips can be created to target genes hypothesized to be involved in a specific cancer (e.g., the lymphochip for studying lymphoma, Alizadeh et al., 2000)) or can be quite general (one recent chip from a commercial vendor contains over 12,000 genes).

There are many questions that can be addressed with this new technology, among them:

- What genes or combinations of genes (what genetic profiles) differentiate normal subjects from cancer patients?
- Can genetic profiles be used to define more useful subsets of specific cancers (replacing histology or standard laboratory measurements, for example)?
- Can genetic profiles be used to develop targeted therapy against the gene products (proteins) expressed by individual patients?

If the analyses discussed in earlier sections of this chapter have been called exploratory, it should be clear that with thousands of variables on a much smaller number of patients (these chips are not cheap), the analysis of microarray data is *highly* exploratory. Any analysis of these data is subject to extreme problems of multiple comparisons and must be confirmed on independent data sets before being given credence.

The question of differentiating normals from cancer patients, called "class prediction" by Golub et al. (1999), can be approached for each gene using familiar statistics (Rosner, 1986) such as the χ^2 (for categorical outcomes, gene on or off) or the t-test or Wilcoxon test (for measured expression ratios). To account for the fact that thousands of such statistical tests will be done, a p-value <0.001 or less might be used instead of the usual 5% level. Regression techniques (logistic regression for categorical outcomes, simple linear regression for measured outcomes) could be used to determine if combinations of genes predict whether a sample is from the normal or the cancer class, but the number of genes involved make this mathematically impossible. A common solution to this problem is through a data reduction technique such as principal components (Quackenbush, 2001), which replaces the original set of thousands of variables with a much smaller set (typically 10 to 50) of linear combinations of the original variables, chosen to capture most of the variability in the sample. Ordinary regression techniques (or neural networks, Khan et al., 2001) can then be applied to this reduced number of variables. While such techniques might predict well whether a sample is from a normal or a cancer patient and might (if validated) be used in diagnosis, the resulting regression equation is not easily interpretable (especially with neural networks).

The question of finding subsets of cancer patients based on genetic profiles, called class discovery by Golub et al. (1999), is much harder to address. Statistical techniques called clustering are often used in this context. Perhaps the most common such clustering algorithm is hierarchical clustering. While there are many variations, most are based on distances between gene expression ratios for patients (in 12,000 space, quite a generalization from distances in a plane, or 2 space!). The two closest patients are clustered together, and a new profile is defined (by averaging or other ways) for the two-patient cluster, and the algorithm repeats until all patients are in one cluster. The result can be depicted in a tree-like structure known as a dendogram. An example using patients with multiple myeloma, as well as a few patients with a pre-myeloma condition known as monoclonal gamopathy of undetermined significance (MGUS) and a few samples from myeloma cell lines (Zhan et al., 2002), is illustrated in Figure 9.12. The investigators identified four clusters, denoted MM1–MM4, and hypothesized that these clusters represented patients with a decreasing prognosis. The fact that the MGUS patients clustered with MM1 and the cell lines (presumably from patients with advanced disease) with MM4 bolstered their conclusions. However, further follow-up for survival and independent confirmation is needed. It

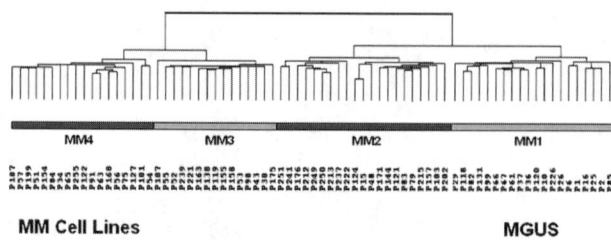

Figure 9.12. A dendogram from a hierarchical clustering of samples from myeloma patients as well as patients with MGUS and samples from several myeloma cell lines. Four groups are identified, with MGUS patients clustered with the best prognosis group (MM1) and the cell lines with the worst group (MM4). (From Zhan et al., *Blood*, 99:1745–1757, 2002. With permission.)

also should be pointed out that the hierchical clustering algorithm always finds clusters, by definition, whether there really are important groupings or not. Other clustering routines require a prespecification of the number of clusters (usually not known, thus arbitrary) and are extremely computationally intensive (thus often requiring a preliminary data reduction step using principal components or similar methods).

Perhaps the most promising aspect of genetic profiling involves development of targeted therapy. One can foresee the day when a patient will be screened for 12,000 genes and treated for the specific genetic abnormalities of his or her tumor. Cancers will be defined, staged, and treated according to their genetics, not their anatomic site or appearance under a microscope. Already several new agents are available that target specific gene products (from over expression of certain genes) involved in one or more cancers, including Herceptin (her-2 neu, in breast cancer, lung cancer, other sites) and Gleevec (c-KIT, in chronic myelogenous leukemia, gastrointestinal stromal tumors, other sites), with more on the way. Of course, the new treatments will need to be tested using the methods for clinical trials described in this book.

9.6 Meta-Analysis

The term meta-analysis seems to have been used in various ways, so at the outset let us state that we are discussing the statistical analysis of data from multiple randomized cancer clinical trials. The purposes of such meta-analyses are many, but include the testing of a null hypothesis about a given treatment in a given cancer, the estimation of the treatment effect, and the exploration of the treatment effect in subsets of patients. The fundamental reason for the growth in interest in meta-analyses is that most cancer clinical trials are too small, so that there is little power to detect clinically meaningful differences, little precision in the estimation of such differences, and almost no value in doing subset analyses (see Chapter 8). The combination of trials into a single analysis is meant to overcome these difficulties caused by small sample sizes for individual trials, but meta-analyses are no panacea, as we shall see.

9.6.1   Some principles of meta-analysis

As with any statistical analysis, a meta-analysis can be done well or done poorly. Too often results from an arbitrary selection of tangentially related published results are thrown together and termed a meta-analysis. Conclusions from such poorly done analyses are clinically uninterpretable. Principles for a valid meta-analysis include the following:

- All trials must be included, published or not. Identification of all such trials may be the most difficult part of a meta-analysis. Including only those trials that were published runs the risk of the well-known bias toward the publication of positive trials.
- The raw data from each trial must be retrieved and reanalyzed. This allows a common endpoint to be estimated, with standard errors, from each trial. Published data are almost never sufficient for this purpose since different studies will have used different endpoint definitions and will have presented different endpoints in the results sections of manuscripts. Use of the raw data gives the opportunity to employ a uniform set of inclusion criteria and to update the survival results, which besides resulting in more mature data also reduces the bias resulting from trials that stopped early in one-sided monitoring situations (Green, Fleming, Emerson, 1987).
- One must be wary of lumping fundamentally different interventions into one meta-analysis. Treatment regimens often differ in basic ways that could affect efficacy, such as dose, dose intensity, dose modifying agents, or route and timing of administration. Truly disparate interventions should not be forced into a single measure of treatment benefit. Each trial should be presented in summary form and the overall analysis (if any!) should be done by stratifying on the trials, not by collapsing over trials.

- Some measure of the quality of the trials should be incorporated into the analysis. Sensitivity analyses using different weights for each trial (including leaving some trials out altogether) should be performed.

9.6.2 An example meta-analysis: Portal vein infusion

We will discuss several aspects of meta-analysis in the context of a specific example concerning the value of portal vein infusion of 5-fluorouracil (5-FU) after surgery for colorectal cancer. A more detailed exposition can be found in Crowley (1994). The liver is a frequent site of failure after resection in colorectal cancer patients, and metastases reach the liver via the portal vein. Thus Taylor and colleagues at the University of Liverpool performed a randomized trial of perioperative portal vein infusion of 5-FU vs. surgery alone for the treatment of non-metastatic colorectal cancer (Taylor, Rowling, and West 1979; Taylor, Machin, and Mullee 1985). The experimental arm consisted of the infusion of 1 gram of 5-FU daily by catheter into the portal vein for the first 7 postoperative days (heparin was also given to prevent thrombosis). Eligible patients included those with Dukes' A, B, or C colorectal cancer. The result was a dramatic difference in favor of 5-FU infusion via the portal vein vs. controls, both in survival and in the incidence of hepatic metastases as a site of first failure. There was a 50% reduction in the hazard rate for the experimental group and a 4% incidence of liver metastases against 17% in the control group, but with a total sample size of less than 250 evaluable patients for this adjuvant trial, the confidence limits were rather wide, and the authors wisely called for confirmatory trials.

Since then nine such confirmatory trials have been completed. The results of these trials can best be described as mixed; some show an effect on liver metastases but little or no effect on survival, some show a survival benefit but no difference in liver metastases, some show neither, and some claim to show both. The largest trial was performed by the NSABP (Wolmark, Rockette, and Wickerham, 1990; Wolmark, Rockette, and Fisher, 1993). Approximately 750 eligible patients were randomized to the same two arms as in the Liverpool trial, with small survival differences emerging at about 30 months but no differences in the incidence of liver metastases. The authors attribute any treatment effect to a systemic one, not one localized to the liver. In an attempt to sort out the issues, a formal meta-analysis was performed by the Liver Infusion Meta-analysis Group (1997). We review the issues faced by the authors of this effort as a way to illustrate the promise and problems of meta-analyses.

Inclusion of trials

A great deal of effort went into identifying trials for the portal vein infusion meta-analysis, as attested to by the inclusion of a trial presented only in abstract form. But are there trials (most likely negative) that have not even been presented in abstract form? While inclusion of all trials is the best way to avoid publication bias, it does increase the likelihood that trials of highly variable quality will be assembled for analysis. A related issue is whether the initial trial should be included in the meta-analysis, since in cases such as this one where a positive trial is the catalyst for confirmatory trials, the first study almost certainly overestimates the treatment benefit. The Liver Infusion Meta-Analysis Group (LIMG) addressed this issue by providing analyses both including and excluding the Taylor trial.

Use of raw data

The LIMG gathered raw data from each investigator. This allowed them to define relative risk as a common measure of treatment benefit and to calculate standard errors of the estimate from each trial. The incidence of liver metastases is subject to the problem of competing risks (Chapter 8), however, and having the raw data does not solve that problem. Some of the heterogeneity in eligibility criteria in these trials (e.g., the inclusion of Dukes' A patients or not) can be handled (through stratified analyses) only if the raw data are analyzed. Several of the trials excluded treatment violations from their reports, but the intent-to-treat analysis was restored in the meta-analysis. In fact, all patients, eligible or not, were included, apparently in the belief that it is better to guard against the possible biases introduced by inappropriate or selective enforcement of eligibility criteria than to restrict the variability by excluding patients not likely to benefit from treatment.

Lumping interventions

All of the trials delivered 5-FU via the portal vein for 1 week, starting with surgery. There were variations in the dose of 5-FU, but most would probably regard these as minor. Thus the trials included in the meta-analysis can be argued to be testing a comparable intervention. This is in stark contrast to many of the other such efforts with which we have been involved. A recent literature-based meta-analysis we reviewed compared single agent vs. combination chemotherapy in advanced non-small cell lung cancer, without regard to which single agent, which combination, or which doses. Other recent examples address the value of chemotherapy in head and neck cancer without regard to which agents, and the possible benefit of radiotherapy in limited small cell lung cancer, without regard to timing (concomitant or sequential), dose, or fractionation. It is doubtful whether any formal analysis of existing trials can sort out such complex issues.

Quality of trials

Our own review of the portal-vein infusion trials revealed considerable heterogeneity with respect to their quality. Some of the deficiencies can be rectified in a meta-analysis of the raw data, some cannot. The sample size was inadequate for all but extremely unrealistic differences in all but one of the trials and most were reported too early (a few had no follow-up data on some patients at the time of publication). While meta-analysis does result in larger numbers and can present updated survival data, in at least one trial no such updates were possible (the trial organization having terminated).

The most serious problems with the individual studies involved the timing of randomization and exclusions from analysis. As stated in Chapter 3, randomization should take place as close in time as possible to the point where treatments first diverge. In trials of portal vein infusion via catheter placed at surgery, there is the option of randomizing preoperatively or intraoperatively. Preoperative randomization was done in about half of the trials, and resulted in from 2 to 38% of patients declared ineligible at surgery (because of metastatic disease not detected before surgery, or an inability to perform a curative resection, for example). There is the possibility that a retrospective review of such cases for ineligibility could be biased due to knowledge of the treatment assignment. Intraoperative randomization in the other trials resulted in ineligibility rates (largely for reasons known in principle before randomization) ranging from 2 to 14%. While all ineligibles were included in the meta-analysis, eliminating such biases, one still wonders about the overall quality of some of the studies, and whether the ineligible patients were followed with the same rigor as the eligible ones.

Taylor reported the exclusion from the analysis of 7% of patients in whom a catheter could not be placed, which as we have noted in Chapters 3 and 7 destroys the balance created at randomization and introduces biases in the analysis. Only patients randomized to portal vein infusion have the chance to be excluded as protocol violations, and they could well have a different prognosis from the remainder of patients. In other trials this was either not done or happened in only a few cases. Again, meta-analysis using all the data can in theory rectify such problems, but Taylor reported that the patients excluded due to protocol violations were lost to follow-up.

9.6.3 Conclusions from the portal vein meta-analysis

The LIMG concluded from their meta-analysis that there was a benefit for portal vein infusion over observation (relative risk $= 0.86$, $p = 0.006$) but noted that the strength of that conclusion depended heavily on whether or not Taylor's original trial was included in the meta-analysis. They called for more randomized evidence. Our conclusion from a more informal review of the individual trials is that the usefulness of this approach is unproven. Combining nine trials of uneven quality did not result in one good trial. The only trial of adequate size demonstrated a very small, late-appearing improvement in survival, and no effect on liver metastases. Since adjuvant therapy with 5-FU and levamisole starting 1 month after surgery has been shown to be of benefit over observation at least for Dukes' C patients (Moertel et al., 1990), our review suggests that the relevant question is not about infusion but whether early systemic therapy, beginning right after surgery, adds benefit to conventional adjuvant therapy. This is being tested in a current intergroup trial being coordinated by the Eastern Cooperative Oncology Group (INT-0136), which recently closed short of its accrual goal, but which nonetheless should shed light on this issue when published.

9.6.4 Some final remarks on meta-analysis

Our inclusion of this topic in a chapter on exploratory analyses is an indication of our belief that the importance of meta-analyses lies mainly in exploration, not confirmation. In settling therapeutic issues, a meta-analysis is a poor substitute for one large, well-conducted trial. In particular, the expectation that a meta-analysis will be done does not justify designing studies that are too small to detect realistic differences with adequate power. Done well, a meta-analysis is a good review of existing data, and can provide an idea of the plausible magnitude of treatment benefit and generate hypotheses about treatment effects in subsets. However, there is a tendency to view the results of meta-analyses as being more definitive than they really are (Machtay, Kaiser, and Glatstein, 1999). As pointed out by Kassirer (1992), there is a near certainty that the studies collected for a meta-analysis are heterogeneous in their designs, and thus should not be thought of as providing estimates of a single quantity. The statistical techniques for accounting for this variability are controversial (see Marubini and Valsecchi, 1995 for a discussion). The quality of each trial needs to be taken into account, at least informally. With a very large meta-analysis, one also needs to keep in mind that not all statistically significant results are clinically meaningful.

9.7 Concluding remarks

One approach to cancer clinical trials, espoused by Richard Peto (Peto et al., 1976), is for the large, simple trial. There is much to commend this attitude, and we are sympathetic with the goal of designing clinical trials that are large enough to yield definitive answers to important clinical questions. Each secondary objective with its associated additional data requirements jeopardizes the ability to answer the primary question, and eventually the trial submerges of its own weight (see Chapter 6). Yet, one does want to learn something even from negative trials, so the urge to add limited secondary objectives is almost irresistible. We have tried to illustrate here, in the context of exploratory analyses using survival data, what might be learned from a trial or sequence of trials beyond answers to the primary treatment questions, and what the limitations are of such explorations. Further, we have tried to indicate that performing one large trial well is much to be preferred over combining several smaller ones.

CHAPTER 10

Summary and Conclusions

- *The grand thing is to be able to reason backwards.*
- *There is nothing more deceptive than an obvious fact.*
- *The temptation to form premature theories upon insufficient data is the bane of our profession.*
- *It is an error to argue in front of your data. You find yourself insensibly twisting them round to fit your theories.*

–**Sherlock Holmes**

Sherlock Holmes had it right. Reasoning backward from data to truth is full of traps and pitfalls. Statistics helps us to avoid the traps and to reason correctly. The main points we have tried to make in this book about such reasoning can be summarized briefly as follows:

- Clinical research searches for answers in an heterogeneous environment. Large variability, little understood historical trends, and unquantifiable but undoubtedly large physician and patient biases for one or another treatment are all indications for carefully controlled, randomized clinical trials.
- Statistical principles (and thus statisticians) have a large role (but certainly not the only role) in the design, conduct, and analysis of clinical trials.
- Careful attention to design is essential for the success of such trials. Agreement needs to be reached among all parties as to the objectives, endpoints, and definitions thereof, population to be studied and thus the eligibility criteria for the trial, treatments to be studied, and potential benefits of treatment to be detected with what limits of precision or statistical error probabilities (defining sample size).
- Two-arm trials have the virtue of a high likelihood of being able to answer one question well. Multi-arm trials should only be conducted with adequate sample size to protect against multiple comparisons and multiple other problems, and should not

be based on untested and unlikely assumptions regarding how treatments will behave in combinations.
- The analysis of trials as they unfold should be presented only to a select, knowledgeable few who are empowered to make decisions, using statistical guidelines, as to whether the results are so convincing that accrual should be stopped, that the trial should be reported early, or that other fundamental changes should be made.
- Careful attention to the details of data quality, including clear and concise protocols, data definitions, forms and protocols; quality control and quality assurance measures; and data base management is crucial to the success of trials.
- All completed trials should be reported in the literature, with a thorough accounting of all patients entered and a clear statistical analysis of all eligible patients on the arm to which they were assigned.
- There is no substitute for a randomized trial of adequate sample size with clinical endpoints for answering questions about the benefit of cancer treatments. Historical controls are completely unreliable, retrospective analyses of groups defined by their response or their attained dose are subject to irreparable biases, and the use of short-term endpoints of little clinical relevance can lead to seriously flawed conclusions.
- The protocol-stated analysis of the primary endpoint should result in an unassailable conclusion of a clinical trial. Any other analyses are secondary. The data should be explored to generate hypotheses for future research; this is a familiar province of the statistician, but be aware that there is more art (and thus less reproducibility) than science in this endeavor. Meta-analyses should be viewed as exploratory, and as supplements to but not as substitutes for large randomized trials.
- Clinical trials are a complex undertaking and a fragile enterprise. Every complication, every extra data item, every extra arm should be viewed with the suspicion that their addition might jeopardize the whole trial. Make sure one important question is answered well, then see what else might be learned.

Recently we were asked to write a mission statement for the SWOG Statistical Center. Here is our view:

> The primary mission of the Southwest Oncology Group Statistical Center is to make progress in the prevention and cure of cancer through clinical research. The mission is accomplished through the conduct of important trials and through translation of biologic concepts. Quality

SUMMARY AND CONCLUSIONS

research, quality data, and publication of results are critical to the effort. The Statistical Center contributes through:

Study Design. The Statistical Center has a fundamental role in clarifying study objectives and in designing statistically sound studies to meet those objectives.

Protocol Review. The Statistical Center reviews all protocols for logical consistency and completeness, in order that study conduct not be compromised through use of an inaccurate protocol document.

Data Quality Control and Study Monitoring. The Statistical Center continually enters, forwards to study coordinators, reviews, corrects, updates, and stores data from all active Southwest Oncology Group studies, in order that study results not be compromised by flawed data and that studies be monitored for patient safety.

Analysis and Publication. The Statistical Center is responsible for statistical analysis and interpretation of all Southwest Oncology Group coordinated studies and all Southwest Oncology Group data base studies.

Statistical Research. The Statistical Center has an active research program addressing unresolved design and analysis issues important to the conduct of cancer clinical trials and to ancillary biologic studies.

We hope that this book has contributed to an understanding of how we conduct ourselves in fulfillment of this mission.

Bibliography

Advanced Colorectal Meta-Analysis Project, Modulation of fluorouracil by levcovrin in patients with advanced colorectal cancer: Evidence in terms of response rate. *Journal of Clinical Oncology*, 10:896–903, 1992.

Al-Sarraf, M., LeBlanc, M., Giri, P.G.S., Fu, K.K., Cooper, J., Vuong, T., Forastiere, A.A., Adams, G., Sakr, W.A., Schuller, D.E., and Ensley, J.F., Chemoradiotherapy versus radiotherapy in patients with advanced nasopharyngeal cancer: Phase III randomized intergroup study 0099, *Journal of Clinical Oncology*, 16:1310–1317, 1998.

Alberts, D.S., Green, S., Hannigan, E.V., O'Toole, R., Stock-Novak, D., Anderson, P., Surwit, E.A., Malviya, V.K., Nahhas, W.A., and Jolles, C.J., Improved therapeutic index of carboplatin plus cyclophosphamide versus cisplatin plus cyclophosphamide: Final report by the Southwest Oncology Group of a phase III randomized trial in stages III and IV ovarian cancer, *Journal of Clinical Oncology*, 10:706–717, 1992.

Alizaeh, A.A., Eisen, M.B., Davis, R.E., Ma, C., Lossos, I.S., Rosenwald, A., Boldrick, J.C., Sabet, H., Tran, T., Yu, X., Powell, J.I., Yang, L., Marti, G.E., Moore, T., Hudson, J.Jr., Lu, L., Lewis, D.B., Tibshirani, R., Sherlock, G., Chan, W.C., Greiner, T.C., Weisenburger, D.D., Armitage, J.O., Warnke, R., Levy, R., Wilson, W., Grever, M.R., Byrd, J.C., Botstein, D., Brwon, P.O., and Staudt, L.M., Distinct types of diffuse large B-cell lymphoma identified by gene expression profiling, *Nature*, 403:503–511, 2000.

Altaman, L., US Halts Recruitment of Cancer Patients for Studies, Pointing to Flaws in Oversight, *New York Times*, Wed. March 30, p. A-12, 1994.

Altman, D.G., Schultz, K.F., Moher, D., Egger, M., Davidoff, F., Elbourne, D., Gøtzsche, P.C., and Lang, T., The revised CONSORT statement for reporting randomized trials: Explanation and elaboration, *Annals of Internal Medicine*, 134 v8: 663–694, 2001.

Anderson, G.L., LeBlanc, M., Liu, P.-Y., and Crowley, J., Choosing the test statistic for a clinical trial when the randomization uses covariates. Under revision, 2002.

Anderson, J.R., Cain K.C., and Gelber R.D., Analysis of survival by tumor response, *Journal of Clinical Oncology*, 1:710–719, 1983.

Anderson, P.K., Conditional power calculations as an aid in the decision whether to continue a clinical trial, *Controlled Clinical Trials*, 8:67–74, 1987.

Antman, K., Crowley, J., Balcerzak, S.P., Rivkin, S.E., Weiss, G.R., Elias, A., Natale, R.B., Cooper, R.M., Barlogie, B., Trump, D.L., Doroshow, J.H.,

Aisner, J., Pugh, R.P., Weiss, R.B., Cooper, B.A., Clamon, G.H., and Baker, L.H., An intergroup phase III randomized study of doxorubicin and dacarbazine with or without ifosfamide and mesna in advanced soft tissue and bone sarcomas, *Journal of Clinical Oncology*, 11:1276–1285, 1993.

Armitage, P., Data and safety monitoring in the Alpha and Concorde trials. *Controlled Clinical Trials*, 20:207–228, 1999.

Balcerzak, S., Benedetti, J., Weiss, G.R., and Natale, R.B., A phase II trial of paclitaxel in patients with advanced soft tissue sarcomas: A Southwest Oncology Group study, *Cancer*, 76:2248–2252, 1995.

Barlogie, B., Anderson, K., Berenson, J., Crowley, J., Cunningham, D., Gertz, M., Henon, P., Horowitz, M., Jagannath, S., Powles, R., Reece, D., Reiffers J., Salmon, S., Tricot, G., and Vesole, D., In Dicke, K. and Keeting A. (Eds.), *Autologous Marrow and Blood Transplantation. Proceedings of the Seventh International Symposium*. Arlington, Texas, pp. 399–410, 1995.

Bartlett, R., Rolo., D., Cornell, R., Andrews, A., Dillon, P., and Zwischenberger, J., Extracorporeal circulation in neonatal respiratory failure: A prospective randomized study, *Pediatrics*, 76:476–487, 1985.

Battaille, R., Durie, B.G.M., and Grenier, J., Serum beta-2 microglobulin and survival duration in multiple myeloma: A simple reliable marker for staging, *British Journal of Haematology*, 55:439–447, 1983.

Benedetti, J.K., Liu, P.-Y., Sather, H., Seinfeld, H., and Epson, M., Effective sample size for censored survival data, *Biometrika*, 69:343–349, 1982.

Berlin, J., Stewart, J.A., Storer, B., Tutsch, K.D., Arzoomanian, R.Z., Alberti, D., Feierabend, C., Simon, K., and Wilding, G., Phase I clinical and pharmacokinetic trial of penclomedine using a novel, two-stage trial design for patients with advanced malignancy, *Journal of Clinical Oncology*, 16: 1142–1149, 1998.

Bernard, C.L., *Introduction à l'Etude de la Médecine Expérimentale*, 1866, reprinted, Garnier-Flammarion, London 1966.

Bernstein, D., and Lagakos, S., Sample size and power determination for stratified clinical trials, *Journal of Statistical Computations and Simulation*, 8:65–73, 1978.

Blackwelder, W.C., "Proving the null hypothesis" in clinical trials, *Controlled Clinical Trials*, 3:345–353, 1982.

Blumenstein, B.A., The relational database model and multiple multicenter clinical trials, *Controlled Clinical Trials*, 10:386–406, 1989.

Boissel, J.-P., Impact of randomized clinical trials on medical practices, *Controlled Clinical Trials*, 10:120S–134S, 1989.

Bonadonna, G., and Valagussa, P., Dose-response effect of adjuvant chemotherapy in breast cancer, *New England Journal of Medicine*, 34:10–15, 1981.

Breiman, L., Friedman, J.H., Olshen, R.A., and Stone, C.J., *Classification and Regression Trees*, Wadsworth International Group, Belmont, CA, 1984.

Breslow, N., and Crowley, J., Large sample properties of the life table and PL estimates under random censorship, *Annals of Statistics*, 2:437–453, 1972.

Brookmeyer, R., and Crowley, J., A confidence interval for the median survival time, *Biometrics* 38:29–41, 1982.

Bryant, J., and Day, R., Incorporating toxicity considerations into the design of two-stage phase II clinical trials, *Biometrics*, 51:1372–1383, 1995.

Budd, G.T., Green, S., O'Bryan, R.M., Martino, S., Abeloff, M.D., Rinehart, J.J., Hahn, R., Harris, J., Tormey, D., O'Sullivan, J., and Osborne, C.K., Short-course FAC-M versus 1 year of CMFVP in node-positive, hormone receptor-negative breast cancer: An intergroup study, *Journal of Clinical Oncology*, 13:831–839, 1995.

Bunn, P.A., Crowley, J., Kelly, K., Hazuka, M.B., Beasley, K., Upchurch, C., and Livingston, R., Chemoradiotherapy with or without granulocyte-macrophage colony-stimulating factor in the treatment of limited-stage small-cell lung cancer: A prospective Phase III randomized study of the Southwest Oncology Group, *Journal of Clinical Oncology*, 13:1632–1641, 1995.

Byar, D.P., Simon, R.M., Friedewalde, W.T., Schlesselman, J.J., DeMets, D.L., Ellenberg, J.H., Gail, M.H., and Ware, J.H., Randomized clinical trials: Perspectives on some recent ideas, *New England Journal of Medicine*, 295:74–80, 1976.

Chang, M., Therneau, T., Wieand, H.S., and Cha, S., Designs for group sequential Phase II clinical trials, *Biometrics*, 43: 865–874, 1987.

Chang, M.N., and O'Brien P.C., Confidence intervals following group sequential tests, *Controlled Clinical Trials*, 7:18–26, 1986.

Chen, T., and Simon, R., Extension of one-sided test to multiple treatment trials, *Controlled Clinical Trials*, 15:124–134, 1994.

Christian, M.C., McCabe, M.S., Korn, E.L., Abrams, J.S., Kaplan, R.S., and Friedman, M.A., The National Cancer Institute audit of the National Surgical Adjuvant Breast and Bowel Project Protocol B-06, *New England Journal of Medicine*, 333:1469–1474, 1995.

Ciampi, A., Thiffault, J., Nakache, J.-P., and Asselain, B., Stratification by stepwise regression, correspondence analysis and recursive partitioning, *Computational Statistics and Data Analysis*, 4:185–204, 1986.

Clark, D.A., Stinson, E.B., Griepp, R.B., Schroeder, J.S., Shumway, N.E., and Harrison, D.C., Cardiac transplantation in man, VI. Prognosis of patients selected for cardia transplantation, *Annals of Internal Medicine*, 75:15–21, 1971.

Collins, J.M., Innovations in Phase I design: Where do we go next? *Clinical Cancer Research*, 6:3801–3802, 2000.

Collins, J.M., Zaharko, D.S., Dedrick, R.L., and Chabner, B.A., Potential roles for preclinical pharmacology in phase I clinical trials, *Cancer Treatment Reports*, 70:73–80, 1986.

Collins, J.M., Grieshaber, C.K., and Chabner, B.A., Pharmacologically guided Phase I clinical trials based upon preclinical drug development, *Journal of the National Cancer Institute*, 82:1321–1326, 1990.

Conaway, M.R., and Petroni, G.R., Bivariate sequential designs for phase II trials, *Biometrics*, 51:656–664, 1995.

Conaway, M., and Petroni, G., Designs for phase II trials allowing for a trade-off between response and toxicity, *Biometrics*, 52: 1375–1386, 1996.

Concorde Coordinating Committee, Concorde: MRC/ANRS randomized double-blind controlled trial of immediate and deferred zidovudine in symptom-free HIV infection, *Lancet*, 343:871–881, 1994.

Cook, R.J., and Farewell, V.T., Guidelines for monitoring efficacy and toxicity response in clinical trials, *Biometrics*, 50:1146–1152, 1994.

Cooper, R., Holland, J., and Glidewell, O., Adjuvant chemotherapy of breast cancer, *Cancer*, 44:793–798, 1979.

Coronary Drug Research Project Research Group, Influence of adherence to treatment and response of cholesterol on mortality in the coronary drug project, *New England Journal of Medicine*, 303:1038–1041, 1980.

Cox, D.R., Regression models and life-tables (with discussion), *Journal of the Royal Statistical Society*, Series B 34:187–220, 1972.

Crowley, J., Perioperative portal vein chemotherapy, in *ASCO Educational Book*, 30th Annual Meeting, Dallas, TX, 1994.

Crowley, J., and Breslow, N., Statistical analysis of survival data, *Annual Review of Public Health*, 5:385–411, 1984.

Crowley, J., Green, S., Liu, P.-Y., and Wolf, M., Data monitoring committees and early stopping guidelines: The Southwest Oncology Group experience, *Statistics in Medicine*, 13:1391–1399, 1994.

Crowley, J., LeBlanc, M., Gentleman, R., and Salmon, S., Exploratory methods in survival analysis, in Koul, H.L. and Deshpande, J.V., Eds., *Analysis of Censored Data*, IMS Lecture Notes-Monograph Series Hayward, CA, 27:55–77, 1995.

Crowley, J., LeBlanc, M., Jacobson, J., and Salmon. S.E., Some exploratory methods for survival data, in Lin, D.-Y. and Fleming, T.R., Eds., *Proceedings of the First Seattle Symposium on Biostatistics*, Springer-Verlag. New York, 1997, 199–229.

DeMets, D.L., Fleming, T.R., Whitley, R., Childress, J.F., Ellenberg, S.S., Foulkes, M., Mayer, K.H., O'Fallon, J., Pollard, R.B., Rahal, J.J., Sande, M., Straus, S., Walters, L., and Whitley-Williams, P., The data and safety monitoring board and acquired immune deficiency syndrome (AIDS) trials, *Controlled Clinical Trials*, 16:408–421, 1995.

De Moulin, D., *A Short History of Breast Cancer*, Kluwer, Dordrecht, Germany, 1989.

Dees, E.C., Whitfield, L.R., Grove W.R., Rummel, S., Grochow, L.B., and Donehower, R.C., A phase I and pharmacologic evaluation of the DNA intercalator CI-958 in patients with advanced solid tumors, *Clinical Cancer Research*, 6:3801–2, 2000.

Diem, K., and Lentner, C. (Eds.), *Scientific Tables*, Geigy, J.R., Basel, Switzerland, 1970.

Dimond, E.G., Kittle, C.F., and Crockett, J.E., Comparison of internal mammary artery ligation and sham operation for angina pectoris, *American Journal of Cardiology*, 5:483–486, 1960.

Draper, N.R., and Smith, H., *Applied Regression Analysis*, Wiley, New York, 1968.

Duffy, D.E., and Santner, T.J., Confidence intervals for a binomial parameter based on multistage tests, *Biometrics*, 43:81–94, 1987.

Durie, B.G.M., and Salmon, S.E., A clinical system for multiple myeloma. Correlation of measured myeloma cell mass with presenting clinical features, response to treatment and survival, *Cancer*, 36:842–854, 1975.

Durie, B.G.M., Dixon, D.O., Carter, S., Stephens, R., Rivkin, S., Bonnet, J., Salmon, S.E., Dabich, L., Files, J.C., and Costanzi, J., Improved survival duration with combination induction for multiple myeloma: A Southwest Oncology Group study, *Journal of Clinical Oncology*, 4:1227–1237, 1986

Duvillard, E.E., *Analyse et tableaux de l'influence de la petite vérole sur la mortalité à chaque âge, et de celle qu'un préservatif tel que la vaccine peut avoir sur la population et la longevité.* Imprimerie Imperiale, Paris, 1806.

Echt, D., Liebson, P., Mitchell, L., Peters, R., Obias-Manno, D., Barder, A., Arensberg, D., Baker, A., Friedman, L., Greene, H., Hutcher, M., Richardson, D., and the CAST investigators. Mortality and morbidity in patients receiveing ecainide, flecainide or placebo: The Cardiac Arrythmia Suppression Trial, *New England Journal of Medicine*, 324:781–788, 1991.

Ederer, F., Jerome Cornfield's contributions to the conduct of clinical trials, *Biometrics* (Suppl.) 38:25–32, 1982.

Eisenhauer, E.A., O'Dwyer, P.J., Christian, M., and Humphrey, J.S., Phase I clinical trial design in cancer drug development, *Journal of Clinical Oncology*, 18:684–692, 2000.

Ellenberg, S., Randomization designs in comparative clinical trials, *New England Journal of Medicine*, 310:1404–1408, 1984.

Ellenberg, S.S., Finkelstein, D.M., and Schoenfeld, D.A., Statistical issues arising in AIDS clinical trials, *Journal of the American Statistical Association*, 87:562–569, 1992.

Faraggi, D., LeBlanc, M., and Crowley, J., Understanding neural networks using regression trees: An application to multiple myeloma survival data, *Statistics in Medicine*, 20:2965–2976, 2001.

Farewell, V., and Matthews, D., *Using and Understanding Medical Statistics*, third ed., Karger, Basel, 1996.

Fisher B., Winds of change in clinical trials — from Daniel to Charlie Brown, *Controlled Clinical Trials*, 4:65–74, 1983.

Fisher, R., Gaynor, E., Dahlberg, S., Oken, M., Grogan, T., Mize, E., Glick, J., Coltman, C., and Miller, T., Comparison of a standard regimen (CHOP) with three intensive chemotherapy regimens for advanced non-Hodgkin's lymphoma, *New England Journal of Medicine*, 328:1002–1006, 1993.

Fleiss, J.L., *Statistical Methods for Rates and Proportions,* second ed., John Wiley & Sons, New York, 1981.

Fleiss, J.L., Tytun, A., and Ury, H.K., A simple approximation for calculating sample sizes for comparing independent proportions, *Biometrics*, 36:343–346, 1980.

Fleming, I.D., Cooper, J.S., Henson, D.E., Hutter, R.V.P., Kennedy, B.J., Murphy, G.P., O'Sullivan, B., Sobin, L.H., and Yarbro, J.W., (Eds.) *AJCC Cancer Staging Manual*, 5th ed, Lippincott, Williams and Wilkens, Philadelphia, 1997.

Fleming, T., One sample multiple testing procedures for Phase II clinical trials, *Biometrics*, 38:143–151, 1982.

Fleming, T.R., Evaluating therapeutic interventions: Some issues and experiences, *Statistical Science*, 7:428–456, 1992.

Fleming, T.R., Interpretation of subgroup analyses in clinical trials, *Drug Information Journal*, 29:1681S–1687S, 1995.

Fleming, T., Green, S., and Harrington, P., Considerations for monitoring and evaluating treatment effects in clinical trials, *Controlled Clinical Trials*, 5:55–66, 1984.

Freeman, T., Vawtner, D., Leaverton, P., Godbold, J., Hauser, R., Goetz, C., and Olanow, C.W., Use of placebo surgery in controlled trials of a cellular based therapy for Parkinson's disease, *New England Journal of Medicine*, 341:988–992, 1999.

Frei, E. III, Holland, J.F., Schneiderman, M.A., Pinkel, D., Selkirk, C., Freireich, E.J., Silver, R.T., Gold, C.L., and Regelson, W., A comparative study of two regimens of combination chemotherapy in acute leukemia, *Blood*, 13:1126–1148, 1958.

Frytak, S., Moertel, C., O'Fallon, J., Rubin, J., Creagan, E., O'Connel, M., Schutt, A., and Schwartau, N., Delta-9-Tetrahydrocannabinol as an antiemetic for patients receiving cancer chemotherapy, *Annals of Internal Medicine*, 91:825–830, 1979.

Gail, M.H., Statistics in action, *Journal of the American Statistical Association*, 91:1–13, 1996.

Gandara, D.R., Crowley, J., Livingston, R.B., Perez, E.A., Taylor, C.W., Weiss, G., Neefe, J.R., Hutchins, L.F., Roach, R.W., Grunberg, S.M., Braun, T.J., Natale, R.B., and Balcerzak, S.P., Evaluation of cisplatin in metastatic non-small cell lung cancer: A phase III study of the Southwest Oncology Group, *Journal of Clinical Oncology*, 11:873–878, 1993.

Gehan, E., A generalized Wilcoxon test for comparing arbitrarily singly-censored samples, *Biometrika*, 52:203–223, 1965.

Gentleman, R., and Crowley, J., Local full likelihood estimation for the proportional hazards model, *Biometrics*, 47:1283–1296, 1991a.

Gentleman, R., and Crowley, J., Graphical methods for censored data, *Journal of the American Statistical Association*, 86:678–682, 1991b.

George, S., A survey of monitoring practices in cancer clinical trials, *Statistics in Medicine*, 12:435–450, 1993.

Gil Deza, E., Balbiani, L., Coppola, F. et al., Phase III study of Navelbine (NVB) versus NVB plus cisplatin in non-small cell lung cancer (NSCLC) stage IIIB or IV, ASCO Abstract, *Proceeding of ASCO*, 15:394 (#193), 1996.

Gilbert, J.P., McPeek, B., and Mosteller, F., Statistics and ethics in surgery and anesthesia, *Science* 198:684–689, 1977.

Goldberg, K.B., and Goldberg, P. (Eds.) *Four patients in tamoxifen treatment trial had died of uterine cancer prior to BCPT, The Cancer Letter*, April 29, 1994.

Goldie, J.H., Coldman, A.J., and Gudauskas, G.A., Rationale for the use of alternating non-cross-resistant chemotherapy, *Cancer Treatment Reports*, 66:439–449, 1982.

Golub, T.R., Slonim, D.K., Tamayo, P., Huard, C., Gaasenbeck, M., Mesirov, J.P., Coller, H., Loh, M.L., Dowving, J.R., Caligiuri, M.A., Bloomfield, C.D., and Lander, E.S., Molecular classification of cancer: Class discovery and class prediction be gene expression monitoring, *Science* 286:531–537, 1999.

Goodman, S.N., Zahurak, M.L., and Piantadosi, S., Some practical improvements in the continual reassessment method for phase I studies, *Statistics in Medicine*, 14:1149–1161, 1995.

Gooley, T., Martin, P., Fisher, L., and Pettinger, M., Simulation as a design tool for Phase I/II clinical trials: An example from bone marrow transplantation, *Controlled Clinical Trials*, 15:450–462, 1994.

Gooley, T., Leisenring, W., Crowley, J., and Storer, B., Estimation of failure probabilities in the presence of competing risks: New representations of old estimators, *Statistics in Medicine*, 18:695–706, 1999.

Gordon, R., *The Alarming History of Medicine*, St. Martin's Press, New York, 1993.

Gray, R.J., A class of K-sample tests for comparing the cumulative incidence of a competing risk, *The Annals of Statistics*, 161141–1154, 1988.

Green, S., Overview of phase II clinical trials, in Crowley, J. Ed., *Handbook of Statistics in Clinical Trials*, Marcel Dekker, New York, 93–103, 2001.

Green, S., and Crowley, J., Data monitoring committees for Southwest Oncology Group trials, *Statistics in Medicine*, 12:451–455, 1993.

Green, S., and Dahlberg, S., Planned versus attained design in Phase II clinical trials, *Statistics in Medicine*, 11:853–862, 1992.

Green, S., Factorial designs with time-to event endpoints, in Crowley, J. Ed., *Handbook of Statistics in Clinical Trials*, Marcel Dekker, New York, 161–171, 2001.

Green, S.J., Fleming, T.R., and O'Fallon, J.R., Policies for study monitoring and interim reporting of results, *Journal of Clinical Oncology*, 5:1477–1484, 1987.

Green, S.J., Fleming, T.R., and Emerson, S., Effects on overviews of early stopping rules for clinical trials, *Statistics in Medicine*, 6:361–367, 1987.

Green, S., and Weiss, G., Southwest Oncology Group standard response criteria, endpoint definitions and toxicity criteria, *Investigational New Drugs*, 10:239–253, 1992.

Harrington, D., Crowley, J., George, S., Pajak, T., Redmond, C., and Wieand, S., The case against independent monitoring committees, *Statistics in Medicine*, 13:1411–1414, 1994.

Harrington, D., Fleming, T., and Green, S., Procedures for serial testing in censored survival data, in Crowley, J.J. and Johnson R.A. (Eds.), *Survival Analysis*, IMS Lecture Notes Monograph Series, CA, Hayward, 2:269–286, 1982.

Hawkins, B.S., Data monitoring committees for multicenter clinical trials sponsored by the National Institutes of Health: Roles and membership of data monitoring committees for trials sponsored by the National Eye Institute, *Controlled Clinical Trials*, 12:424–437, 1991.

Haybittle, J.L., Repeated assessments of results in clinical trials of cancer treatment, *British Journal of Radiology*, 44:793–797, 1971.

Hellman, S., and Hellman, D.S., Of mice but not men: Problems of the randomized clinical trial, *New England Journal of Medicine*, 324:1585–1589, 1991.

Henderson, I.C., Hayes, D., and Gelman, R., Dose-response in the treatment of breast cancer: A critical review, *Journal of Clinical Oncology*, 6:1501–1515, 1988.

Hill, A.B., *Principles of Medical Statistics*, Lancet, London, 1937.

Hill, A.B., Memories of the British streptomycin trial in tuberculosis, *Controlled Clinical Trials*, 11:77–79, 1990.

Hogan, J.W., and Laird, N.M., Mixture models for the joint distribution of repeated measures and event times, *Statistics in Medicine*, 16:239–257, 1997.

Hryniuk, W., and Levine, M.N., Analysis of dose intensity for adjuvant chemotherapy trials in stage II breast cancer, *Journal of Clinical Oncology*, 4:1162–1170, 1986.

Hsieh, F.-Y., Crowley, J., and Tormey, D.C., Some test statistics for use in multistate survival analysis, *Biometrika*, 70:111–119, 1983.

Huff, D., *How to Lie with Statistics*. Norton, New York, 1954.

Jacobson, J.L., Hussein, M., Barlogi, B., Durie, B.G.M., and Crowley, J.J., Beta 2 microglobulin (B2m) and albumin define a new staging system for multiple myeloma: The Southwest Oncology Group (SWOG) experience, *Blood*, 98:#657, 155a, 2001.

Jennison, C., and Turnbull, B.W., Confidence intervals for a binomial parameter following a multistage test with application to MIL-STD 105D and medical trials, *Technometrics*, 25:49–58, 1983.

Kalbfleisch, J.D., and Prentice, R.L., *The Statistical Analysis of Failure Time Data*, Wiley, New York, 1980.

Kaplan, E.L., and Meier, P., Nonparametric estimation from incomplete observations, *Journal of the American Statistical Association*, 53:457–481, 1958.

Kassirer, J.P., Clinical trials and meta-analysis: What they do for us. (editorial), *New England Journal of Medicine*, 325:273–274, 1992.

Kelly, K., Crowley, J., Bunn, P.A., Hazuka, M., Beasley, K., Upchurch, C., Weiss, G., Hicks, W., Gandara, D., Rivkin, S., and Livingston, R., Role of recombinant interferon alfa-2a maintenance in patients with limited-stage small-cell lung cancer responding to concurrent chemoradiation: A Southwest Oncology Group study, *Journal of Clinical Oncology*, 13:2924–2930, 1995.

Khan, J., Wei, J.S., Ringner, M., Saal, L.H., Ladanyi, M., Westerman, F., Berthold, F., Schwab, M., Antonescu, C.R., Peterson, C., and Meltzer, P.S., Classification and diagnostic prediction of cancers using gene expression profiling and artificial neural networks, *Nature Medicine*, 7:673–679, 2001.

Kies, M.S., Mira, J., Chen, T., and Livingston, R.B., Value of chest radiation therapy in limited small cell lung cancer after chemotherapy induced complete disease remission (for the Southwest Oncology Group) (abstract), *Proceedings of the American Society of Clinical Oncology*, 1:141 (C-546) 1982.

Kies, M.S., Mira, J., Crowley, J., Chen, T., Pazdur, R., Grozea, P., Rivkin, S., Coltman, C., Ward, J.H., and Livingston, R.B., Multimodal therapy for limited small cell lung cancer: A randomized study of induction combination chemotherapy with or without thoracic radiation in complete responders; and with wide field versus reduced-field radiation in partial responders: A Southwest Oncology Group study, *Journal of Clinical Oncology*, 5: 592–600, 1987.

Klimt, C.R., Varied acceptance of clinical trial results, *Controlled Clinical Trials*, 10 (Supplement):1355–141S, 1989.

Lamm, D.L., Blumenstein, B.A., Crawford, E.D., Crissman, J.D., Lowe, B.A., Smith, J.A., Sarosdy, M.F., Schellhammer, P.F., Sagalowsky, A.I., Messing, E.M., Loehrer, P., and Grossman, H.B., Randomized intergroup comparison of bacillus Calmette-Guerin immunotherapy and mitomycin C chemotherapy prophylaxis in superficial transitional cell carcinoma of the bladder: A Southwest Oncology Group study, *Urologic Oncology*, 1:119–126, 1995.

Lan, K., and DeMets, D., Discrete sequential boundaries for clinical trials, *Biometrika*, 70: 659–663, 1983.

Lan, K., Simon, R., and Halperin, M., Stochastically curtailed test in long-term clinical trials, *Sequential Analysis*, 1:207–219, 1982.

Lancaster, H.O., *Quantitative Methods in Biological and Medical Sciences*, Springer-Verlag, New York, 1994.

Laurie, J.A., Moertel, C.G., Fleming, T.R., Wieand, H.S., Leigh, J.E., Rubin, J., McCormack, G.W., Gerstner, J.B., Krook, J.E., Malliard, J., Twito, D.I., Morton, R.F., Tschetter, L.K., and Barlow, J.F., Surgical adjuvant therapy of large-bowel carcinoma: An evaluation of levamisole and the combination of levamisole and fluorouracil, *Journal of Clinical Oncology*, 7:1447–1456, 1989.

LeBlanc, M., and Crowley, J., Relative risk trees for censored survival data, *Biometrics*, 48:411–425, 1992.

LeBlanc, M., and Crowley, J., Survival trees by goodness of split, *Journal of the American Statistical Association*, 88:457–467, 1993.

LeBlanc, M., and Crowley, J., Using the bootstrap for estimation in group sequential design: An application to a clinical trial for nasopharyngeal cancer, *Statistics in Medicine*, 18:2635–2644, 1999.

LeBlanc, M., Jacobson, J., and Crowley, J., Partitioning and peeling for constructing prognostic groups, *Statistical Methods in Medical Research*, 11:1–28, 2002.

Leichman, C.G., Fleming, T.R., Muggia, F.M., Tangen, C.M., Ardalan, B., Doroshow, J.H., Meyers, F.J., Holcombe, R.F., Weiss, G.R., Mangalik, A., and MacDonald, J.S., Phase II study of fluorouracil and its modulation in advanced colorectal cancer: A Southwest Oncology Group study, *Journal of Clinical Oncology*, 13:1301–1311, 1995.

Lind, J. *A Treatise of the Scurvy*, Sands, Murray, and Cochran, Edinburgh, 1753.

Liu, P.-Y., and Dahlberg, S., Design and analysis of multiarm clinical trials with survival endpoints, *Controlled Clinical Trials*, 16:119–130, 1995.

Liu, P.-Y., Dahlberg, S., and Crowley, J., Selection designs for pilot studies based on survival endpoints, *Biometrics*, 49:391–398, 1993.

Liu, P.-Y., LeBlanc, M., and Desai M., False positive rates of randomized Phase II designs, *Controlled Clinical Trials*, 20:343–352, 1999.

Liu, P.-Y., Voelkel, J., Crowley, J., and Wolf, M. Sufficient conditions for treatment responders to have longer survival than non-responders, *Statistics and Probability Letters*, 18:205–208, 1993.

Liu, P.-Y, Tsai, W.-Y., and Wolf, M., Design and analysis for survival data under order restrictions: A modified ordered logrank test, manuscript, 1996.

Liver Infusion Meta-Analysis Group, Portal vein infusion of cytotoxic drugs after colorectal cancer surgery: A meta-analysis of 10 randomised studies involving 4000 patients, submitted to *Journal of National Cancer Institute*, 89:497–505, 1997.

Macdonald, J.S., Smalley, S.R., Benedetti, J., Hundahl, S.A., Estes, N.C., Stemmermann, G.N., Haller, D.G., Ajani, J.A., Gunderson, L.L., Jessup, J.M., and Martenson, J.A., Chemoradiotherapy after surgery compared with the surgery alone for adenocarcinoma of the stomach or gastroesophageal junction, *New England Journal of Medicine*, 345:725–730, 2001.

Machtay, M., Kaiser, L.R., and Glatstein, E., Is meta-analysis really metaphysics? *Chest*, 116:539–544, 1999.

Mackillop, W.J., and Johnston, P.A., Ethical problems in clinical research: The need for empirical studies of the clinical trials process, *Journal of Chronic Diseases*, 39:177–188, 1986.

Macklin, R., The ethical problems with sham surgery in clinical research, *New England Journal of Medicine*, 341:992–996, 1999.

Mantel, N., Evaluation of survival data and two new rank order statistics arising in its consideration, *Cancer Chemotherapy Reports*, 50:163–170, 1966.

Margolin, K.M., Green, S., Osborne, K., Doroshow, J.H., Akman, S.A., Leong, L.A., Morgan, R.J., Raschko, J.W., Somlo, G., Hutchins, L., and Upchurch, C., Phase II trial of 5-fluorouracil and high-dose folinic acid as first- or second-line therapy for advanced breast cancer, *American Journal of Clinical Oncology*, 17:175–180, 1994.

Marubini, E., and Valsecchi, M.G., *Analysing Survival Data from Clinical Trials and Observational Studies*, Wiley, New York, 1995.

McCracken, D., Janaki, L.M., Crowley, J., Taylor, S.A., Giri, P.G., Weiss, G.B., Gordon, J.W., Baker, L.H., Mansouri, A., and Kuebler, J.P., Concurrent chemotherapy/radiotherapy for limited small-cell carcinoma: A Southwest Oncology Group study, *Journal of Clinical Oncology*, 8:892–898, 1990.

McFadden, E.T., LoPresti, F., Bailey, L.R., Clarke, E., and Wilkins, P.C., Approaches to data management, *Controlled Clinical Trials*, 16:30S–65S, 1995.

Meier, P., Statistics and medical experimentation, *Biometrics*, 31:511–529, 1975.

Meyers, P., Schwartz, C., Bernstein, M., Betcher, D., Conrad, E., Ferguson, W., Gebhardt, M., Goodman, M., Goorin, A., Grier, H., Harris, M., Healy, J., Huvos, A., Kleinerman, E., Krailo, M., Link, M., Montebello, J., Nieder, M., Sato, J., Siegal, G., Weiner, M., Wells, R., Wold, L., and Womer, R., Addition of ifosfamide amd muramyl tripeptide to cisplatin, doxorubicin and high-dose methotrexate improves event free survival (EFS) in localized osteosarcoma (OS), *Proceedings of ASCO*, 20:367a (#1463), 2001.

Miller, T.P., Crowley, J.J., Mira, J., Schwartz, J.G., Hutchins, L., Baker, L., Natale, R., Chase, E.M., and Livingston, R.B., A randomized trial of chemotherapy and radiotherapy for stage III non-small cell lung cancer, *Cancer Therapeutics*, 1:229–36, 1998.

Mira, J.G., Kies, M.S., and Chen, T., Influence of chest radiotherapy in response, remission duration, and survival in chemotherapy responders in localized small cell lung carcinoma: A Southwest Oncology Group Study, *Proceedings of the American Society of Clinical Oncology*, 3:212 (C-827), 1984.

Moertel, C.G., Fleming, T.R., MacDonald, J.S., Haller, D.G., Laurie, J.A., Goodman, P.J., Ungerleider, J.S., Emerson, W.A., Tormey, D.C., Glick, J.H., Veeder, M.H., and Mailliard, J.A., Levamisole and fluorouracil for adjuvant therapy of resected colon carcinoma, *New England Journal of Medicine*, 322:352–358, 1990.

Moher D., Schultz, K.F., and Altman, D.G., The CONSORT statement: Revised recommendations for improving the quality of reports of parallel-group randomized trials. *Annals of Internal Medicine*, 134 (v8): 657–662, 2001.

Moinpour, C., Feigl, P., Metch, B., Hayden, K., Meyskens, F., and Crowley, J., Quality of life end points in cancer clinical trials: Review and recommendations, *Journal of the National Cancer Institute*, 81:485–496, 1989.

Moinpour, C., Triplett, J., McKnight, B., Lovato, L., Upchurch, C., Leichman, C., Muggia, F., Tanaka, L., James, W., Lennard, M., and Meyskens, F., Challenges posed by non-random missing quality of life data in an advanced-stage colorectal cancer clinical trial, *Psycho-Oncology*, 9:340–354, 2000.

Moinpour, C. M., Costs of quality of life research in Southwest Oncology Group trials, *Monographs of the Journal of the National Cancer Institute*, 20:11–16, 1996.

Møller, S., An extension of the continual reassessment methods using a preliminary up-and-down design in a dose finding study in cancer patients, in order to investigate a greater range of doses, *Statistics in Medicine*, 14: 911–922, 1995.

Monro, A., Collections of blood in cancerous breasts, in Monro A., *The Works of Alexander Monro*, Ch Elliot, Edinburgh, 1781.

Muggia, F.M., Liu, P.-Y., Alberts, D.S., Wallace, D.L., O'Toole, R.V., Terada, K.Y., Franklin, E.W., Herrer, G.W., Goldberg, D.A., and Hannigan, E.V., Intraperitoneal mitoxantrone or floxuridine: Effects on time-to-failure and survival in patients with minimal residual ovarian cancer after second-look laparotomy – a randomized Phase II study by the Southwest Oncology Group. *Gynecologic Oncology*, 61:395–402, 1996.

Norfolk, D., Child, J.A., Cooper, E.H., Kerrulsh, S., and Milford-Ward, A., Serum β_2 microglobulin in myelomatosis: Potential value in stratification and monitoring, *British Journal of Cancer*, 42:510–515, 1980.

O'Brien, P., Procedures for comparing samples with multiple endpoints, *Biometrics*, 40:1079–1087, 1984.

O'Quigley, J., Dose finding designs using continual reassessment methods, in Crowley, J. Ed., *Handbook of Statistics in Clinical Trials*, Marcel Dekker, New York, NY, 35–72, 2001.

O'Quigley, J., Pepe, M., and Fisher, L., Continual reassessment method: A practical design for Phase I clinical trials, *Biometrics*, 46:33–48, 1990.

Passamani, E., Clinical trials – are they ethical? *New England Journal of Medicine* 324:1589–1592, 1991.

Peters, W., Rosner, G., Vredenburg, J., Shpall, E., Crump, M., Richardson, P., Marks, L., Cirrincione, C., Wood, W., Henderson, I., Hurd, D., and Norton, L., A prospective, randomized comparison of two doses of combination alkylating agents as consolidation after CAF in high-risk primary breast cancer involving ten or more axillary lymph nodes: Preliminary results of CALGB 9082/SWOG 9114/NCIC MA-13, *Proceedings of the American Society of Clinical Oncology*, 18:Abstract #2, 1999.

Peterson, B., and George, S.L., Sample size requirements and length of study for testing interaction in a $2 \times k$ factorial design when time to failure is the outcome, *Controlled Clinical Trials*, 14:511–522, 1993.

Peto, R., and Peto, J., Asymptotically efficient rank invariant test procedures, *Journal of the Royal Statistical Society*, Series A 135:185–198, 1972.

Peto, R., Pike, M.C., Armitage, P., Breslow, N.E., Cox, D.R., Howard, S.V., Mantel, N., McPherson, K., Peto, J., and Smith, P.G., Design and analysis of randomized clinical trials requiring prolonged observation of each patient, I. Introduction and design, *British Journal of Cancer*, 34:585–612, 1976.

Pocock, S.J., and Simon, R., Sequential treatment assignment with balancing for prognostic factors in the controlled clinical trial, *Biometrics*, 31:103–115, 1975.

Prentice, R.L., Linear rank tests with right censored data, *Biometrika*, 65:167–179, 1978.

Prentice, R.L., Surrogate endpoints in clinical trials: Discussion, definition and operational criteria, *Statistics in Medicine*, 8:431–440, 1989.

Prentice, R.L., Kalbfleisch, J.D., Peterson, A.V., Jr., Flournoy, N., Farewell, V.T., and Breslow, N.E., The analysis of failure times in the presence of competing risks, *Biometrics*, 34:541–554, 1978.

Pritza, D.R., Bierman, M.H., and Hammeke, M.D., Acute toxic effects of sustained-release verapamil in chronic renal failure, *Archives of Internal Medicine*, 151:2081–2084, 1991.

Quackenbush, J., Computational analysis of microarray data, *Nature Reviews*, 2:418–427, 2001.

Redmond, C., Fisher, B., and Wieand, H.S., The methodologic dilemma in retrospectively correlating the amount of chemotherapy received in adjuvant therapy protocols with disease-free survival, *Cancer Treatment Reports*, 67:519–526, 1983.

Rivkin, S.E., Green, S., Metch, B., Glucksberg, H., Gad-el-Mawla, N., Constanzi, J.J., Hoogstraten, B., Athens, A., Maloney, T., Osborne, C.K., and Vaughn, C.B., Adjuvant CMFVP versus melphalan for operable breast cancer with positive axillary nodes: 10-year results of a Southwest Oncology Group study, *Journal of Clinical Oncology*, 7:1229–1238, 1989.

Rivkin, S.E., Green, S., Metch, B., Jewell, W., Costanzi, J., Altman, S., Minton, J., O'Bryan, R., and Osborne, C.K., One versus 2 years of CMFVP adjuvant chemotherapy in axillary node-positive and estrogen receptor negative patients: A Southwest Oncology Group study, *Journal of Cinical Oncology*, 11:1710–1716, 1993.

Rivkin, S.E., Green, S., Metch, B., Cruz, A.B., Abeloff, A.M., Jewell, W.R., Costanzi, J.J., Farrar, W.B., Minton, J.P., and Osborne, C.K., Adjuvant CMFVP versus tamoxifen versus concurrent CMFVP and tamoxifen for postmenopausal, node-positive and estrogen-receptor positive breast cancer patients: A Southwest Oncology Group study, *Journal of Clinical Oncology*, 12:2078–2085, 1994.

Rivkin, S.E., Green, S., O'Sullivan, J., Cruz, A., Abeloff, M.D., Jewell, W.R., Costanzi, J.J., Farra, W.B., and Osborne, C.K., Adjuvant CMFVP plus ovariechtomy for premenopausal, node-positive and estrogen receptor-positive breast cancer patients: A Southwest Oncology Group study, *Journal of Clinical Oncology*, 14:46–51, 1996.

Rockhold, F.W., and Enas, G.G., Data monitoring and interim analysis in the pharmaceutical industry: ethical and logistical considerations, *Statistics in Medicine*, 12:471–479, 1993.

Rosner, B., *Fundamentals of Biostatistics*, second ed. Duxbury, Boston, 1986.

Royall, R., Ethics and statistics in randomized clinical trials, *Statistical Science*, 6:52–88, 1991.

Salmon, S.E., Haut, A., Bonnet, J.D., Amare, M., Weick, J.K., Durie, B.G.M., and Dixon, D.O., Alternating combination chemotherapy and levamisole improves survival in multiple myeloma: A Southwest Oncology Group study, *Journal of Clinical Oncology*, 1:453–461, 1983.

Salmon, S.E., Tesh, D., Crowley, J., Saeed, S., Finley, P., Milder, M.S., Hutchins, L.F., Coltman, C.A., Jr., Bonnet, J.D., Cheson, B., Knost, J.A., Samhouri, A., Beckord, J., and Stock-Novack, D., Chemotherapy is superior to sequential hemibody irradiation for remission consolidation in multiple myeloma: A Southwest Oncology Group study, *Journal of Clinical Oncology*, 8:1575–1584, 1990.

Salmon, S.E., Crowley, J., Grogan, T.M., Finley, P., Pugh, R.P., and Barlogie, B., Combination chemotherapy, glucocorticoids, and interferon alpha in the treatment of multiple myeloma: A Southwest Oncology Group study, *Journal of Clinical Oncology*, 12:2405–2414, 1994.

Salmon, S.E., Crowley, J.J., Balcerzak, S.P., Roach, P.W., Taylor, S.A., Rivkin, S.E., and Samlowski, W., Interferon versus interferon plus prednisone remission maintenance therapy for multiple myeloma: A Southwest Oncology Group study, *Journal of Clinical Oncology*, 16:890–896, 1998.

Sasieni, P.D., and Winnett, A., Graphical approaches to exploring the effects of prognostic factors on survival, in Crowley, J. (Ed.), *Handbook of Statistics in Clinical Trials*. Marcel Dekker, New York, NY, 433–456, 2001.

Schemper, M., and Smith, T.L., A note on quantifying follow-up studies of failure time, *Controlled Clinical Trials*, 17:343–346, 1996.

Schoenfeld, D., Sample-size formula for the proportional-hazards regression model, *Biometrics*, 39:499–503, 1983.

Schumacher, M., Holländer, N., Schwarzer, G., and Saurbrei, W., Prognostic factor studies, in Crowley, J. (Ed.), *Handbook of Statistics in Clinical Trials*, Marcel Dekker, New York, NY, 321–378, 2001.

Segal, M.R., Regression trees for censored data, *Biometrics*, 44:35–48, 1988.

Sessa, C., Capri, G., Gianni, L., Peccatori, F., Grasselli, G., Bauer,J., Zucchetti, M., Vigano, L., Gatti, A., Minoia, C., Liati, P., Van den Bosch, S., Bernareggi, A., Camboni, G., and Marsoni, S., Clinical and pharmacological phase I study with accelerated titration design of a daily times five schedule of BBR3436, a novel cationic triplatinum complex, *Annals of Oncology*, 11:977–983, 2000.

Silverman, W.A., Doctoring: From art to engineering, *Controlled Clinical Trials*, 13:97–99, 1992.

Silverman, W.A., and Chalmers, I., Sir Austin Bradford Hill: An appreciation, *Controlled Clinical Trials*, 13:100–105, 1991.

Simon, R., How large should a Phase II trial of a new drug be? *Cancer Treatment Reports*, 71:1079–1085, 1987.

Simon, R., Optimal two-stage designs for Phase II clinical trials, *Controlled Clinical Trials*, 10:1–10, 1989.

Simon, R., Practical aspects of interim monitoring of clinical trials, *Statistics in Medicine*, 13:1401–1409, 1994.

Simon, R., Freidlin, B., Rubinstein, L., Arbuck, S., Collins, J., and Christian, M., Accelerated titration designs for phase I clinical trials in oncology, *Journal of the National Cancer Institute*, 89:1138–1147, 1997.

Simon, R., and Ungerleider, R., Memorandum to Cooperative Group Chairs, 1992.

Simon, R., and Wittes, R. E., Methodologic guidelines for reports of clinical trials (editorial), *Cancer Treatment Reports*, 69:1–3, 1985.

Simon, R., Wittes, R., and Ellenberg, S., Randomized Phase II clinical trials, *Cancer Treatment Reports*, 69:1375–1381, 1985.

Slud, E., Analysis of factorial survival experiments, *Biometrics*, 50:25–38, 1994.

Smith, J., *Patenting the Sun: Polio and the Salk Vaccine*, William Morrow and Co., New York, 1990.

Smith, J.S., Remembering the role of Thomas Francis, Jr. in the design of the 1954 Salk vaccine trial, *Controlled Clinical Trials*, 13:181–184, 1992.

Spiegelhalter, D.J., Freedman, L.S., and Blackburn, P.R., Monitoring clinical trials: Conditional or predictive power? *Controlled Clinical Trials*, 7:8–17, 1986.

Storer, B., Design and analysis of Phase I clinical trials, *Biometrics*, 45:925–938, 1989.

Storer, B., Choosing a Phase I design, in *Handbook of Statistics in Clinical Oncology*, Crowley, J. (Ed.), Marcel Dekker, New York, 2001.

Streptomycin in Tuberculosis Trials Committee of the Medical Research Council, Streptomycin treatment of pulmonary tuberculosis, *British Medical Journal*, 2:769–782, 1948.

Stuart, C.P., and Guthrie, D. (Eds.), *Lind's Treatise on Scurvy*, University Press, Edinburgh, 1953.

Stuart, K.E., Hajdenberg, A., Cohn, A., Loh, K.K., Miller, W., White, C., and Clendinnin, N.J., A phase II trial of Thymitaq^{TM} (AG337) in patients with hepatocellular carcinoma (HCC), *Proceedings of the American Society of Clinical Oncology*, 15:202 (#449), 1996.

Sylvester, R., Bartelink, H., and Rubens, R., A reversal of fortune: Practical problems in the monitoring and interpretation of an EORTC breast cancer trial, *Statistics in Medicine*, 13:1329–1335, 1994.

Tang, D.-I., Gnecco, C., and Geller, N., Design of group sequential clinical trials with multiple endpoints, *Journal of the American Statistical Association*, 84:776–779, 1989.

Taylor, I., Machin, D., and Mullee, M., A randomized controlled trial of adjuvant portal vein cytotoxic perfusion in colorectal cancer, *British Journal of Surgery*, 72:359–363, 1985.

Taylor, I., Rowling, J., and West, C., Adjuvant cytotoxic liver perfusion for colorectal cancer, *British Journal of Surgery*, 66:833–837, 1979.

Thall, P., and Estey, E., Graphical methods for evaluating covariate effects in the Cox model, in Crowley, J. (Ed.) *Handbook of Statistics in Clinical Trials*, Marcel Dekker, New York, NY, 411–432, 2001.

Thall, P., and Russell, K., A strategy for dose-finding and safety monitoring based on efficacy and adverse outcome in phase I/II clinical trials, *Biometrics*, 54:251–265, 1998.

Therasse, P., Arbuck, S., Eisenhauer, E., Wanders, J., Kaplan, R., Rubinstein, L., Verweij, J., Van Glabbeke, M., van Oosterom, T., Christian, M., and Gwyther, S., New guidelines to evaluate the response to treatment in solid tumors, *Journal of the National Cancer Institute*, 92:205–216, 2000.

Thomas, L., *The Youngest Science*, Viking Press, New York, 1983.

Tibshirani, R.J., and Hastie, T., Local likelihood estimation, *Journal of the American Statistical Association*, 82:559–567, 1987.

Troxel, A.B., Harrington, D.P., and Lipsitz, S.R., Analysis of longitudinal data with non-ignorable non-monotone missing values, *Applied Statistics*, 47:425–438, 1998.

Ulm, K., Hekarda, H., Gerein, P., and Berger, U., Statistical methods to identify prognostic factors, in Crowley, J. (Ed.), *Handbook of Statistics in Clinical Trials*, Marcel Dekker, New York, NY, 379–395, 2001.

Volberding, P.A., Lagakos, S.W., Koch, M.A., and the AIDS Clinical Trials Group of the National Institute of Allergy and Infectious Disease. Zidovudine in asymptomatic human immunodeficiency virus infection, *New England Journal of Medicine*, 322:941–949, 1990.

Walsh, T., Noonan, N., Hollywood, D., Kelly, A., Keeling, N., and Hennessy. T., A comparison of multimodal therapy and surgery for esophageal adenocarcinoma, *New England Journal of Medicine*, 335:462–467, 1996.

Walters, L., Data monitoring committees: The moral case for maximum feasible independence, *Statistics in Medicine*, 12:575–580, 1993.

Wei, L.J., and Durham, S., The randomized play-the-winner rule in medical trials, *Journal of the American Statistical Association*, 73:830–843, 1978.

Weick, J.K., Kopecky, K.J., Appelbaum, F.R., Head, D.R., Kingsbury, L.L., Balcerzak, S.P., Mills, G.M., Hynes, H.E., Welborn, J.L., Simon, S.R., and Grever, M., A randomized investigation of high-dose versus standard dose cytosine arabinoside with daunorubicin in patients with previously untreated acute myeloid leukemia: A Southwest Oncology Group study, *Blood*, 88:2841–2851, 1996.

Wolff, J., *Lehre von den Krebskrankheiten von den ältesten Zeiten bis zur Gegenwart*, 4 Teile in 5Bde.Jena: G Fischer, 1907–1928.

Wolmark, N., Rockette, H., and Fisher, B., Adjuvant therapy for carcinoma of the colon: A review of NSABP clinical trial, in Salmon, S, (Ed.), *Adjuvant Therapy of Cancer*, vol. 7, Lippincott, Philadelphia, 300–307, 1993.

Wolmark, N., Rockette, H., and Wickerham, D.L., Adjuvant therapy of Dukes' A, B and C adenocarcinoma of the colon with portal-vein fluorouracil hepatic infusion: Preliminary results of National Surgical Adjuvant Breast and Bowel Project C-02, *Journal of Clinical Oncology*, 8:1466–1475, 1990.

Zee, B., Melnychuk, D., Dancey, J., and Eisenhauer, E., Multinomial Phase II cancer trials incorporating response and early progression, *Journal of Biopharmaceutical Statistics*, 9:351–363, 1999.

Zelen, M., A new design for randomized clinical trials, *New England Journal of Medicine*, 300:1242–1246, 1979.

Zhan, F., Hardin, J., Bumm, K., Zheng, M., Tiang, E., Wilson, C., Crowley, J., Barlogie, B., and Shaughnessy, J., Molecular profiling of multiple myeloma, *Blood*, 99:1745–1757, 2002.

Zubrod, C.G., Schneiderman, M., Frei, M. III, Brindley, C. et al., Appraisal of methods for the study of chemotherapy of cancer in man: Comparative therapeutic trial of nitrogen mustard and thiophosphoramide, *Journal of Chronic Diseases*, 11:7–33, 1960.

Zubrod, C.G., Clinical trials in cancer patients: An introduction, *Controlled Clinical Trials*, 3:185–187, 1982.

Index

A

Accelerated titration design, 51
Accrual rate
    data monitoring committees, 104
    esophageal cancer trials, 100
    Phase II trials, 60
        standard design, 54–55, 56, 58
    Phase III trials, 72
        continuation from Phase II, 167
        problems caused by reporting primary, 166
        stopping equivalence trial for positive results, 118
Accuracy, 137
Adaptive allocation, 64
Adjuvant chemotherapy, 136
Adriamycin
    multi-arm trials, 81
    multiple myeloma trials, 210
    soft-tissue sarcoma trials, 196–199
Advanced breast cancer prestudy form, 142, see also Breast cancer; SWOG 8811
Advanced disease trial, 16
Adverse Drug Reaction reports, 146
Age, 63, 202
AIDS research, 207
Alternative hypothesis, 24, see also Null hypothesis
Area under the curve (AUC)
    interim analysis, 101
    Phase I trials, 51
    Phase III trials, 27–28, 29
Asymmetric testing, 101
AUC, see Area under the curve

B

Bacillus-Calmette-Guerin (BCG), 112
Background, 129, see also Protocol development
Bayesian methods, 50
BCG, see Bacillus-Calmette-Guerin (BCG)
BCNU, 210, see also Multiple myeloma
Bell-shaped curve, 16
Bias
    clinical trials, 233
    competing risks, 189
    data monitoring committees, 111
    dose intensity analysis, 200
    early studies, 123, 124
    endpoint in clinical trials, 44
    meta-analysis, 227, 229, 230
    multi-arm trials, 94
    outcome analyses, 196
    Phase I/II trials, 52
    Phase II trial, 23
    Phase III trials, 23, 32, 33
        blinding designs, 68
        randomization, 64, 65
    protocol development, 134
    reporting of results, 170, 171, 173, 174
    survival distributions, 182
Biased coin, 12–13, 14
Biblical trials, 79
Binomial distribution, 14, 15, 22
Biologic agents, 52–53
Bisantrene, 80
Bladder cancer, 112
Bleomycin, 81
Blinding, 67–69, 106
Bonadonna–Valagussa approach, 199, 200

Bone lesions, 148
Bone marrow transplants, 184, 185, 186
Bonferroni correction, 83
Brain radiotherapy (RT), 83, 94, see also Radiotherapy
Breast cancer
    data management/quality control, 124, 125, 126
    dose intensity analyses, 199–202
    EORTC study and interim analysis, 98, 100
    history of clinical trials, 2
    multi-arm trials, 80
    Phase II trials, 55
    phase III trials, 8, 65, 66
    stopping early for negative results, 115
    survival distributions, 182, 183
Bubble sort approach, 84

C

CA-125 antigen, 12, 13
CAF regimen, see Cyclophosphamide/adriamycin/5-fluorouracil (CAF) regimen
CALGB, see Cancer and Leukemia Group B
Cancer and Leukemia Group B (CALGB), 115
Cancer Therapy Evaluation Program (CTEP), 47
Carboplatin
    ovarian cancer
        stopping equivalence trial, 115, 117–118, 119
        Southwest Oncology Group, 8
    Phase II trials, 59–60
    Phase III trials, 24, 25
Cardiac Arrhythmia Suppression Trial (CAST), 4, 207
CAST, see Cardiac Arrhythmia Suppression Trial
Categorical data, 11–12, 14
Censoring
    data management/quality control, 123
    endpoint in clinical trials, 45
    estimates of competing risks, 191–192
    measurement data, 12
    Phase III trials, 30–31, 32, 34, 35

Central Limit Theorem, 16, 26
Charts, 149
Checklist, 143, 160–161
Chemoradiation, 205
Chemotherapy
    multi-arm trials, 81, 82
    Phase III trials, 9, 65, 66
Children's Cancer Group INT-133, 81, 89, 94
Chi-square (χ^2), 25–26, 27, 214
Chi-square (χ^2) distribution, 26, 27, 28, 29
Chi-square (χ^2) statistic, 219–220
Cisplatin
    design of clinical trials, 60
    interim analysis, 100
    lung cancer trials, 8–9, 115, 116
    multi-arm trials, 80
    outcome as response, 24, 25
    ovarian cancer trials, 8, 115, 117–118, 119
Class discovery, 225
Class prediction, 225
Clinical judgment, 146
Clinical research associates, 151
Clinical trials
    examples, 7–9
    history, 1–6
    Southwest Oncology group, 6–7
Closure, see also Stopping rules
    making final report public, 167
    standard design of Phase II trials, 57–58
    trials
        data monitoring committee, 103, 106, 109
        interim analysis, 100
Clustering, 225
CMF regimen, 98, 100, 199
CMFVP
    dose intensity analyses, 199
    Phase III trials, 8, 65, 66
    survival distributions for breast cancer, 182, 183
Coding, 138, 139
Coin flips, 12–13, 14, 16
Colon cancer, 65, 173, 174
    Dukes' C, 203, 204, 228
Colorectal cancer, 82, 203–204, 228
Common Toxicity Criteria (CTC), 47, 135
Competing risks, 188–194

INDEX

Complete response (CR)
  categorical data for clinical trials, 12
  identification for SWOG 8811, 136
  Phase II IND trial, 19
  stopping equivalence trial for positive results, 117
  timing of randomization in multi-arm trials, 93
Completeness, data, 139–140
Compliance, 67, 145, 169, 200, see also Noncompliance
Computed tomography (CT), 124
Computer software, 151
Computers, 153–154
Conditional power approach, 101, 102
Conduct, data monitoring committees, 109–110
Confidence interval
  interpretation of results of Phase II/Phase III trials, 176–177
  Phase II IND trial, 22
  Phase III trials, 28, 33, 74
  report reliability and reporting summary statistics, 174–175
Confidence levels, 49
Confidential information, 106–107
Confidentiality, 110
Conflict of interest, 108
CONSORT statement, 166
Contingency tables, 26, 35, 36
Continual reassessment methods (CRM), 50, 51
Continuity-corrected Chi-square (χ^2), 26
Control arms, 60
Controlled trials, 3, 80–81
Cornfield, Jerome, 4
Coronary Drug Research Project, 200
Cost, 47, 67
Cox model
  exploratory analyses, 210
  identification of prognostic factors, 212, 213, 214, 218
  interpretation of results of one- or two-sided tests, 176
  reporting summary statistics, 172
Cox regression model, see Proportional hazards model
CR, see Complete response
Criteria, model-based, 50

CRM, see Continual reassessment methods
CT, see Computed tomography
CTC, see Common Toxicity Criteria
CTEP, see Cancer Therapy Evaluation Program
Cumulative incidence curve, 190–193
Cumulative survival, 31, 32, see also Survival
Cyclophosphamide
  breast cancer trials, 202
  EORTC study and interim analysis, 98, 100
  multi-arm trials, 81, 94
  multiple myeloma trials, 210
  outcome as response in Phase III trials, 24
  ovarian cancer trials, 8, 115, 117–118, 119
Cyclophosphamide/adriamycin/5-fluorouracil (CAF) regimen, 55–56
Cystic fibrosis, 205
Cytarabine, 81
Cytoxan, 59–60

D

Dacarbazine, 54
Data and Safety Monitoring Committee (DSMC), 111
Data base management, 151–154
Data collection
  data base management, 152–154
  data management/quality control, 136–143
Data coordinator, 144, 145–146
Data entry, 152–154
Data evaluation, 145–148
Data flow, 144–145
Data forms, 140–143
Data items, 137–140
Data management/quality control
  appendix: examples, 155–163
  data base management, 151–154
  data collection, 136–143
  protocol development, 128–136
  protocol management and evaluation, 143–149
  quality assurance audits, 149–150

training, 150–151
why worry, 123–128
Data monitoring committee
    activities, 112–122
    composition, 107–113
    protocol management/evaluation, 147
    rationale and responsibilities, 103–107
    reporting outcome, 167
Data quality, 234
Data reduction technique, 225
Data submission instructions, 134–135
Data transmission, 152–154
Date stamp, 144
Death, 188, 190–194
Decision making, 23, 57, 106
Decision rules, 61
Dendogram, 225, 226
Density, 14, 16, 18
Design
    clinical trials
        careful attention, 233
        detectable differences or estimate precision, 43
        eligibility, treatments, endpoints, 42
        endpoints, comments, 44–48
        objectives, 42
        Phase I trials, 48–53
        Phase II trials, 53–62
        Phase III trials, 62–76
        sample size calculations, 43–44
        treatment assignment, 43
    study and reporting required information, 168
Deterrents, 145
Dexamethasone, 81, 121
Diabetic Retinopathy Trial, 5
Diet, 1, 41
Differences, detection, 43
Diphtheria, 181–182
Discipline review, 133
Disease assessment form, 141, 142–143, 149
Disease committee chair, 146
Disease committees, 6–7
Disease–drug combinations, 56
Distant relapse, see Relapse
Distribution, concept, 13–14
DLT, see Dose limiting toxicity

Dornase alfa, 205
Dosage, 50, 90, 138, 168
Dose intensity analyses, 199–203
Dose limiting toxicity (DLT), 48–49, 50
Double review process, 146
Double-blinding, 67
Doxorubicin, 54, 80, 121
Draft forms, 140
Drop-out patterns, 173
Drug, information, 129
DSMC, see Data and Safety Monitoring Committee
DTIC, soft-tissue sarcoma and outcome analyses, 196–199
Dukes' C colon cancer, see Colon cancer
Durable responses, 172
Duration of response, 45, 196
Durie–Salmon stages, 210, 211, 220
Duvillard, E., 2
Dynamic allocation schemes, 63

E

Early termination, 169
Eastern Cooperative Oncology Group, 231
ECMO, see Extracorporeal membrane oxygenation
Edit checks, 152, 153
Effective dose, 49, 51
Efficacy assessment, 52
Efficiency, 50
Electronic data forms, 140–141
Eligibility
    data management/quality control, 138, 139
    designing clinical trials, 42
    multiple myeloma trials, 184–186
    patient registration, 143, 162
    Phase II trial, 20, 23
    protocol development, 129–130
    reporting of results, 168, 169, 171
Encainide, 207
Endpoint
    definitions and protocol development, 132
    designing clinical trials, 42, 44–48
    issues and SWOG 8811, 136
    multiple and interpretation of results, 177–178

INDEX

Phase II trials, 54, 61, 62
Phase III trials, 67, 71, 72–73, 172
reporting required information, 168
reviews, 146
stopping equivalence trial for positive results, 117
Enforcement, 143
EORTC, *see* European Organization for Research and Treatment of Cancer
Equivalence trial
designs of Phase III trials, 73–76
stopping early for positive results, 115, 117–118
Equivocal results, 176, 177
Errors, 91, 132, 227, *see also* Individual entries
Escalation, 48–49, 51
Esophageal cancer, 100
Estimated response probability, 20, 21, 25, 166
Estimation, Phase II trails, 19–23
Ethics
Phase III trials
blinding designs, 68–69
randomization, 64, 67
two-arm designs, 70
rationale/responsibilities of data monitoring committees, 104
Etoposide, 81, 118
European Organization for Research and Treatment of Cancer (EORTC), 46, 98, 100
Evaluability, 138, 139, 162
Evaluation, 109
Evolution, 108–109
Example trials, 7–9
Exceptions, 143–144
Exclusions, 170–171, 230
Expectation reports, 145
Exploratory analyses
analysis of microarray data, 224–226
background and notation, 210–212
forming prognostic groups, 219–224
identification of prognostic factors, 212–218
meta-analysis, 226–232
Exponential distribution, 40
Exponential function, 16

Exponential survival, 16, 71
Extracorporeal membrane oxygenation (ECMO), 64

F

Factorial design, 81, 86, 87–88, 90
Failure, 190–193, 201
False negatives, 29, 205
False positives, 176, 206
Fax transmission, 153
Fetal nigral transplantation, 68
Fibonacci design, 48
Filing, forms, 144
Finasteride, 8
Fisher's exact test, 26
Flecainide, 207
Flow sheets, 141, 156
Floxuridine, 59, 60
5-Fluorouracil (5-FU)
background of trial and protocol development, 129
breast cancer trials, 126, 128, 202
colon cancer trials, 173, 174, 203, 204
interim analysis, 98, 100
multi-arm trials, 82
Phase II trials, 7, 55
portal vein infusion and meta-analysis, 228
screening in multi-arm trials, 91–92
Folinic acid, 55, 129
Follow-up, 169, 189
form, 158
Form content, 141
Forms
data entry and data base management, 153
data management/quality control, 140
missing data and reporting summary statistics, 172
protocol development, 135
protocol management/evaluation, 145
Four-arm trial, 80, 86, 87, 90
Francis, Thomas, Jr., 5–6
Fraud detection, 150
5-FU, *see* 5-Fluorouracil
Full likelihood estimate, 215

G

Galen, 1
Gastric cancer, 205
Gastro-esophageal (GE) tumors, 205
Gaussian distribution, 16
GE, see Gastro-esophageal tumors
Gender, 203, 204
Genes, 224
Genetic profiling, 224–226
Gleevec, 226
Global test, 83, 84, 88, 176
GM-CSF, see Granulocyte/macrophage colony-stimulating factor
Goals, 104, 128
Gold treatment, 3
Goldie–Coldman hypothesis, 210
Granulocyte/macrophage colony-stimulating factor (GM-CSF), 118, 120
Granulocytopenia, 120
Guidelines, 128, 141

H

Harm, potential, 105, see also Data monitoring committee
Hart, Phillip D'Arcy, 3
Hazard function, 15–16, 18, 212
Hazard rate, see Hazard function
Hazard ratio
    Phase II trials, 59, 60
    Phase III trials, 71, 72
    power in multi-arm trials, 85
    report reliability and reporting summary statistics, 174
Hazards, cause-specific, 193–194
Heart transplantation, 195–196
Hepatocellular carcinoma, 170
Herceptin, 226
Hierarchical clustering, 225
Hierarchical data bases, 152
High-dose therapy, 186–188
Hill, Sir Austin Bradford, 3
Histograms, 20, 21
Historical background, 182, 183
Humoralistic bases, 2
Hyperfractionation, 97

Hypothesis
    generation, 234
    testing, Phase III trials
        response as outcome, 24–30
        survival as outcome, 30–37

I

Ifosfamide
    multi-arm trials, 81, 89–90
    soft-tissue sarcoma and outcome analyses, 196–199
Inaccuracies, 138
INC, see Increasing
Inclusion criteria, 227
Inclusion of trials, 229
Increasing (INC) response, 12, 19
IND, see Investigational New Drugs
Induction therapy, 118
Infection endpoint, 118, 120
Information, reporting required, 168–170
Informed consent, 130
Institutional Review Boards, 7
Instructions, data forms, 141
Intensity summary, 202
Intent-to-treat principle, 170, 171, 229
Interaction, multi-arm trials, 86–90
Interferon, 118, 120
Interim analysis
    data monitoring committee reporting, 167
    planned, 97–103
    report reliability and reporting summary statistics, 174
    reporting required information, 168
    stopping trials, 112, 113, 114, 117, 118
Interim data, 105
Interpretations, data forms, 142
Interval intensity, 202
Investigational New Drugs (IND), 19

K

K tests, 83
Kaplan–Meier (K–M) estimate, 31, 123, 188, 191
K–M, see Kaplan–Meier estimate
Knowledge, requirement, 107–108

INDEX

L

Leiomyosarcoma, 23
Leucovorin, 91
Leukemia, 4
Levamisole, 203, 204, 230
Limitations, clinical trials, 2–3
Links, establishing, 151
Liver Infusion Meta-analysis Group, 228, 229
Local relapse, see Relapse
Logical completeness, 142
Logistic model, 50
Logrank statistic, 219, 220
Logrank test
    data management/quality control, 124, 125, 126
    interpretation of results of one- or two-sided tests, 176
    Phase III trials, 35, 36
    power in multi-arm trials, 85
    proportional hazards model and statistical concepts, 38–39
LPAM, 199, 200, 201
Lumping interventions, 229–230
Lung cancer, 97, 115, 116, 124, see also Non-small-cell lung cancer; Small-cell lung cancer
Lymphoma trials, 81, see also Non-Hodgkin's lymphoma

M

Maintenance therapy, 93
Margins, form design, 140
Maximum tolerated dose (MTD), design
    Phase I trials, 48–49, 53
        newer, 49–52
    Phase I/II trials, 52
Mayo Clinic, 203
MDR, see Multi-Drug Resistance gene
Measurable disease, 148
Measurement data, 12
Measurement error, 148, see also Errors
Median hazard, 16, 18
Median survival time, 33, see also Survival
Medical emergencies, 69
Melphalan, 8, 94, 124, 210
Menopause, 202

Mesna, 196–199
Meta-analysis
    portal vein infusion, 228–231
    principles, 226–228
Metastatic disease, 189–190
Methotrexate, 81, 98, 100, 202
MGUS, see Monoclonal gamopathy of undetermined significance
Microarray data, 224–226
Mitomycin C
    lung cancer trials, 115, 116
    non-small cell, 8–9
    multi-arm trials, 80, 90
    stopping trials for positive results, 112
Mitoxantrone, 59–60, 80
Model choice, 216–218
Monitoring, 104
Monoclonal gamopathy of undetermined significance (MGUS), 225, 226
MTD, see Maximum tolerated dose
MTP, 89–90, 94
Multi-arm trials
    interaction, 86–90
    interpretation of results, 177
    other model assumptions, 90
    power, 84–85
    significance level, 83
    timing of randomization, 92–94
    to screen or not to screen, 90–92
    types, 80–82
Multi-Drug Resistance gene (MDR), 13
Multi-drug resistance, 121
Multiple myeloma
    analysis of microarray data, 225
    background and notation, 210
    emergency stopping based on unexpected toxic deaths, 121
    forming prognostic groups, 219–222
    historical survival data and bias identification, 182–186
    identification of prognostic factors, 213–218
Multivariate model, 212, 218
Myelocytic leukemia, 82, see also Leukemia

N

Nasopharyngeal cancer, 114

NASS, see No assessment, inadequate assessment
National Cancer Institute (NCI), 3, 110
National Surgical Adjuvant Breast and Bowel Program (NSABP), 4, 228
NCI, see National Cancer Institute
NCCTG, 104
Negative results, 115, 176
Neural networks, 218, 225
No assessment, inadequate assessment (NASS), 19
Noncompliance, 93, 118, 120, see also Compliance
Non-Hodgkin's lymphoma, 4, 81, 92
Noninferiority trials, 73–76
Non-small cell lung cancer, 8, 81, 133, see also Lung cancer
Normal distribution
   Phase II trial, 21, 22
   Phase III trials, 29
   statistical concepts for clinical trials, 16, 39
North Central Cancer Treatment Group, 203
Notes, data forms, 140
Notice of Death, 142, 143, 159, see also Death
Notices of events, 145
NSABP, see National Surgical Adjuvant Breast and Bowel Program
Null hypothesis
   interpretation of results, 176–177
   meta-analysis, 226
   Phase II trials, 54
     standard design, 55, 56, 58
   Phase III trials, 73, 75, 76
     outcome as response, 24, 25, 27, 28
     survival as outcome, 34, 36, 37
     two-arm designs, 69–70
     stopping equivalence trial for positive results, 117
Numerical methods, 2

O

Objectives, clinical trials, 11, 42, 128, 168
OCR, see Optical character recognition
Off-treatment notices, 142
One-sided test
   interim analysis, 101
   interpretation of results, 175–176
   Phase III trials, 25, 29
Optical character recognition (OCR), 153
Order restrictions, 80
Ordered hypothesis, 175, see also Hypothesis
Osteogenic sarcoma, 81
Outcome
   analysis pitfalls, 195–203
   data management/quality control, 138, 141
   data review and rationale/responsibilities of data monitoring committees, 106
   measures
     classification, 11
     probability and statistical concepts, 12–13
   problems caused by reporting primary, 166
   selection of stratification factors and randomization, 63
Outside information, 106
Ovarian cancer
   Phase II trials, design 59, 60
     outcome as response, 24
   stopping equivalence trial for positive results, 115, 117–118, 119
   trials of Southwest Oncology Group, 8

P

Paclitaxel, 19, 20, 22, 23, 60
Pairwise comparisons, 80, 84, 91
PALA, see N-Phosphonoacetyl-L-aspartate disodium
Paper charts, 144
Parkinson's disease, 68
Partial response (PR), 12, 19, 124, 136
Pathology, 133
   material, 145
Patients
   characteristics, 169
     table, 147–148
   consent and timing of randomization, 66–67

INDEX 261

data evaluation and protocol management/evaluation, 145–146
data management/quality control, 140, 141
follow-up, 2
removal from trial and protocol development, 131
PBI, *see* Prophylactic brain irradiation
PCP, *see* Prochlorperazine
Pediatric Oncology Group, 6
Peeling, 222–223
Penicillin, 3
PGDE, *see* Pharmacokinetically guided dose escalation
p-Glycoprotein, 121
Pharmacokinetically guided dose escalation (PGDE), 51
Phase I trials
  considerations for biologic agents, 52–53
  newer designs, 49–52
  – Phase II designs, 52
  traditional designs, 48–49
Phase II trials
  estimation, 19–23
  objectives, 11
  reporting after closure, 167
  results reporting, 170
  Southwest Oncology Group, 7
  summary statistics reporting, 172
  surrogate endpoints, 208
Phase II–III screening design, 91
Phase III trials
  bias identification for multiple myeloma, 182–183, 184, 185
  hypothesis testing
    response as outcome, 24–30
    survival as outcome, 30–37
  objectives, 11
  overseeing by data monitoring committees, 110
  reporting
    mature data, 166
    results, 171
    summary statistics, 172
  Southwest Oncology Group, 8
  temptation to skip, 60
L-Phenylalanine mustard, 124, 125, 126

N-Phosphonoacetyl-L-aspartate disodium (PALA), 91
Pilot studies, 61
Pitfalls
  competing risks, 188–194
  historical controls, 181–188
  outcome by outcome analyses, 195–203
  subset analyses, 203–206
  surrogate endpoints, 206–208
Placebos, 67, 200–201
Platinum, 60
Pneumonia, 3
Pocock–Simon approach, 63–64
Portal infusion therapy, 203–204, 228–231
Positive results
  interpretation of results of Phase II/III trials, 176
  stopping trials early, 112–114
  equivalence, 115, 117–118
Power, 84–85, 176, 204–205
PR, *see* Partial response
Precision, 22
Prednisone, 81, 94, 202, 210
Principle components technique, 225, 226
Probability, 12, 14, 20, 24
Problems, 146, 148–149
Prochlorperazine (PCP), 67–68
Prognostic factors, 212–218
Prognostic groups, 219–224
Progression-free survival, 172, *see also* Survival
Prophylactic brain irradiation (PBI), 81, 89
Proportional hazards assumption, 71, 176
Proportional hazards model, 37–39, 86, 212
Prostate cancer, 8, 134
Protocol
  coordinator, 7
  development, 128–136
  deviations and reporting results, 169
  management/evaluation, 143–149
Publishing, results, 148, 234
Pulmonary function tests, 136
p-Value
  analysis of microarray data, 225
  bladder cancer trials, 114
  interpretation of results, 175

Phase III trials, 28, 35, 73, 74, 75
   study and interim analysis, 100, 102

Q

QOL, see Quality of life
Quality assurance audits, 149–150
Quality of life (QOL)
   data management/quality control, 138
   endpoint in designing clinical trials, 47–48
   reporting summary statistics, 172, 173, 174
   two-arm designs of Phase III trials, 69
Quality of trials, 230–231
Quinine, 121

R

Race, 63–64
Radiotherapy (RT), 9, 100, 114, 118, 167
   films, 145
Randomization
   designing clinical trials, 43
   history of clinical trials, 4–5
   multi-arm trials, 82
   Phase II trials, 58–61
   Phase III trials, 23
      design, 62–69
      survival as outcome, 30
   reporting required information, 168
Randomized block design, 63
Randomized consent designs, 66–67
Raw data, 227, 229
RECIST, see Response Evaluation Criteria in Solid Tumors
Recurrence-free survival, 112, 113, see also Survival
Recursive partitioning, 219, 220, 221
Registration, 143–144, 162
   instructions, 134
Regression model, 213, 214, 217, 218
Regression techniques, 225
Regression tree, 220, 221, 222
Regulatory requirements, 135
Relapse, 136, 188
Relational model, 152
Reliability, 23, 174
Remote data entry, 153

Reports, generation, 146
Responders–non-responders comparison, 195–199
Response
   data management/quality control, 139–140
   endpoint in designing clinical trials, 45–46
   outcome in Phase III trials, 24–30
   problem resolution in SWOG 8811, 149
Response Evaluation Criteria in Solid Tumors (RECIST), 12, 46, 124
Response probability, 56, 73, 102, 170–171
Response tables, 147, 163
Responsibilities, data monitoring committees, 103–107
Results
   publication and protocol management/evaluation, 148
   reporting
      analyses, 170–178
      rationale/responsibilities of data monitoring committees, 106
      required information, 168–170
      timing, 166–167
Reviews, 144–145, 148
RT, see Radiotherapy

S

Safety issues, 136
Salk vaccine, 5
Sample size
   adequacy, 234
   calculation, 39–40, 43–44
   equivalence/noninferiority trials, 76
   history of clinical trials, 4
   multi-arm trials, 84
   Phase I trials, 49
   Phase II trials
      design, 58–59, 60
      IND trial, 20, 21
      pilot studies and design, 61
      standard design, 57–58
   Phase III trials, 29, 64, 71–72
   reporting required information, 168
Sarcoma
   Phase II trials, 54

Phase II IND trial, 19, 20, 22, 23
surrogate endpoints in trials, 207
sb2m
    forming prognostic groups, 219, 220, 221, 222
    identification of prognostic factors, 213–217
Scale of measurement, 212, 213–216, 217
Scatterplot, 216
Screening design, 81–82, 90–92, see also Multi-arm trials
Secondary analysis, 178
Selection designs, 58
Self-report, 47–48
Sensitivity analyses, 228
Serum β_2 microglobulin, 210
Sham surgery, 68–69, see also Surgery
Significance level
    interim analysis, 98, 100, 101
    multi-arm trials, 83, 86, 88
    Phase III trials, 29, 70
Simulation studies, 50, 82, 88
Single-arm trials, 43, 54, see also Two-arm trials; Multi-arm trials
Single-blinding, 67
Single-institution studies, 54
Single-stage designs, 61
Six-arm trial, 79
Small-cell lung cancer, see also Lung cancer; Non-small-cell lung cancer
    historical survival data and bias identification, 186–188
    radiotherapy and final report, 167
    stopping trials based on toxicity and noncompliance, 118, 120
Solid Tumor Committee, 6
Sorting, forms, 144
Southwest Oncology Group (SWOG)
    clinical trials, 6–7, see also SWOG
    history of clinical trials, 4
    interim analysis, 98, 99
    rationale/responsibilities of data monitoring committees, 104
    standard design of Phase II trials, 54–58
Special instructions, 135
Spending function approach, 101–102
STA, see Stable response
Stable (STA) response, 12, 19

Stage definitions, 129
Staging system, 210, 219
Standard therapy, 8
Standardization, 137–140, 142
Standards, 150
Starting dosage, 51, see also Dosage
Statistic, 13
Statistical center, 145, 150
Statistical concepts
    characterization, 11–18
    Phase II trial–estimation, 19–23
    Phase III trial–hypothesis testing, 23–37
    proportional hazards model, 37–39
    protocol development, 133
    role in clinical trials, 233
    sample size calculations, 39–40
Stepwise strategy, 218
Stochastic curtailment approach, see Conditional power approach
Stopping rules, 100, 104–105, 108, see also Closure
Storer design, 50, 51
Stratification factors, 62–63, 130
Streptomycin, 3
Study amendment, 149
Study calendar, 132, 155
Study coordinators, 151
Subjective judgment, 46–47
Subset analyses, 203–206
Summary statistics, 172–175
Summary tables, 147, 151–152
Surgery, 1, 133
Surrogate endpoints, 206–208
Survival
    disease-free and dose intensity analyses, 199, 200
    endpoint in designing clinical trials, 44, 45
    forming prognostic groups, 219
    identification of prognostic factors, 214, 215
    multi-arm trials, 84, 91, 93
    multiple myeloma, 210, 211
    Phase II trials, 7, 54
    Phase III trials, 23, 69, 71–72
    primary endpoint in breast cancer trials, 206–207
Survival by response, 195–199
Survival curve

multiple myeloma and historical data,
  182–183, 184, 185
outcome analyses, 197
Phase III trials, 32, 33–34, 172
statistical concepts for clinical trials,
  14–15, 16, 17
Survival distributions
  breast cancer trials, 182, 183
    data management/quality control,
      124, 125, 126
  interaction in multi-arm trials, 86, 87
Survival endpoint, 59, 119
Survival tables, 147
Survival time, 30, 31, 32
SWOG 7436, 124
SWOG 7827, 65, 66, 201–202
SWOG 7924, 167
SWOG 8203, 80
SWOG 8229, multiple myeloma
  background and notation, 210, 211
  exploratory analyses, 213–218
  forming prognostic groups, 220–222
  timing of randomization in multi-arm
    trials, 94
SWOG 8269, 186–188
SWOG 8300, 8, 83, 89
SWOG 8412, 8, 24, 115, 117–118, 119
SWOG 8516, 81, 92
SWOG 8600, 82
SWOG 8616, 196
SWOG 8624, 210, 223
SWOG 8738, 8, 80, 90, 115, 116
SWOG 8795, 112–114
SWOG 8811, breast cancer
  additional comments on protocol
    development, 136
  background of trial, 129
  data management/quality control,
    126, 142
  example trials, 7
  objectives of trial, 128
  protocol management/evaluation, 147,
    148–149
  standard design of Phase II trials, 55,
    57–58
  stratification factors, 131
  study calendar, 132
  trials and eligibility criteria, 130
SWOG 8812, 118, 120
SWOG 8835, 59–60

SWOG 8892, 114
SWOG 8905, 91, 92, 173, 174
SWOG 9008, 205
SWOG 9028, 121
SWOG 9106, 59–60
SWOG 9134, 19
SWOG 9217, 8
SWOG 9623, 115, 117
SWOG 9805, 82
SWOG leukemia committee, 93
SWOG treatment protocols, 128–135
SWOG, see Southwest Oncology Group
Symptom distress, 173, 174

T

Taxane, 60
Test of interaction, 178
Test statistic, 13, 25–26, 28, 35
Tetrahydrocannabinol, 67–68
Thalidomide, 3
Thall/Russell approach, 53
THC, see Tetrahydrocannabinol
Theotepa, 60
Thrombocytopenia, 120
Thymidylate synthetase inhibitor, 170
Time to death, 14, 44–45
Time to event data, 12, 14
Time to failure, 45, 197
Time to progression, 45, 46
Timing of randomization
  meta-analysis of portal vein infusion,
    230
  multi-arm trials, 92–94
  Phase III trials, 65–67
Timing of report, 167
Toxicity
  breast cancer trials, 128
  data management/quality control, 141
  endpoint in designing clinical trials,
    47
  interim analysis, 101
  lung cancer trials, 115
  Phase I trials, 49, 53
  Phase II trials, 7, 62
  protocol development, 131–132, 135
  protocol management/evaluation, 139,
    147, 157, 162
  reporting results, 169, 170, 172
Training, 138, 150–151

Treatment
    data management/quality control, 138
    designing clinical trials, 42, 44–45
    interaction in multi-arm trials, 86
    modification and protocol
        development
    Phase II trials, 55–56
    Phase III trials, 23, 24
    protocol development, 131–132
    regimens difference and meta-
        analysis, 227
    reporting results, 168, 169
    summary table, 148, 155, 157
True response probability, 20, 22, 25, 55
True survival times, 35
t-Test, 225
Tuberculosis, 3
Tumor markers, 207
Tumor response, 7
Two by two (2×2) contingency table, 25, 26, 35, 36
Two-arm trials
    interim analysis, 98
    Phase II trials, 60, 69
    Phase III trials, 65, 66
    sample size calculations, 40
    virtues, 233–234
Two-phase designs, 52
Two-sided test, 25, 101, 175–176
Two-stage design, 19
Type I error, 27, 28, 37, 98, *see also* Errors
Type II error, 29, *see also* Errors

U

UGDP, *see* University Group Diabetes Project

Unidimensional measurements, 46
University Group Diabetes Project (UGDP), 4

V

Validation, 222–223
Variables, data management/quality control, 137, 139
Verapamil, 121
Vested interest, 107–108
Vincristine
    breast cancer trials, 202
    emergency stopping based on unexpected toxic deaths, 121
    multi-arm trials, 81, 94
    multiple myeloma trials, 210

W

Warning messages, 140–141
WBCs, *see* White blood cells
Web entry, 154
Wei–Durham design, 64
White blood cells (WBCs), 130
WHO, *see* World Health Organization
Wilcoxon test, 35, 36
Wilms' tumor, 5
World Health Organization (WHO), 46

Z

Zubrod, Gordon, 4